Cardiac Rehabilitation,
Adult Fitness,
and Exercise Testing

Cardiac Rehabilitation, Adult Fitness, and Exercise Testing

Paul S. Fardy, Ph.D.

President, Cardiac Pulmonary Consultants, Inc.
Gary, Indiana

Frank G. Yanowitz, M.D.

Associate Professor of Medicine
University of Utah, School of Medicine
Medical Director, The Fitness Institute
LDS Hospital
Salt Lake City, Utah

Philip K. Wilson, Ed.D.

Professor
Director, Human Performance Laboratory
College of Health, Physical Education
* and Recreation*
University of Wisconsin-LaCrosse
La Crosse, Wisconsin

Second Edition

LEA & FEBIGER
Philadelphia
1988

Lea & Febiger
600 Washington Square
Philadelphia, PA 19106-4198
U.S.A.
(215) 922-1330

Library of Congress Cataloging-in-Publication Data

Fardy, Paul S.
  Cardiac rehabilitation, adult fitness, and exercise
testing.

  Wilson's name appears first on the earlier edition.
  Includes bibliographies and index.
  1. Heart—Diseases—Patients—Rehabilitation.
2. Exercise tests. 3. Physical fitness. 4. Community
health services—Planning. I. Yanowitz, Frank G.
II. Wilson, Philip K. III. Title. [DNLM: 1 Exercise
Test. 2. Heart Diseases—rehabilitation. 3. Physical
Fitness. WG 200 F221c]
  RC682.F37   1987   616.1'206   87-22837
  ISBN 0-8121-1104-4

PRINTED IN THE UNITED STATES OF AMERICA

Print No. 4   3   2   1

To our children
Stephen, Beth Ann, Patrick,
Andrew, Peter, Barrie Anne,
Michelle, Kristy, Michael

Preface

Since the publication of the 1st edition of *Cardiac Rehabilitation, Adult Fitness, and Exercise Testing*, the number of such programs has increased substantially. Hospital-based programs have increased in number and size as administrators and hospital boards have looked eagerly at new outpatient programs, particularly those that complement services already provided. The interest in programs has been particularly accentuated by the advent of diagnosis-related groups (DRGs), which have, in most cases, reduced income and caused hospitals to trim costs.

Physician-owned and/or -operated, free-standing facilities have grown even more rapidly than hospital programs. Declining income and increased competition among physicians have created an upsurge of entrepreneurial interest in the medical community. The entrepreneurial spirit is very apparent in the development of medical and quasimedical programs such as physical rehabilitation, cardiac and pulmonary rehabilitation, health, fitness, wellness, and sports medicine programs. Perhaps most striking is the growth of comprehensive facilities that combine several of these programs.

The benefits of exercise, either for patients or the general populace, are still being argued. Data from prospective studies to prove that physical activity prolongs life and reduces the occurrence or recurrence of coronary heart disease have not resolved the issue. The probability of a clinical trial to conclusively answer the question is remote because of the cost and complexity of such an undertaking. Nevertheless, considerable retrospective and epidemiologic data suggest decreased mortality with increased physical activity, and in addition, numerous studies demonstrate improved mental and physical well-being as well as other therapeutic benefits of regular exercise.[2–4]

Perhaps the most important programmatic change witnessed in recent years is the acceptance, integration, and application of exercise combined with other life-style management programs such as weight control, nutrition, smoking cessation, and stress management. The multifaceted and multipurpose approach seems correct. Of significance to this is the recognition that life-style programs are more than education classes. Increased didactic knowledge is beneficial but is only the first step in getting people to adopt better living habits.

In the 2nd edition the authors have updated information and added considerable new material. The most substantive changes include a new chapter on cardiovascular anatomy and physiology; a comprehensive presentation of cardiovascular assessment and treatment; a new and comprehensive chapter on exercise testing; updated and new material on the business of cardiac rehabilitation, adult fitness, and exercise testing; information on integration of fitness and rehabilitation programs; a new chapter on phase II cardiac rehabilitation; a new chapter on patient education and behavior modification; and a fresh look at future perspectives.

Alternative rehabilitation programs are also discussed. The traditional approach of continually monitored and supervised exercise is presented along with nontraditional programs that enable greater numbers to participate and simultaneously reduce program costs. Program design is discussed to ensure that programs are safe and beneficial.

The 2nd edition contains 16 chapters, which are grouped in five sections as follows: (I) Foundational Information (Chapters 1 and 2); (II) Evaluation and Exercise Prescription (Chapters 3 through 6); (III) Administrative Concerns (Chapters 7 through 11); (IV) Inpatient, Outpatient, Adult Fitness Exercise, and Life-style Management Programs (Chapters 12 through 15); (V) Current and Future Perspectives (Chapter 16).

The authors hope that the reader finds this volume to be a logical progression and comprehensive treatment of cardiac rehabilitation, adult fitness, and exercise testing. The authors consider this text to be an in-depth presentation of the subject matter that takes the reader through the need, planning, implementation, and benefits of these programs. It is intended that the book serve as a reference for professionals in the field and as a textbook for those training in their careers. We wish all of you the best and hope that the information contained here will serve you along the way.

PSF., FGY., PKW.

REFERENCES

1. Fitch, E.: Healthcare marketing: more than the doctor ordered. *Advertising Age,* Dec. 15, 1986, p. S-1.
2. Paffenbarger, R.S., Jr.: Exercise in the primary prevention of coronary heart disease. *In* Heart Disease and Rehabilitation. Edited by M.L. Pollock and D.H. Schmidt. New York, John Wiley & Sons, 1986.
3. Fox, S.M., III: Relationship of activity habits to coronary heart disease. *In* Exercise Testing and Exercise Training in Coronary Heart Disease. Edited by J.P. Naughton, H.K. Hellerstein, and I.C. Mohler. New York, Academic Press, 1973.
4. Haskell, W.L.: Mechanisms by which physical activity may enhance the clinical status of cardiac patients. *In* Heart Disease and Rehabilitation. Edited by M.L. Pollock and D.H. Schmidt. New York, John Wiley & Sons, 1986.

Contents

FOUNDATIONAL INFORMATION

1

INTRODUCTION

"Americans know more today about how to make a living than how to live" (Henry David Thoreau). Thoreau's remarks of 150 years ago are probably truer today than ever before. However, the picture isn't entirely bad. Mortality in the United States from coronary heart disease (CHD) continues to decline,[1] and interest in the benefits of exercise and maintaining a healthier life-style continues to increase as does the need for well-thought-out professionally supervised programs with realistic goals. Unfortunately, programs that promise unattainable benefits whose methods are likely unsafe and whose basis is primarily monetary gain are still in abundance.

The American public is, in fact, more sophisticated today than ever before concerning factors that impact on its health. But, confusion remains over numerous claims and counter claims on the best way to improve one's health, prevent chronic degenerative diseases associated with an unhealthy life-style, and live longer and live better. Those who are seriously and knowledgeably involved in the health, physical fitness, preventive medicine, and rehabilitation professions have made considerable progress in providing appropriate direction, but there is still a long way to go.

Although improvement in life-style is not limited to increased physical activity, regular exercise is probably the focal point and motivator for other behavioral programs in many if not most rehabilitation and fitness centers. Exercise should not be regarded as a panacea, but it does offer benefits that are not characteristic of other life-style interventions. Group dynamics, sociability, relatively quick feedback on improvement, good feelings about self, more pep and energy, and looking and feeling better are typical reasons for people choosing to exercise. And, because people are choosing to exercise more, the need persists for knowledgeable professional direction, particularly in those persons with diagnosed heart disease or who are of increased risk for CHD.

This opinion is supported in the Report of the Inter-Society Commission for Heart Disease Resources.[2]

> Regular exercise, particularly those forms of endurance exercise which enhance cardiovascular fitness, may have a role to play in the prevention of atherosclerotic diseases. It is important to emphasize, however, that exercise is not free of danger both to the muscoloskeletal and the cardiovascular systems. This is particularly true for middle-aged individuals—especially coronary prone persons—who suddenly take up vigorous exercise after years of minimal physical activity. Physicians and other professionals need aid in guiding a concerned public to avoid these problems. (p. 89)

If exercise is accepted as a beneficial therapeutic intervention that can play a significant role in preventive medicine and rehabilitation, then we need to focus our energies on providing proper guidance. This requires establishing and promoting professionally sound programs, appropriate training of personnel, and making the

3

public more knowledgeable. There must also be a balance between the Spartan philosophy, which emphasized physical prowess, and the Athenian philosophy, which stressed cultural development. If humans are to flourish, then cultural, spiritual, and physical maturation are all important. As George Sheehan proposes, "man is an animal" and physically we should endeavor to satisfy that part of ourselves. But, as Sheehan points out, we are also children who need to play, and we are culturally and intellectually curious.[3] Plato identified this in *The Republic* in promoting a balanced life-style, one that continues to grow until death.[4]

IDENTIFYING TODAY'S HEALTH PROBLEMS

If longevity in the United States is an indication of health, then the clinical advances of the past 50 years have had equivocal results. The average person lives significantly longer today compared to 50 years ago, with life expectancies of 75 and 54 years, respectively,[5] although this change is greatly affected by decreased mortality at childbirth and from childhood diseases. Changes in longevity for the adult who attains 40 years of age have been appreciably less over this period of time (Fig. 1–1 and Table 1–1).[6,7]

Compared to the United States, life expectancy is greater in many other countries, none of which are considered more medically advanced (Table 1–2).[8] This fact is particularly perplexing considering the vast sums of money that are spent annually on health care, approximately $400 billion, including $85 billion for cardiovascular disease.[9] The comparatively low life expectancy in the United States is even more astonishing in view of the drastic reduction or elimination of many death-causing infectious diseases. Apparently, mortality from infectious diseases has been replaced by that from chronic degenerative diseases.

The leading cause of mortality today in the United States, as well as throughout the advanced countries of the world, continues to be cardiovascular diseases (Fig. 1–2),

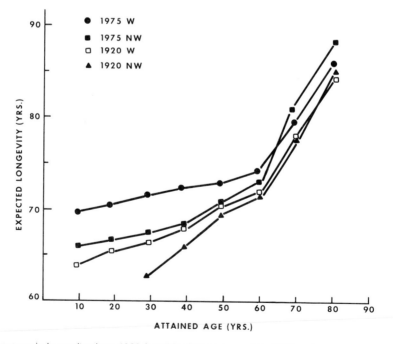

Fig. 1–1.   Increase in longevity since 1920 for white (W) and nonwhite (NW) males.

Table 1–1. Comparisons in Longevity for Adults Who Attain 40 Years of Age in 1920, 1975, and 1981

Year	Whites (%)	Blacks (%)
1920	68	65
1975	72	68
1981	77	73

Statistical Abstracts of United States, 1983.

with the most prevalent being from myocardial infarction (Fig. 1–3). CHD manifests after continued exposure to a variety of harmful agents or risk factors, such as diets high in saturated fat, cholesterol, and calories; sedentary living; increased mental and emotional stress; and cigarette smoking. The result of these harmful factors can be as great as a thirtyfold increase in risk of CHD (Fig. 1–4). In addition, mortality rates per 100,000 in females have plateaued since 1960, whereas mortality rates in males have decreased significantly.[5] Thus, it appears that the major determinants of longevity are a product of twentieth century life-style, the basis of which is cultural rather than medical. Rehabilitation and primary prevention programs, therefore, should emphasize improving life-style.

In the United States, cardiovascular diseases account for 48% of total mortality.[9] Of these, approximately 55% are attributed to myocardial infarction (Fig. 1–3). More alarming is the conspicuous absence of any prior indication of CHD in almost 50% of those who died suddenly.[10,11] Additional evidence of the insidiousness of the disease is that almost 25% of heart attacks go undetected, "silent infarcts,"[12] and go untreated unless noted during a subsequent examination. It is estimated that more than 63 million Americans have some form of cardiovascular disease (Fig. 1–5).[9] Moreover, while victims of CHD are usually thought to be older citizens, approximately 20% of mortalities and more than 50% of CHD prevalence are under the age of 65, and 6% of mortalities and 10% of CHD prevalence are under 44 years of age.[5,9,13]

The economics of heart disease are equally dismal. The cost of cardiovascular

Table 1–2. A Comparison of Longevities by Sex Among Countries (1980)

Males		Females	
Country	Life Expectancy (Years)	Country	Life Expectancy (Years)
Iceland	73.6	Iceland	80.5
Japan	73.6	Netherlands	79.5
Greece	73.1	Norway	79.3
Sweden	72.8	Sweden	79.1
The Netherlands	72.5	Switzerland	79.1
Norway	72.4	France	79.1
Switzerland	72.3	Japan	79.1
Israel	72.2	Canada	78.9
Canada	71.4	Hong Kong	78.3
Denmark	71.2	Australia	78.2
Hong Kong	71.2	Finland	78.0
Australia	71.0	United States	77.8
Italy	71.0	Italy	77.7
Costa Rica	71.0	Greece	77.6
France	70.8	Denmark	77.4
United Kingdom	70.7	Fed. Rep. Germany	76.8
United States	70.1	United Kingdom	76.8
Fed. Rep. Germany	69.9	New Zealand	76.4
Luxembourg	69.9	Austria	76.1
Ireland	69.8	Costa Rica	76.0
New Zealand	69.8	Israel	75.8
Finland	69.2	Luxembourg	75.3

World Health Organization, 1982 to 1984.

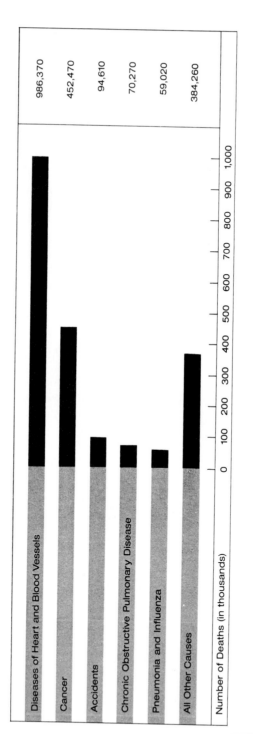

Diseases of Heart and Blood Vessels	986,370
Cancer	452,470
Accidents	94,610
Chronic Obstructive Pulmonary Disease	70,270
Pneumonia and Influenza	59,020
All Other Causes	384,260

Number of Deaths (in thousands)

Fig. 1–2. Leading causes of death. United States, 1984 estimate. National Center for Health Statistics, U.S. Public Health Service, DHHS.

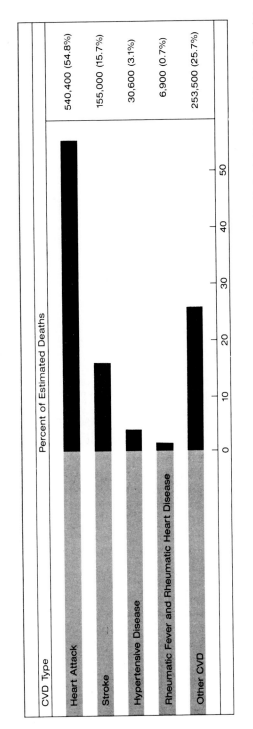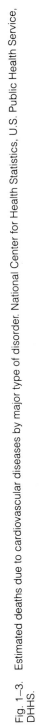

CVD Type	Percent of Estimated Deaths
Heart Attack	540,400 (54.8%)
Stroke	155,000 (15.7%)
Hypertensive Disease	30,600 (3.1%)
Rheumatic Fever and Rheumatic Heart Disease	6,900 (0.7%)
Other CVD	253,500 (25.7%)

Fig. 1–3.   Estimated deaths due to cardiovascular diseases by major type of disorder. National Center for Health Statistics, U.S. Public Health Service, DHHS.

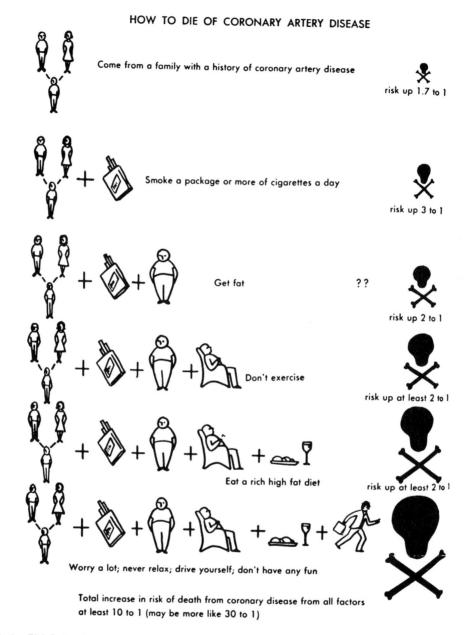

HOW TO DIE OF CORONARY ARTERY DISEASE

Come from a family with a history of coronary artery disease — risk up 1.7 to 1

Smoke a package or more of cigarettes a day — risk up 3 to 1

Get fat — ?? — risk up 2 to 1

Don't exercise — risk up at least 2 to 1

Eat a rich high fat diet — risk up at least 2 to 1

Worry a lot; never relax; drive yourself; don't have any fun

Total increase in risk of death from coronary disease from all factors at least 10 to 1 (may be more like 30 to 1)

Fig. 1–4. Risk factors in coronary artery disease.

disease in this country is estimated at $85 billion for 1987 (Fig. 1–6), which includes the cost for approximately 200,000 bypass procedures.[5,9] This figure does not take into consideration job training, reinvestment in training replacements, and lost capital from those who depend on the occupation of the victim. The loss of manpower is estimated at 62 million man days/

year,[5,9] as a result of 16.4 million Americans who have limited physical activity from heart disease.[5] The drain on our economic resources plus the psychologic and social trauma experienced by the victim, family, and friends, emphasize the need for a carefully planned strategy of prevention and rehabilitation.

While heart attacks account for approx-

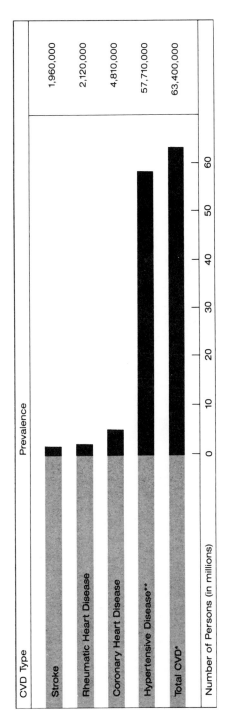

CVD Type	Prevalence
Stroke	1,960,000
Rheumatic Heart Disease	2,120,000
Coronary Heart Disease	4,810,000
Hypertensive Disease**	57,710,000
Total CVD*	63,400,000

Number of Persons (in millions)

Fig. 1–5. Estimated prevalence of the major cardiovascular diseases. United States, 1984 estimate. (Reproduced with permission, 1987 Heart Facts. American Heart Association.)

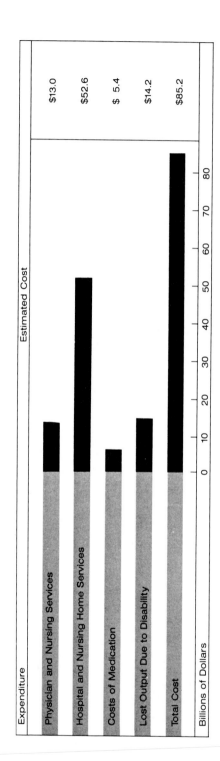
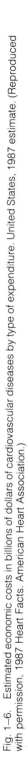

Expenditure	Estimated Cost
Physician and Nursing Services	$13.0
Hospital and Nursing Home Services	$52.6
Costs of Medication	$ 5.4
Lost Output Due to Disability	$14.2
Total Cost	$85.2

Billions of Dollars

Fig. 1–6.   Estimated economic costs in billions of dollars of cardiovascular diseases by type of expenditure. United States, 1987 estimate. (Reproduced with permission, 1987 Heart Facts. American Heart Association.)

imately half a million deaths each year, another million will have survived the initial event.[9] The majority of survivors are less than 65 years of age and are potentially productive members of society. For them, a well-planned program of physical and psychosocial rehabilitation is essential for returning to an active and productive life. The prognosis for conservatively treated cardiac patients is variable and depends, in part, on severity of the infarct and age;[14,15] 25% to 30% of a typical employed male population die within 5 years of the acute episode and usually from a recurring infarct.[16]

Exercise intervention in some form is well accepted today by the medical community as an integral component of rehabilitation and secondary prevention programs.[17] Data on patient safety are encouraging,[18–20] equipment used in rehabilitation programs continues to get better, and our experience with exercise has increased the quality and quantity of programs. Data from numerous exercise and life-style modification programs support cardiac rehabilitation as a needed, safe, and worthwhile service.[21,22] Exercise is fun, it provides positive reinforcement of getting better, and it has been shown time and again to enhance the quality if not the quantity of life.[21–23]

Endorsements and statements of support by professional associations such as the American Association of Cardiovascular and Pulmonary Rehabilitation, American Heart Association,[24] American College of Sports Medicine,[25] American College of Cardiology, and the American Medical Association[26–27] have also been helpful in establishing acceptance of cardiac rehabilitation. As a result, the number of rehabilitation programs has escalated significantly in the past 5 years, especially the number of freestanding, physician-directed and -owned facilities. All of this has occurred in spite of the fact that there are still no long-term prospective data from randomized controlled studies that show decreased mortality from regular exercise. Past experiences have shown that these studies are extremely expensive and are difficult to control. The ethical and financial impediments of getting several thousand postinfarct patients into a controlled clinical trial today are so overwhelming as to make the possibility of future studies virtually nonexistent.

CHD AND OCCUPATIONAL–LEISURE TIME PHYSICAL ACTIVITY

The impact of occupational physical activity on incidence and mortality of CHD has been widely reported. These studies have consistently reported that the frequency of heart disease is less in more active populations,[28–33] and that survival from myocardial infarct during the initial months following the event is lower among less active workers.[34,35] Unfortunately, the physical demands of modern-day jobs continue to decrease in our highly automated society.[36] Since physical work time and energy expenditure have been on the decline with the advent of technological developments, there is greater interest today in the potential prophylactic benefits of exercise programs at work and leisure-time physical activity, which has also been associated with increased fitness and decreased incidence of CHD.[37–40]

PHYSICAL ACTIVITY AND CHD RISK FACTORS

The inverse relationship between decreased CHD and increased physical activity has also been concluded from numerous studies that show favorable risk factor modification has a concomitant effect on lowering CHD incidence and mortality. However, a cause-and-effect relationship has yet to be demonstrated, even though the majority of evidence substantiates an improvement in most risk factors with increased physical activity.

Cholesterol

The majority of evidence indicates that persons and societies who consume large amounts of saturated fats and cholesterol have a greater risk of CHD.[7,41–43] In recent years, interest in total cholesterol (TC) measurement has been replaced with measurement of the cholesterol fractions, LDLC (low-density lipoprotein cholesterol) and HDLC (high-density lipoprotein cholesterol). It has been suggested that the ratio of TC to HDLC is the best predictor of developing CHD.[42] This ratio, TC/HDL, should be less than 5.0 in males and less than 4.5 in females.[42] The problem with any ratio, however, is that it gives no indication by itself of the absolute values. Is 350:70 the same as 200:40? It is suggested, therefore, that if the TC/HDL ratio is used, absolute values also be indicated.

LDLC seems to be the major culprit for CHD,[42] and HDLC appears to have some protective capability.[42,44] Consequently, exercise training is generally assessed in its relation to both LDLC and HDLC. To date, the preponderance of evidence is that exercise, especially in conjunction with a low-fat diet, reduces LDLC[45–47] and results in increased HDLC.[48–51]

The exact mechanism whereby cholesterol fractions impact CHD, either positively or negatively, remains partially unknown. However, this research has gained more attention with the National Institutes of Health (NIH) study on cholesterol lowering[52] and the awarding of the 1985 Nobel Prize for Medicine for work in the area of cholesterol metabolism.

Triglycerides

A lipid profile obtained on a patient with known or suspected CHD should also contain a triglyceride level. Although elevated triglycerides are generally associated with increased risk of CHD, controversy remains as to whether triglycerides act independently from cholesterol.[7,53] Regardless, triglycerides do provide important dietary information for counseling patients and demonstrate greater acute changes than cholesterol does.[54,55] Elevated triglycerides, especially with type IV hyperlipoproteinemia, are related to obesity and are altered significantly by dietary caloric restrictions.[56] Triglyceride levels are also more susceptible to change than cholesterol as a result of acute exercise.[57] Therefore, it is especially important that a 12- to 14-hour fast and refraining from physical activity precede the drawing of blood.

To lower cholesterol and triglycerides it is advised that exercise be accompanied by a low-fat diet. It is also suggested that lipid levels be obtained at the beginning, middle, and end of the intervention program. This will help to better establish the effectiveness of the program and perhaps to get more aggressive in those cases where no changes have occurred.

Hypertension

Although the evidence is inconclusive, there is considerable interest in the relationship between hypertension and physical activity. Both systolic and diastolic blood pressure have been observed to increase with age in developed countries,[58,59] while this has not been the case in undeveloped countries,[60] where among other differences in life-style, the level of physical activity is generally higher. Unfortunately, other factors are present in those societies that are likely to confound this relationship. Consequently, in order to assess the effect of exercise on blood pressure, comparisons are usually made within populations preceding and following intervention. The findings from blood pressure studies generally support a lower blood pressure in more active individuals[61–63] and lowered blood pressure in response to regular exercise.[64–66]

A similarity to lipid research is that much remains unknown about hypertension. What are its causes, and why is there generally lowering of blood pressure with diet and exercise? It is known that blood pressure is related to obesity, so that reduction in body weight usually is accompanied by decrease in blood pressure.[67] It is also known that blood pressure is related to blood volume, thereby explaining the association with sodium, which has the capacity to retain water and thereby increase blood volume. Decreases in blood pressure are probably also related to lowered sympathetic adrenergic activity, which results in less constriction in peripheral blood vessels and reduced peripheral resistance.[60,68] Since blood pressure is also related to stress, it is possible that exercise can reduce hypertension through an increase in opiate-acting endorphins.[69,70] More studies are needed to clarify this hypothesis.

PHYSICAL ACTIVITY AND OTHER PROPHYLACTIC MECHANISMS

Regular physical activity also benefits a variety of other cardiovascular mechanisms. For example, myocardial function can be enhanced with vigorous exercise.[71,72] The coronary arteries might also be improved with systematic exercise. Coronary vasodilation, as well as increased vessel size and number have been reported.[73–76] Other studies have evaluated the effect of regular exercise on hemodynamic, metabolic, electrocardiographic, and neurohormonal factors. Data from these investigations have shown overwhelmingly the possibility of preventive mechanisms including increased myocardial efficiency, and decreased heart rate, electrocardiogram (ECG) abnormalities, cardiac sympathetic tone, and myocardial oxygen demand.[71,72,77–81] A summary of cardiovascular and other adaptive responses is presented in Table 1–3.

Implementing Exercise Programs

A rapid growth has occurred in both hospital-based and freestanding cardiac rehabilitation programs. This trend will probably continue with an even greater number of centers being started outside of the hospital. The number of physical fitness programs, health clubs, wellness centers, and spas will most likely continue to increase as well.

In most instances, the quality of these programs is also on the rise. Undergraduate and graduate professional programs are recognizing and emphasizing alternative educational opportunities in health and fitness, as well as clinical applications of exercise. Professional associations such

Table 1–3. Mechanisms by Which Physical Activity May Reduce the Occurrence or Severity of Coronary Heart Disease[a]

Physical Activity May:	
Increase	*Decrease*
Coronary collateral vascularization	Serum lipid levels
Coronary artery size	Triglycerides
Myocardial efficiency	Cholesterol
Efficiency of peripheral blood distribution and return	Glucose intolerance
Electron transport capacity	Obesity-adiposity
Fibrinolytic capability	Platelet stickiness
Red blood cell mass and blood volume	Arterial blood pressure
Thyroid function	Vulnerability to dysrhythmias
Growth hormone production	Neurohormonal overreaction
Tolerance to stress	"Strain" associated with
Prudent living habits	psychic "stress"
Joie de vivre	

[a]From Fox, S.M., III: Relationship of activity habits to coronary heart disease. *In* Exercise Testing and Exercise Training in Coronary Heart Disease. Edited by J.P. Naughton, H.K. Hellerstein, and I.C. Mohler. Orlando, Fla., Academic Press, 1973.

as the American College of Sports Medicine and the American Heart Association are developing standards to ensure some level of quality control among allied health professionals involved in cardiac rehabilitation. In spite of these steps, more work is needed to better prepare students and to further enhance programs.

One of the greatest needs remains in the preparation of medical students, who, in general, are still inadequately educated in exercise physiology, cardiac rehabilitation, nutrition, and preventive medicine. Consequently, the exercise specialist and the physician need to be closely allied for the conduct of these programs. More accredited programs for physicians need to be sponsored to promote a better understanding of prevention and rehabilitation. Today, the best way to improve health, physical fitness, rehabilitation, and prevention programs is still through the cooperative efforts of the exercise physiologist or other allied health professionals and the physician. This formula still offers the greatest chance for prudent, safe, and effective programs.

REFERENCES

1. Kannel, W.: Epidemiologic insights into atherosclerotic cardiovascular diseases from the Framingham Study. *In* Heart Disease and Rehabilitation. Edited by M.L. Pollock and D.H. Schmidt. New York, John Wiley & Sons, 1986.
2. Report of the Inter-Society Commission for Heart Disease Resources. Primary prevention of the atherosclerotic diseases. Circulation, *42*(A55):71, 1967.
3. Sheehan, G.A.: This Running Life. New York, Simon & Schuster, 1980.
4. Plato: The Republic. New York, Great Books, Encyclopaedia Britannica, 1952.
5. National Data Book and Guide to Sources, Statistical Abstract of the United States, 1985. 105th Ed. Washington, D.C., United States Department of Commerce, Bureau of Census, 1985.
6. Life Insurance Fact Book. Washington, D.C., American Council of Life Insurance, 1977.
7. Blackburn, H.: Progress in the epidemiology and prevention of coronary heart disease. *In* Progress in Cardiology. Edited by P.N. Yu and J.F. Goodwin. Philadelphia, Lea & Febiger, 1974.
8. Selected World Demographic Indicators by Countries, 1950–2000. UN Population Division Working Paper No. 55, 1975.
9. Heart Facts. Dallas, American Heart Association, 1987.
10. Gordon, T., and Kannel, W.B.: Preventive Mortality from CHD: Framingham Study. JAMA, *215*:1617, 1971.
11. Shurtleff, D.: Some Characteristics Related to the Incidence of Cardiovascular Disease and Death: Framingham Study; 18 Year Follow-up. Washington, D.C., U.S. Government Printing Office, Dept. of H.E.W. Publication Number (NIH) 74–599, 1974.
12. Margolis, J.R., et al.: Clinical features of unrecognized myocardial infarction—Silent and symptomatic: 18 year follow-up. Framingham Study. Am. J. Cardiol., *32*:1, 1973.
13. Daniel, A.: Coronary heart disease: An overview. *In* Heart Disease and Rehabilitation. Edited by M.L. Pollock and D.H. Schmidt. New York, John Wiley & Sons, 1986.
14. Helander, S., and Levander, M.: Primary mortalty and 5 year prognosis of cardiac infarction: Study which considers in particular how prognosis is affected by comparison of materials as regards to age and sex of patients and severity of infarction. Acta Med. Scand., *163*:289, 1959.
15. Seigel, D.G., and Loncin, H.: A critique of studies of long-term survivorship of patients with myocardial infarction. Am. J. Public Health, *58*:1348, 1968.
16. Kavanagh, T., and Shephard, R.J.: Importance of physical activity in post-coronary rehabilitation. Am. J. Phys. Med., *52*:304, 1973.
17. Shephard, R.J.: Cardiac rehabilitation in prospect. *In* Heart Disease and Rehabilitation. Edited by M.L. Pollock and D.H. Schmidt. New York, John Wiley & Sons, 1986.
18. Meyer, G.C.: Telemetry electrocardiographic monitoring in cardiac rehabilitation: How long? How often? *In* Cardiac Rehabilitation: Exercise Testing and Prescription. Edited by L.K. Hall. Jamaica, New York, Spectrum Publications, 1984.
19. Haskell, W.L.: Cardiovascular complications during exercise training of cardiac patients. Circulation, *57*:920, 1978.
20. VanCamp, S.P. and Peterson, R.A.: Cardiovascular complications of outpatient cardiac rehabilitation programs. JAMA, *256*:1160, 1986.
21. Roman, O.: Do randomized trials support the use of cardiac rehabilitation? J. Cardiac Rehabil., *5*:93, 1985.
22. Kallio, V., et al.: Reduction in sudden deaths by a multifactoral intervention programme after acute myocardial infarction. Lancet, *2*:1091, 1979.
23. Shephard, R.J.: The value of exercise in ischaemic heart disease—a cumulative analysis. J. Cardiac Rehab., *3*:294, 1983.
24. Exercise Standards Book. Dallas, American Heart Association, 1979.
25. Guidelines for Exercise Testing and Prescription. American College of Sports Medicine. 3rd Ed. Philadelphia, Lea & Febiger, 1986.
26. American Medical Association, Council on Sci-

entific Affairs: Physician-supervised exercise programs in rehabilitation of patients with coronary heart disease. JAMA, *245*:1463, 1981.

27. Hellerstein, H.K.: Cardiac rehabilitation: A retrospective view. *In* Heart Disease and Rehabilitation. 2nd Ed. Edited by M.L. Pollock and D.H. Schmidt. New York, John Wiley & Sons, 1986.

28. Paffenbarger, R.S., et al.: Epidemiology of exercise and coronary heart disease. Clin. Sports Med., *3*:297, 1984.

29. Paffenbarger, R.S., and Hyde, R.T.: Exercise in the prevention of coronary heart disease. Prev. Med., *13*:3, 1984.

30. Paffenbarger, R.S., Jr.: Exercise in the primary prevention of coronary heart disease. *In* Heart Disease and Rehabilitation. Edited by M.L. Pollock and D.H. Schmidt. New York, John Wiley & Sons, 1986.

31. Fox, S.M., III: Relationship of activity habits to coronary heart disease. *In* Exercise Testing and Exercise Training in Coronary Heart Disease. Edited by J.P. Naughton, H.K. Hellerstein, and I.C. Mohler. Orlando, Fla., Academic Press, 1973.

32. Paffenbarger, R.S., et al.: Work-energy level, personal characteristics, and fatal heart attack: A birth-cohort effect. Am. J. Epidemiol., *105*:200, 1977.

33. Brand, R.J., et al.: Work activity and fatal heart attacks studied by multiple logistic risk analysis. Am. J. Epidemiol., *110*:52, 1979.

34. Rose, G.: Physical activity and coronary heart disease. Proc. R. Soc. Med., *62*:1183, 1969.

35. Kannel, W.B., Sortie, P., and McNamara, P.: The relation of physical activity to risk of coronary heart disease. The Framingham Study. *In* Coronary Heart Disease and Physical Fitness. Edited by O.A. Larsen and R.O. Malmborg. Copenhagen, Munksgaard, 1971.

36. Shephard, R.J.: The working capacity of the older employee. A.M.A. Arch. Environ. Health., *18*:982, 1969.

37. Morris, J.N., et al.: Vigorous exercise in leisure-time and the incidence of coronary heart-failure disease. Lancet, *1*:333, 1973.

38. Morris, J.N., et al.: Vigorous leisure-time: Protection against coronary heart-disease. Lancet, *2*:1207, 1980.

39. Paffenbarger, R.S., Jr., Wing, A.L., and Hyde, R.T.: Chronic disease in former college students. XVI. Physical activity as an index of heart attack risk in college alumni. Am. J. Epidemiol., *108*:161, 1978.

40. Paffenbarger, R.S., Jr., et al.: Physical activity, all-cause mortality, and longevity of college alumni. N. Engl. J. Med., *314*:605, 1986.

41. Keys, A.: Coronary heart disease in seven countries. Circulation *41*(Suppl. 1):1, 1970.

42. Kannel, W.B., Castelli, W.P., and Gordon, T.: Cholesterol in the prediction of atherosclerotic heart disease: New perspectives based on the Framingham Study. Ann. Intern. Med., *90*:85, 1979.

43. Gordon, T., et al.: Lipoproteins, cardiovascular disease and death: The Framingham Study. Arch. Intern. Med., *141*:1128, 1981.

44. Miller, N.E., et al.: The Thromso Heart Study: High density lipoprotein and coronary heart disease: A prospective case control study. Lancet, *1*:965, 1977.

45. Joseph, J.J., and Bena L.L.: Cholesterol reduction—a long term intense exercise program. J. Sports Med. Phys. Fitness, *17*:163, 1977.

46. Kallio, V., et al.: Reduction of sudden deaths by a multifactorial intervention programme after acute myocardial infarction. Lancet, *2*:1091, 1979.

47. Vermuelen, A., Lie, K.I., and Durrer, D.: Effects of cardiac rehabilitation after myocardial infarction: Changes in coronary risk factors and long-term prognosis. Am. Heart J., *105*:798, 1983.

48. Blackburn, H.: Physical activity and coronary heart disease: A brief update and population view. Part I. J. Cardiac. Rehab., *3*:101, 1983.

49. Wood, P.D., et al.: Increased exercise level and plama lipoprotein concentrations: A one-year randomized, controlled study in sedentary, middle-aged men. Metabolism, *32*:31, 1983.

50. Rotkis, T.C.,et al.: Relationship between high density lipoprotein cholesterol and weekly running mileage. J. Cardiac Rehab., *2*:109, 1982.

51. Rotkis, T.C., et al.: Increased high-density lipoprotein cholesterol and lean weight in endurance trained women runners. J. Cardiac Rehab., *4*:62, 1984.

52. Lipid Research Clinics Program: The Lipids Research Clinics coronary primary prevention trial results. II. The relationship of reduction in incidence of coronary heart disease to cholesterol lowering. JAMA, *251*:365, 1984.

53. Gordon, T., et al.: High density lipoprotein as a protective factor against coronary heart disease. The Framingham Study. Am. J. Med., *62*:707, 1977.

54. Carlson, L.A., and Bottinger, L.E.: Ischemic heart-disease in relation to fasting values of plasma triglycerides and cholesterol. Stockholm prospective study. Lancet, *1*:865, 1972.

55. Carlson, L.A., and Ericsson, M.: Quantitative and qualitative serum lipoprotein analysis. Part 2. Studies in male survivors of myocardial infarction. Atherosclerosis, *21*:435, 1975.

56. Dietary Management of Hyperlipoproteinemia: A Handbook for Physicians. National Heart and Lung Institute, Bethesda, Md., 1971.

57. Holloszy, J., Skinner, J., and Toro, G.: Effect of a six-month program of exercise on the serum lipids of middle-aged men. Am. J. Cardiol., *14*:753, 1964.

58. Blood pressure of adults by age and sex (United States) 1960–1962. U.S. Dept. of H.E.W., Public Health Services and Mental Health Administration, National Center for Health Statistics, Series II, No. 4, June, 1964.

59. Fardy, P.S., et al.: An assessment of the influence of habitual physical activity, prior sport participation, smoking habits, and aging upon indices of cardiovascular fitness: Preliminary report of a cross sectional and retrospective study. J. Sports Med. Phys. Fitness, *16*:77, 1976.

60. Epstein, F.H., and Eckhoff, R.D.: The epide-

miology of high blood pressure-geographic distributions and etiological factors. *In* The Epidemiology of Hypertension. Edited by J. Stamler and R. Stamler. Orlando, Fla., Grune & Stratton, 1967.

61. Blair, S.N., et al.: Physical fitness and incidence of hypertension in healthy normotensive men and women. JAMA, *252*:487, 1984.

62. Morris, J.N.: Epidemiology and cardiovascular diseases of middle-age. Part I. Mod. Concepts Cardiovasc. Dis., *29*:625, 1960.

63. Paffenbarger, R.S., Jr., et al.: Physical activity and incidence of hypertension in college alumni. XX. Am. J. Epidemiol., *117*:245, 1983.

64. Boyer, J.L., and Kasch, F.W.: Exercise therapy in hypertensive men. JAMA, *211*:1668, 1970.

65. Fitzgerald, W.: Labile hypertension and jogging: New diagnostic tool or spurious discovery? Br. Med. J., *282*:542, 1981.

66. Wilcox, R.G., et al.: Is exercise good for high blood pressure? Br. Med. J., *285*:767, 1982.

67. Gillum, R.F., et al.: Nonpharmacologic control of hypertension: The independent effects of weight reduction and salt restriction in overweight borderline hypertensive patents. Am. Heart. J., *105*:128, 1983.

68. Duncan, J.J., et al.: The effect of an aerobic exercise program on sympathetic neural activity and blood pressure in mild hypertension. Abstract. Circulation, *68*:285, 1983.

69. Morgan, W.P.: Affective beneficence of vigorous physical activity. Med. Sci. Sports Exer., *19*:94, 1985.

70. Grossman, A.: Endorphins: "Opiates for the masses." Med. Sci. Sports Exerc., *17*:101, 1985.

71. Froelicher, V.F.: The hemodynamic effects of physical conditioning in healthy young, and middle-aged individuals, and in coronary heart disease patients. *In* Exercise Testing and Exercise Training in Coronary Heart Disease. Edited by J.P. Naughton, H.K. Hellerstein, and I.C. Mohler. Orlando, Fla., Academic Press, 1973.

72. Haskell, W.L.: Mechanisms by which physical activity may enhance the clinical status of cardiac patients. *In* Heart Disease and Rehabilitation. 2nd Ed. Edited by M.L. Pollock and D.H. Schmidt. New York, John Wiley & Sons, 1986.

73. Eckstein, R.W.: Effect of exercising and coronary artery narrowing on coronary collateral circulation. Circ. Res., *5*:230, 1957.

74. Scheel, K.W.: The stimulus for coronary collateral growth: Ischemia or mechanical factors. J. Cardiac Rehab., *1*:149, 1981.

75. Kattus, A.A.: The UCLA interdepartmental conference. Diagnosis, medical and surgical management of coronary insufficiency. Ann. Intern. Med., *69*:115, 1968.

76. Lamb, L.E.: Eldminen on Sydamen Asia. Helsinki, Weilin & Boos, 1971.

77. Franks, B.D.: Effects of different types and amounts of training on selected fitness measures. *In* Exercise and Fitness. Edited by B.D. Franks. Chicago, Athletic Institute, 1969.

78. Fardy, P.S.: Left ventricle time component changes in middle-aged men following a twelve week physical training intervention program. J. Sports Med. Phys. Fitness, *13*:219, 1973.

79. Clausen, J.P., and Trap-Jensen, J.: Effects of training on the distribution of cardiac output in patients with coronary artery disease. Circulation, *42*:611, 1970.

80. Lepeschkin, E., and Bruis, O.A.: Effect of physical training on the exercise electrocardiogram. Recent Adv. Stud. Cardiac Struct. Metab., *1*:753, 1970.

81. Noakes, T.D., Higginson, L., and Opie, L.H.: Physical training increases ventricular fibrillation thresholds of isolated rat hearts during normoxia, hypoxia and regional ischemia. Circulation, *67*:24, 1983.

2

ANATOMIC AND PHYSIOLOGIC ASPECTS OF EXERCISE

For the health professional working in cardiac rehabilitation and adult fitness, an understanding of cardiovascular, respiratory, and skeletal muscle structure and function is essential. This chapter discusses anatomic and physiologic aspects of these three organ systems, particularly as they relate to the exercising individual. An outline of the major topics to be considered is presented in Table 2–1.

ANATOMIC COMPONENTS OF THE CARDIOVASCULAR SYSTEM

The three general functions of the cardiovascular system are (1) to deliver oxygen and nutrients to the cells and tissues of the body; (2) to facilitate the removal of carbon dioxide and other waste products pro-

Table 2–1. Anatomic and Physiologic Aspects of Exercise

Anatomic components of the cardiovascular system
  Heart
  Systemic circulation
  Pulmonary circulation
The physiology of exercise
  Skeletal muscle structure and function
  Cardiovascular and pulmonary physiology
    Oxygen uptake
    Heart rate response to exercise
    Stroke volume response to exercise
    Arterial oxygen content
    Oxygen extraction and utilization by
      skeletal muscle
    Myocardial oxygen supply and demand

---

duced by these cells and tissues; and (3) to transport regulatory substances between various regions of the body. A schematic view of the circulation is illustrated in Figure 2–1.[1] The circulation is a continuous circuit involving two major subdivisions, the systemic circulation and the pulmonary circulation, with the heart serving as a muscular pump to provide the necessary pressure for the movement of blood through these two circulations. Resistance to blood flow primarily occurs at the level of the arterioles and capillaries, with the requirement for systolic pressures of approximately 120 mm Hg in the systemic circulation and 20 mm Hg in the pulmonary circulation to drive the blood through these resistance vessels.

The Heart

From a structural point of view, the heart consists of four separate muscular pumps: two primer pumps, the right and left atria, and two power pumps, the right and left ventricles. These are schematically diagrammed in Figure 2–2.[1] Each "side" of the heart serves a major subdivision of the circulation. The right heart receives blood from the inferior and superior vena cava and pumps it into the pulmonary circulation where gas exchange occurs. The left heart pumps oxygenated blood into the high-pressure systemic circulation to serve the organ systems of the body. The atria

PULMONARY CIRCULATION

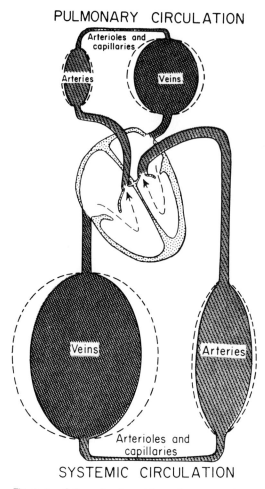

SYSTEMIC CIRCULATION

Fig. 2–1. Schematic view of the pulmonary and systemic circulation. The heart serves as a four-chamber muscular pump to move blood through these two circulations. From Guyton, A.C.: Textbook of Medical Physiology. 6th Ed. Philadelphia, W.B. Saunders, 1981.

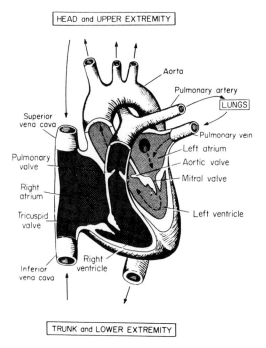

Fig. 2–2. Schematic view of the cardiac chambers and great vessels. From Guyton, A.C.: Textbook of Medical Physiology. 6th Ed. Philadelphia, W.B. Saunders, 1981.

primarily function as reservoirs for returning venous blood during ventricular systole and conduits during ventricular diastole. In addition, atrial contraction just prior to ventricular systole provides a further increment of blood into the ventricles, which enhances the contractile force of ventricular systole.

The heart is composed of two separate syncytia of cardiac muscle, the thin-walled atria and the thick-walled ventricles. The atria and ventricles, the four heart valves, and the two arterial trunks leaving the ventricles are fastened to the fibrous "skeleton" of the heart, which consists of four dense connective tissue rings called annuli fibrosi illustrated in Figure 2–3.[2] The atrial syncytium, aorta, pulmonary artery, and semilunar valves are anchored to the superior surface of the fibrous skeleton, while the ventricular syncytium, mitral, and tricuspid valves originate from the inferior surface.

The two semilunar heart valves (aortic and pulmonary) consist of three symmetric valve cusps, which form a perfect seal when closed, preventing regurgitation of blood back into the ventricles. Behind the valve cusps are outpouchings called sinuses of Valsalva. The ostia for the right and left coronary arteries are located in the anterior two sinuses of Valsalva in the aorta.

The mitral and tricuspid valves are more complex structures. The proximal ends of these valves are attached to the annuli fibrosi of the fibrous skeleton, while the dis-

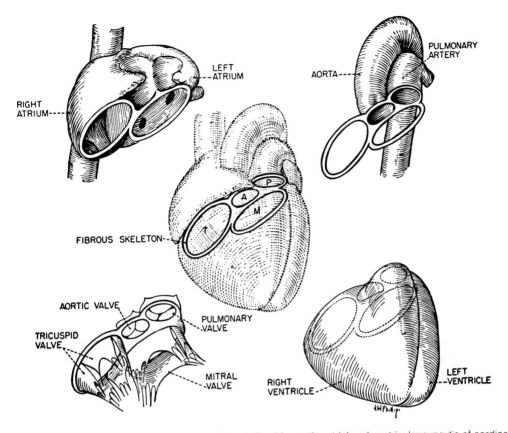

Fig. 2–3. The fibrous skeleton of the heart and its relationships to the atrial and ventricular syncytia of cardiac muscle and the great arteries. From Rushmer, R.F.: Cardiovascular Dynamics. 3rd Ed. Philadelphia, W.B. Saunders, 1970.

tal ends are connected to papillary muscles by fibrous strands called chordae tendineae, as illustrated in Figure 2–4 for the mitral valve.[3] The tricuspid valve has three leaflets of unequal size, while the mitral valve has two leaflets, also of unequal size.

Normal function of these valves requires the intricate interaction of six anatomic structures: the atrial wall, the annuli fibrosi, the valvular tissue, the chordae tendineae, the papillary muscles, and the ventricular wall. Abnormalities involving one or more of these components can lead to valvular regurgitation during ventricular systole. For example, in mitral valve prolapse, which affects approximately 6% of the general population, there is myxomatous degeneration of the valve leaflets, resulting in their prolapse into the left atrium

during ventricular systole. Depending on the severity of the degenerative process, there may or may not be concurrent valvular regurgitation. In contrast, mitral regurgitation may occur in coronary artery disease when the papillary muscles become ischemic or infarcted. Finally, in bacterial endocarditis mitral regurgitation may occur if the chordae tendineae rupture as a result of the infectious process.

The mechanical activities of the heart are initiated and coordinated by an intrinsic electrical system called the specialized conduction system, located within the chambers of heart and illustrated in Figure 2–5.[4] Spontaneously derived electrical impulses originate in a region of pacemaker cells, the sinoatrial (SA) node, located at the junction of the superior vena cava and

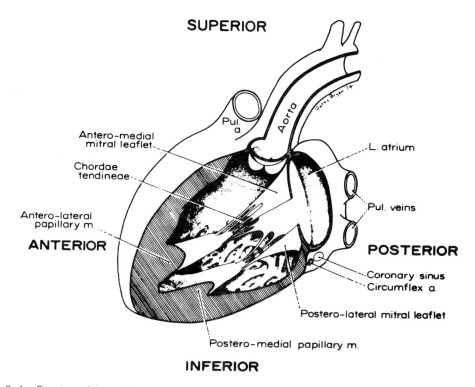

SUPERIOR

Pul.
a.

Aorta

Antero-medial
mitral leaflet

L. atrium

Chordae
tendineae

Antero-lateral
papillary m.

Pul. veins

ANTERIOR

POSTERIOR

Coronary sinus
Circumflex a.

Postero-lateral mitral leaflet

Postero-medial papillary m.

INFERIOR

Fig. 2–4.   Structure of the mitral valve, illustrating the relationships between the papillary muscles, chordae tendineae, and the valve leaflets. Source: From The Heart. 6th Ed. Edited by J.W. Hurst. New York, McGraw-Hill, 1986.

right atrium. These electrical impulses initiate wavefronts of electrical activation, which spread through the atrial musculature causing atrial contraction. Specialized internodal tracts in the right atrium conduct preferentially to the atrioventricular (AV) node, located in the AV junction in close proximity to the tricuspid valve. Electrical impulses conduct slowly through the AV node in order to allow time for atrial systole to contribute to ventricular filling. Distal to the AV node, the electrical signals conduct rapidly through the bundle of His and into the right and left bundle branches, located in the right and left ventricles, respectively. In the ventricles the electrical impulses spread through a network of specialized tissue called Purkinje fibers and finally enter the ventricular muscle fibers. Conduction spreads from endocardium to epicardium and from apex to base, initiating an organized sequence of ventricular

contraction. These electrical events of cardiac excitation and the subsequent recovery from excitation are reflected on the body surface electrocardiogram (ECG), discussed in more detail in Chapter 3.

The heart is richly innervated by the sympathetic and parasympathetic divisions of the autonomic nervous system. Postganglionic sympathetic fibers originate in ganglia located along the right and left cervical sympathetic chains. Cardiac sympathetic receptors are found in the atria, ventricles, and specialized conduction system. These receptors are primarily of the beta-1 adrenergic type, stimulation of which results in increased contractile force (inotropism) and increased heart rate or conduction velocity (chronotropism). Parasympathetic fibers are carried in the right and left vagus nerves and are primarily distributed to the atria, the sinus node, and the AV node. Parasympathetic stimulation results in de-

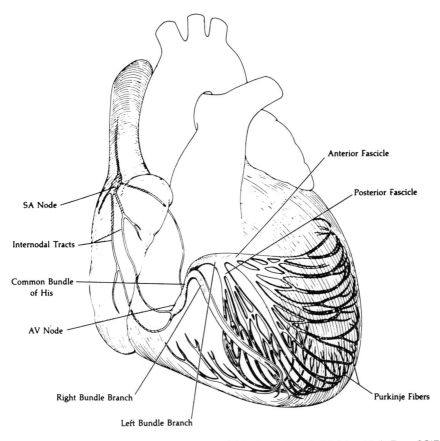

Fig. 2–5.   The specialized cardiac conduction system. AV (atrioventricular), SA (sinoatrial). From SCIENTIFIC AMERICAN Medicine, Section 1, Subsection VI. © 1987 Scientific American, Inc. All rights reserved.

creased contractile force, slowing of the heart rate, and slowing of conduction in the AV node. In addition to these efferent nerves, sensory afferent fibers conduct impulses from various locations in the heart to the central nervous system (CNS). These fibers may become activated under a variety of circumstances including distension of heart chambers and myocardal ischemia.

The Systemic Circulation

The systemic (peripheral) circulation distributes blood to all cells and tissues of the body in order to maintain a biochemical environment for bodily functions at rest and during exercise. Beginning with the aorta, the arteries branch to all regions of the body, transporting blood under high pressures to various tissues and organ systems. The arterioles, or terminal muscular branches of the arteries, are the resistance vessels that serve as control valves regulating blood flow into the various capillary beds, depending on need. An exchange of fluids, nutrients, oxygen, carbon dioxide, and regulatory substances between the interstitial space of tissues and the blood takes place in the capillaries. These are thin-walled tubules with pores through which substances can diffuse in both directions, depending on chemical and hydrostatic gradients. The venules begin at the distal end of the capillaries and join together to form veins that transport blood back to the heart under low pressure.

The coronary arteries originate from the

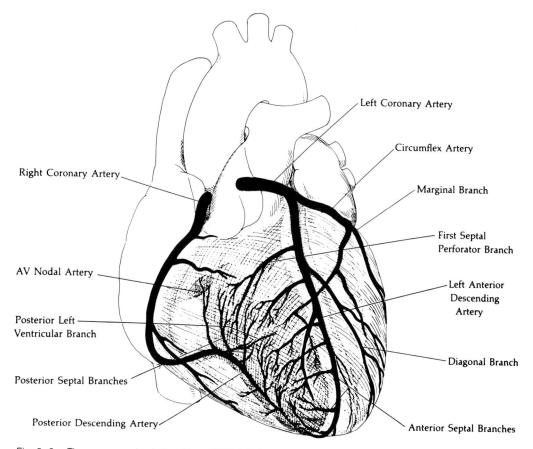

Fig. 2–6.   The coronary circulation. From SCIENTIFIC AMERICAN Medicine, Section 1, Subsection IX.© 1987. Scientific American, Inc. All rights reserved.

ascending aorta immediately above the two anterior cusps of the aortic valve. The distribution of the epicardial branches of the right and left coronary arteries is illustrated in Figure 2–6.[5] The right coronary artery runs in the groove between right atrium and right ventricle, providing branches to the right atrium, the anterior right ventricular wall, and the posterior surface of both ventricles. In approximately 90% of individuals, the right coronary artery provides the blood supply to the AV node and posterior third of the interventricular septum. In these individuals the right coronary artery is called the "dominant" vessel. The left coronary artery has a short *main* branch before bifurcating into a left anterior descending branch, which runs in the anterior groove

between right and left ventricles, and a left circumflex branch, which runs in the groove between left atrium and left ventricle. When the right coronary artery is the dominant vessel, the left circumflex and its branches are limited to the lateral left ventricular wall. In 10% of hearts, however, the left circumflex is the dominant vessel and continues in the left AV groove to supply the posterior ventricular wall, AV node, and posterior third of the interventricular septum. The anterior two thirds of the septum, the right bundle branch and the anterior division of the left bundle branch are supplied by septal perforating branches of the left anterior descending artery.

An understanding of coronary artery anatomy is necessary in order to appreciate the pathologic effects of coronary atherosclerosis on various cardiac structures. Occlusive lesions of the right coronary artery are most likely to affect the AV node, posterior or diaphragmatic (inferior) surfaces of the ventricles and posterior septum. Lesions of the left anterior descending artery affect the anterior left ventricular wall and the anterior two thirds of the interventricular septum. The bundle branches are also vulnerable to lesions of this vessel. Left circumflex lesions affect the lateral wall of the left ventricles and occasionally the posterior septum and AV node. Obstructive lesions of the left main coronary artery are extremely dangerous, since most of the left ventricular myocardium is at risk.

The structure of the arterial wall is diagrammed in Figure 2–7A, illustrating three morphologically distinct layers.[6] The inner layer, or intima, consists of a single lining of endothelial cells bound to the middle muscular layer, the media, by the internal elastic lamina. The media is made up of smooth muscle fibers and varies in thickness, depending on the size of the artery. The outer layer of loose connective tissues is called the adventitia and provides protective and nutritive functions to the artery.

The lesions of atherosclerosis, illustrated in Figure 2–7B to E, primarily involve the intimal lining of large and medium-sized arteries. Initially, smooth muscle cells from the media migrate into the lesion in response to the deposition of cholesterol and cholesterol esters from the circulating

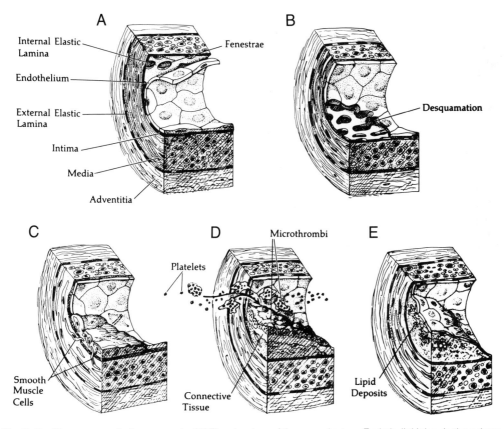

Fig. 2–7.   The process of atherogenesis. (A) The structure of the normal artery. Endothelial injury is the primary stimulus leading to (B) desquamation and (C) smooth muscle cell migration and proliferation. (D) Platelets adhere to the injured endothelium, releasing vasoconstrictive and thrombogenic substances. (E) Lipid deposits, primarily LDL-cholesterol accumulate in the lesions. Ross, R., and Glomset, J.A.: The pathogenesis of arteriosclersis. N. Engl. J. Med., 295:369, 420, 1976.

blood, presumably through a defect in the intimal lining.[6] As the lesion advances in age, there is inflammation and fibrous tissue accumulation, which may be followed by hemorrhage within the atherosclerotic plaque, calcification, cell necrosis, and mural thrombosis, all of which can lead to progressive occlusion of the arterial lumen. Occlusive lesions primarily occur in medium-sized arteries including the coronary, cerebral, renal, and lower extremity arteries.

The Pulmonary Circulation

Unlike the systemic circulation, whose function is to serve the metabolic needs of all cells and tissues in the body, the pulmonary circulation functions primarily to provide gas exchange between the body and the external environment. The pulmonary circulation is part of the respiratory system, which also includes the lungs and the skeletal muscles of respiration. The volume of blood flowing through the lungs from the right heart is comparable to that in the systemic circulation. In contrast to the systemic circulation, however, the pulmonary circulation is a low-pressure, low-resistance system with thinner walled and more distensible arteries than their systemic counterparts. This enables a high-volume pulmonary blood flow through the lungs with right ventricular systolic pressures that are only one fourth that generated by the left ventricle. The uptake of oxygen and the release of carbon dioxide in the lungs occur in the pulmonary capillaries, which are adjacent to the terminal air sacs, the alveoli. The pulmonary capillaries coalesce to from the pulmonary veins, which in turn, join together to form two major pulmonary veins from each lung emptying into the left atrium.

THE PHYSIOLOGY OF EXERCISE

The successful performance of endurance exercise requires the coordinated interaction of three major organ systems: (1) the skeletal muscles, (2) the cardiovascular system, and (3) the respiratory system. As illustrated in Figure 2–8, these three systems are closely coupled to provide homeostatic gas exchange (i.e., oxygen and carbon dioxide) between the external environment and the working muscle fibers.[7] During progressive exercise activities each system adjusts its function on a moment-to-moment basis, according to the metabolic needs of the body, primarily those of the exercising muscles. In addition to the acute response to exercise, the body also adapts more slowly over a period of weeks and months in response to a well-designed exercise program.

It is also important to appreciate that a disturbance or breakdown within one or more of these organ systems may be the cause of an individual's limited exercise tolerance. The workup for suspected disability or exercise intolerance may require a comprehensive assessment of all three organ systems in order to determine the specific mechanisms responsible for the patient's impairment. In the following sections the physiology of exercise is reviewed, beginning with the skeletal muscles and, in turn, considering the cardiovascular and respiratory systems.

Skeletal Muscle Structure and Function

The contraction and relaxation of skeletal muscles provide the underlying basis for all physical activities. Although an understanding of the structural and biochemical mechanisms for these processes is still incomplete, the significant contributions of H.E. Huxley[8,9] and A.F. Huxley[10] and their co-workers have greatly expanded our knowledge of these complex phenomena. Only a brief and simplified description of skeletal muscle is presented here; a more detailed discussion can be found in Astrand and Rodahl's *Textbook of Work Physiology.*[11]

Figure 2–9 presents a schematic diagram

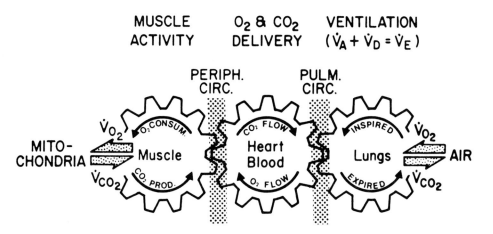

Fig. 2–8.   Homeostatic gas exchange between the outside environment and the skeletal muscle mitochondria. From K. Wasserman, et al. Principles of Exercise Testing and Interpretation. Philadelphia, Lea & Febiger, 1987.

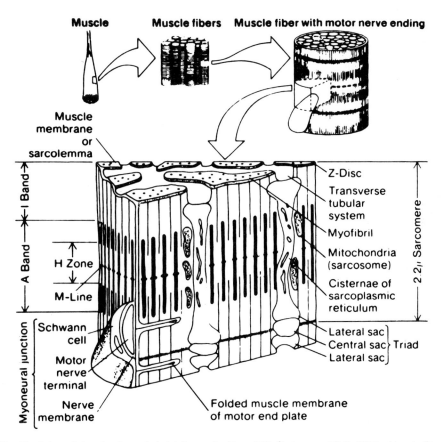

Fig. 2–9.   The intracellular structure of skeletal muscle. From F.D. Carlson and D.R. Wilkie, Muscle Physiology. Englewood Cliffs, N.J, Prentice-Hall, 1974.

of the intracellular structure of a skeletal muscle fiber.[11] Voluntary muscle contractions are under the control of the CNS. Electrical impulses arriving at the myoneural junctions initiate the release of stored calcium ions, Ca^{++}, from the sarcoplasmic reticulum, an elaborate system of tubular sacs, vesicles, and channels surrounding the myofibrils. The Ca^{++} ions, in turn, trigger a chemical interaction between the thin actin and thick myosin filaments within the myofibrils. Muscle shortening occurs when the actin filaments are pulled inward by the sequential chemical interactions with myosin cross bridges. In an isometric contraction there is no change in muscle length, although tension is generated as actin reacts chemically with the myosin cross bridges.

The mechanical events responsible for muscle shortening and tension development require a continuous source of chemical energy in the form of high-energy phosphate compounds. The most important of these compounds, adenosinetriphosphate (ATP), releases energy when the phosphate bonds are broken during a series of reactions called hydrolysis (ADP, adenosinediphosphate; AMP, adenosinemonophosphate):

$$ATP + H_2O \rightarrow ADP + P + energy$$

$$ADP + H_2O \rightarrow AMP + P + energy$$

The free energy liberated in these reactions is used by the cells for muscle contraction and a variety of other biologic processes requiring energy.

In the muscle fibers ATP molecules are continuously resynthesized by several important chemical reactions. An immediate reservoir of high-energy phosphate compounds is available in the form of phosphocreatine (CP), which is in equilibrium with ATP and creatine (C) as indicated by the following reaction:

$$ADP + CP \leftrightarrow ATP + C$$

For sustained skeletal muscle work, however, an adequate supply of ATP can only be provided by the oxidation of foodstuffs consumed in the diet or stored in the body as glycogen and triglycerides. The chemical reactions involved in the oxidation of glucose, glycogen, and fatty acids are part of a process called oxidative phosphorylation.

As indicated in Figure 2–10,[11] the main energy-yielding fuels for the resynthesis of ATP are carbohydrates (muscle glycogen, blood glucose) and fatty acids from triglycerides in stored adipose tissue. In the resting state muscle tissue obtains virtually all of its fuel from circulating fatty acids. During the first several minutes of exercise, stored glycogen in the muscle is utilized for fuel. With continued exercise, however, blood-borne fuels from glucose and fatty acids become increasingly important sources of energy for muscle contraction.

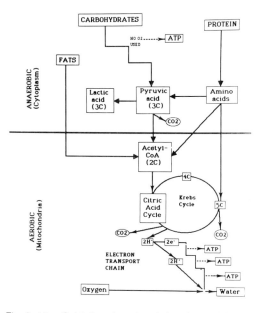

Fig. 2–10. Oxidative phosphorylation. Anaerobic metabolism takes place in the cytoplasm of the muscle cell, where carbohydrates are metabolized to pyruvic acid by a process called glycolysis. In the absence of oxygen, lactic acid is the end product of anaerobic metabolism. Aerobic metabolism occurs in the mitochondria, where the end products are CO_2 and water. Adapted from Astrand, P.O., and Rodahl, K.: Textbook of Work Physiology. 2nd ed. New York, McGraw-Hill, 1977.

Except in starvation states, proteins contribute very little to the total energy expenditure of working muscle fibers.

Oxidative phosphorylation involves an initial anaerobic sequence of reactions that takes place in the cytoplasm of the muscle fibers. During this phase glycogen and glucose are metabolized to pyruvic acid by a process called glycolysis, yielding three moles of ATP for every glucose monomer in glycogen or two ATP for every glucose molecule entering directly from the bloodstream. The availability of oxygen enables pyruvic acid to enter the aerobic phase of oxidative phosphorylation, which takes place in the mitochondria. Initially, pyruvic acid is oxidized to acetyl-CoA, which is also the first step in the metabolism of fatty acids. Acetyl-CoA subsequently enters into a cyclic series of reactions called the Krebs cycle,[11] yielding carbon dioxide and hydrogen. Electrons from hydrogen are transported down an electron-transport chain, releasing energy for the phosphorylation of ADP to ATP. At the end of the chain, the electrons are recombined with hydrogen ions and oxygen to form water. A total of 36 ATP per glucose molecule are synthesized in the mitochondria during aerobic oxidation.

During muscle relaxation newly synthesized ATP molecules are taken up by the myosin filaments, resulting in their detachment from actin and the subsequent release of tension in the muscle fibers. In addition, Ca^{++} ions are released and transported back into the sarcoplasmic reticulum to await the next electrical stimulus for contraction.

There are two major types of muscle fibers with different metabolic and mechanical properties that comprise the various skeletal muscle groups in the human body. Type I, or slow-twitch, fibers have highly developed oxidative enzyme systems and are rich in mitochondria and have a slow contractile response. As a result, these fibers are well suited for sustained aerobic exercise activities. In contrast, the type II,

or fast-twitch, fibers are better designed for strength (isometric) and brief bursts of high-speed activity. These fibers have a well-developed glycolytic enzyme system with a lower mitochondrial content and oxidative activity. Fast-twitch fibers, as named, have a fast contractile response and fatigue rapidly. In addition to these major types of muscle fibers, there are relatively undifferentiated fibers that can be recruited into behaving as type I or type II fibers, according to the particular exercise training program chosen by the individual. For the most part, however, the proportions of type I and II fibers are genetically determined for each individual.[12]

Cardiovascular and Pulmonary Physiology

Oxygen Uptake

It is clear from the preceding discussion that there are two major metabolic requirements for sustained skeletal muscle work: (1) adequate gas exchange between the muscle fibers and the external environment (i.e., the delivery of O_2 and the removal of CO_2) and (2) the availability of combustible materials in the form of glycogen, glucose and fatty acids. Since the ATP yield from aerobic metabolism is more than 10 times that provided by anaerobic glycolysis, the delivery of O_2 to working muscle fibers becomes the single most important determinant of the maximal workload that can be achieved during exercise.

The oxygen transport system involves the coordinated interaction of the cardiovascular and respiratory systems working together as a functional unit to provide the oxygen needs of the body. During incremental exercise there is a near linear relationship between workload and oxygen uptake.[13] Figure 2–11 illustrates this relationship from rest to maximal exercise on a bicycle ergometer or motor-driven treadmill. Oxygen uptake ($\dot{V}O_2$) may be measured in L O_2/min or ml O_2/kg/min, the lat-

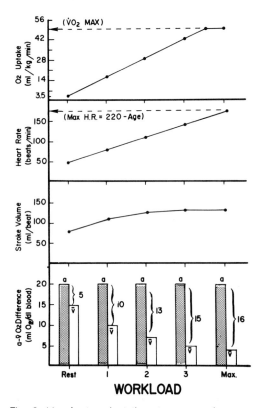

Fig. 2–11. Acute adaptations to progressive exercise. The abscissa indicates the resting state and four incremental levels of exercise to a maximal exercise work load. Oxygen uptake is linear until reaching a plateau at maximal exercise. Heart rate increase is also linear to maximal heart rate (220 minus age). Stroke volume (upright exercise) increases modestly early in exercise and then levels off. The arteriovenous O_2 content difference increases from rest to maximal exercise.

tic acid by muscle cells actually begins to be significant at approximately 50% of $\dot{V}O_2$ max and increases in an exponential-like manner to $\dot{V}O_2$ max.[14] The increase in lactic acid and its subsequent buffering in the muscle cells by the bicarbonate system (HCO_3) results in increased CO_2 efflux from exercising muscles. Since pulmonary ventilation responds primarily to CO_2 production rather than oxygen requirements, the metabolic acidosis of exercise is accompanied by a significant increase in minute ventilation ($\dot{V}E$), which accounts for the subjective experience of dyspnea when exercising close to $\dot{V}O_2$ max.

The determination of $\dot{V}O_2$ max in the exercise laboratory using either direct measurement techniques or estimation methods has become the "gold-standard" approach to evaluating an individual's cardiorespiratory fitness or functional aerobic capacity. Techniques for measuring $\dot{V}O_2$ max are discussed in Chapter 5.

The Fick principle,[15] which relates $\dot{V}O_2$ at any workload to the cardiac output and the arteriovenous O_2 content, can be expressed as follows:

$$\dot{V}O_2 = \dot{Q}_t \times (CaO_2 - C\bar{v}O_2)$$

where $\dot{V}O_2$ is oxygen uptake (ml O_2/min), $\dot{Q}_t$ is cardiac output (L/min), and $CaO_2 - C\bar{v}O_2$ is the arteriovenous oxygen content difference (ml O_2/L of blood). This equation provides a useful starting point for understanding the close coupling of the cardiovascular and respiratory systems to the metabolic activities of working muscle cells. Since cardiac output is the product of heart rate (HR, beats per minute) and stroke volume (SV, ml/beat), the Fick equation can also be expressed as follows:

$$\dot{V}O_2 = (HR \times SV) \times (CaO_2 - C\bar{v}O_2)$$

From this relationship it can be seen that the uptake of oxygen at rest and during exercise is determined by the oxygen transport system, defined by HR, SV, and CaO_2, and the utilization of oxygen, reflected by the arteriovenous O_2 content difference.

ter being more useful when comparing individuals, since it normalizes for differences in body weight. At rest, in the sitting position, $\dot{V}O_2$ is approximately 3.5 ml/kg/min; this resting $\dot{V}O_2$ is conveniently called one metabolic equivalent, or MET. With increasing workloads the $\dot{V}O_2$ rises until a workload is reached beyond which $\dot{V}O_2$ fails to increase ($\dot{V}O_2$ max).

Although a small increment in workload can usually be achieved at $\dot{V}O_2$ max, it is done entirely through anaerobic mechanisms and is associated with a marked increase in lactic acid production (metabolic acidosis of exercise). The production of lac-

During increasing exercise the transport and utilization of O_2 increase appropriately to accommodate the increased demands for O_2 by the exercising skeletal muscles. It has been estimated that at maximal exercise, approximately 90% of the cardiac output is transported to the exercising muscles.[13]

At maximal exercise the Fick equation identifies the four major parameters that combine to determine an individual's physical working capacity:

$$\dot{V}_{O_2}\ \text{max} = (\text{max HR} \times \text{max SV}) \times (\text{max } Ca_{O_2} - \text{min } C\bar{v}_{O_2})$$

$$1 \qquad\qquad 2 \qquad\qquad 3 \qquad\qquad 4$$

These are (1) the maximal heart rate response to exercise, (2) the maximal stroke volume response to exercise, (3) the maximal O_2 content of the arterial blood, and (4) the maximal ability of the exercising muscles to extract O_2 from the blood (which determines the minimal mixed venous O_2 content). Abnormalities in one or more of these parameters are usually associated with decreased exercise tolerance, dyspnea on exertion, and easy fatigability.

Heart Rate Response to Exercise

The heart rate in normal individuals is determined by the rate of discharge of pacemaker cells in the SA node. Although pacemaker cells have an intrinsic frequency of impulse formation, the normal heart rate is primarily influenced by extrinsic controls including the autonomic nervous system, circulating catecholamines, and other biochemical substances produced in the body or administered as drugs. At rest, the heart rate is usually between 60 and 90 beats per minute (bpm) and is predominately under the influence of the parasympathetic nervous system (right and left vagus nerves). During physical activities (Fig. 2–11) or emotionally stimulating events, the heart rate increases, as parasympathetic nervous activity diminishes and sympathetic stimuli and circulating catecholamines increase.

In healthy individuals the maximal rate of discharge of the SA node is age determined and is approximately 220 minus age. There is considerable variation in maximal heart rate among individuals of the same age with a standard deviation of $\pm$ 10 bpm.[11] With aging, therefore, maximal heart rate declines approximately 1 bpm/year. Assuming all other parameters of the Fick equation at maximal exercise remain unchanged, $\dot{V}_{O_2}$ max will decline in proportion to the decline in maximal heart rate.

Several drug-induced or disease-related states can affect pacemaker activity in the SA node and further limit the heart rate response to exercise. Ellestad[16] has coined the term *chronotropic incompetence* to indicate a heart rate response to exercise that is below the 95th percent confidence limits for the age-determined normal values. This may be an early manifestation of coronary artery disease or may reflect other diseases involving the SA node. Atrioventricular nodal heart block may also limit the heart rate response to exercise by blocking some or all of the impulses originating in the SA node from reaching the ventricles. Finally, the commonly used beta-blocking drugs have a profound effect on the SA node, resulting in a slower than normal heart rate response to exercise. All of these factors may result in a decrease in $\dot{V}_{O_2}$ max and contribute to a decline in cardiorespiratory fitness.

Stroke Volume Response to Exercise

The second factor of importance in determining $\dot{V}_{O_2}$ max is the maximal stroke volume during exercise. The stroke volume is the volume of blood ejected from the right and left ventricles during ventricular systole. It is a complex function, depending on at least three different hemodynamic parameters: (1) the preload, (2) the afterload, and (3) the inotropic state or contractility of ventricular muscle. In patients with previous myocardial infarctions, regional ventricular wall-motion abnormalities may further compromise the stroke volume response to exercise.

The *preload* represents the passive filling characteristics of ventricular muscle during diastole that determine the end-diastolic fiber length just prior to ventricular systole. Ventricular filling occurs in two phases. Early filling takes place as soon as the AV valves open at the beginning of diastole when pressures in the atria exceed the ventricular pressures. In late diastole there is a second component to filling resulting from atrial contraction. According to the Frank-Starling Law of the Heart[15] the greater the end-diastolic fiber length (or end-diastolic volume) the greater the contractile force of the subsequent ventricular contraction and the greater the stroke volume. There is also a similar relationship between end-diastolic pressure and stroke volume, since ventricular filling pressures are related to both the diastolic fiber length and the compliance of the ventricular muscle. In the normal heart there is a near-linear increase in stroke volume as end-diastolic volumes increase.

The afterload is a measure of the resistance against which the ventricles contract during systole. In the left ventricle this resistance is determined by several different factors including the systemic vascular resistance, the stiffness of the aortic wall, the mass of blood in the systemic circulation, and the blood viscosity. The afterload affects the rate of ventricular contraction and the extent to which the ventricles empty with each contraction. Increases in stroke volume occur when the afterload is reduced (usually brought about by factors that decrease the systemic vascular resistance). As a result there is more complete emptying of the ventricles during systole.

To some extent the increase in stroke volume during exercise is the result of a decrease in the systemic vascular resistance caused by vasodilation within the exercising skeletal muscles.

The third hemodynamic factor affecting the ventricular stroke volume is the inotropic state or contractility. This parameter is determined by the intrinsic contractile state of the myocardium as well as by extrinsic inotropic stimuli provided by the cardiac sympathetic nerves, circulating catecholamines released from the adrenal medulla, and in some patients, pharmacologic agents such as digitalis glycosides. The increase in stroke volume resulting from these processes is due to an increase in the velocity of fiber shortening and more complete emptying of the ventricles. During exercise, contractility is increased as a result of sympathetic stimulation and increased circulating catecholamines.

The stroke volume response to exercise is curvilinear, with the greatest increase occurring during the transition from rest to moderate exercise in the upright position (Fig. 2–11). When the heart rate exceeds 120 bpm, further increases in stroke volume are minimal, since diastolic filling times become progressively shorter at faster heart rates. During supine exercise the stroke volume changes very little from its resting value. In healthy individuals maximal stroke volume is a function of ventricular diastolic size (preload) and the degree of systolic emptying (contractility and afterload). These parameters can be influence favorably by exercise training, which results in a greater stroke volume at maximal exercise. To some extent, heart size is also under genetic control, which may account for some of the variations in $\dot{V}O_2$ max among similarly trained individuals.

Arterial Oxygen Content

The third important determinant of $\dot{V}O_2$ max is the arterial O_2 content (CaO_2). Together with heart rate and stroke volume, these parameters define oxygen transport to the tissues. At maximal exercise, for example, the quantity of oxygen delivered to the tissues can be calculated as the product of blood flow and arterial O_2 content:

Max O_2 transport (ml O_2/min)

$$= (\text{max HR} \times \text{max SV}) \times \text{max } Ca_{O_2}$$

The factors affecting maximal heart rate and stroke volume have been discussed. The O_2 content of arterial blood is a complex function depending on (1) the arterial partial pressure of O_2 (Pa_{O_2}), (2) the hemoglobin concentration (g/100 ml), and (3) the affinity of hemoglobin for oxygen. Disturbances in one or more of these factors may significantly limit oxygen transport to the tissues.

There are several factors that determine Pa_{O_2}, the first being the concentration of O_2 in the inspired air. Although the fraction of O_2 in the air is always 21%, the O_2 tension or partial pressure (PI_{O_2}) falls with increasing altitude in proportion to the fall in barometric pressure (P_B) according to the following equation:

$$PI_{O_2} = (P_B - 47) \times 0.21$$

where 47 is the vapor pressure (mm Hg) of water at normal body temperature. As a result, the concentration of O_2 in the inspired air, reflectd by PI_{O_2}, becomes significantly reduced when one goes from sea level to increasing altitudes, as illustrated in Figure 2–12.

From the inspired air to the various cells and tissues of the body, the oxygen tension or P_{O_2} drops in a series of steps called the *oxygen cascade*. The initial fall in P_{O_2} from inspired air to pulmonary alveoli, ($PI_{O_2} - PA_{O_2}$), is a function of the magnitude of pulmonary ventilation. PA_{O_2} can be calculated from PI_{O_2}, Pa_{CO_2} and the respiratory exchange ratio (R), which is the ratio of CO_2 output to O_2 uptake ($\dot{V}_{CO_2}/\dot{V}_{O_2}$), according to the following equation:

$$PA_{O_2} = PI_{O_2} - Pa_{CO_2}/R$$

The importance of this relationship becomes apparent when considering the acute adaptation to high altitude. The reduced ambient O_2 pressure illustrated in Figure 2–12 at high altitude causes a stepwise reduction of PA_{O_2} and Pa_{O_2}. The fall in Pa_{O_2} reduces the quantity of arterial O_2 (hypoxemia), which in turn stimulates increased ventilation via the carotid body chemoreceptors. The result of this increased ventilation is a decrease in Pa_{CO_2}, an increase in the respiratory exchange ratio (i.e., CO_2 output), and from the preceding equation, an increase in PA_{O_2}. This feedback mechanism, therefore, compensates for the initial fall in Pa_{O_2} by decreasing the drop in P_{O_2} that occurs from inspired air to alveoli.

The second step in the oxygen cascade is the drop in P_{O_2} from alveolar air to arterial blood, called the A–a P_{O_2} gradient. To a large extent this gradient reflects the adequacy of gas exchange in the lungs. In normal lungs where ventilation and perfusion are well matched and where diffusion across the air–blood barrier is not impaired, the A-a gradient ranges from 12 to 20 mm Hg. Factors that increase the A-a gradient and thereby reduce Pa_{O_2} include right-to-left vascular shunts either in the lungs or the heart, ventilation-perfusion abnormalities found in a variety of pulmonary parenchymal and vascular diseases, and possibly diseases that primarily affect diffusion across the alveolar-capillary membrane. The end result of these pathophysiologic disturbances is a reduction in Pa_{O_2} (arterial hypoxemia).

The third step in the oxygen cascade concerns the actual mechanism by which O_2 is carried in the arterial blood. Oxygen molecules entering the pulmonary capillary blood quickly diffuse into red blood cells and chemically combine with reduced hemoglobin to form oxyhemoglobin. Since each gram of hemoglobin (Hb) can combine with 1.34 ml O_2, the oxygen carrying capacity of arterial blood can be computed as follows:

O_2 Capacity (ml O_2/100 ml)

$$= [\text{Hb}] \text{ (g/100 ml)} \times 1.34$$

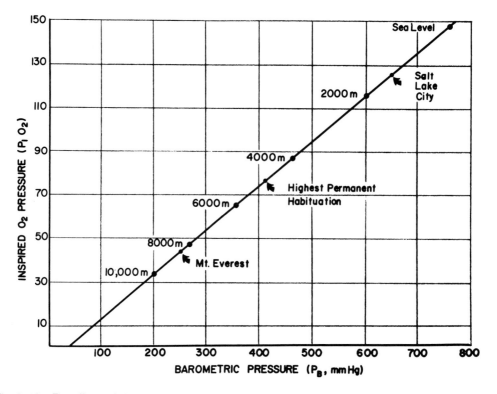

Fig. 2–12.   The effects of altitude on barometric pressure and inspired O_2 pressure.

In a normal individual with approximately 15 g/100 ml blood hemoglobin, the O_2 capacity is 20 ml/100 ml, or 20 vol %.

Not all of the O_2 molecules entering the pulmonary capillary blood are able to combine with hemoglobin. The reversible chemical interaction between oxygen and hemoglobin is defined by the oxygen–hemoglobin dissociation curve, which is illustrated in Figure 2–13. A family of curves depending on pH, temperature, and other factors represent relationships between the partial pressures of O_2 and the percentage of saturation of hemoglobin (SO_2). At sea level, for example, where the PaO_2 is approximately 100 mm Hg, the arterial O_2 saturation, SaO_2, is 97.5%, assuming normal body temperature of 37° C and pH 7.40. The curve's flat upper portion is physiologically advantageous, allowing high oxygen saturations to remain, despite falling arterial PO_2 values. The steep middle segment permits large quantities of O_2

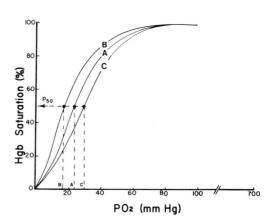

Fig. 2–13.   Oxygen–hemoglobin dissociation curves (A) the normal relationship between PO_2 and hemoglobin saturation. (B) The curve shifts to the left as a result of decreased body temperature, increased pH, or carbon monoxide exposure. (C) The curve shifts to the right as a result of increased body temperature or decreased pH.

to be released in the peripheral capillaries, where P_{O_2} values are much lower, enabling O_2 to diffuse into the cells and tissues of the body.

The affinity of hemoglobin for oxygen is conveniently defined by the P50, which represents the P_{O_2} value where hemoglobin O_2 saturation is 50%. Normally, the P50 is 26.6 mm Hg (curve A, Fig. 2–13). The O_2 affinity of hemoglobin is strongly influenced by a number of factors including body temperature, hydrogen ion (pH), carbon monoxide exposure, and abnormal hemoglobin molecules. Decreased body temperature, increased pH, and carbon monoxide exposure all shift the curve to the left (curve B in Fig. 2–13), enabling more O_2 to be bound to hemoglobin in the lungs but making it more difficult for O_2 to be released at the peripheral tissues (increased affinity, decreased P50). A rightward shift in the oxyhemoglobin dissociation curve (curve C, Fig. 2–13) occurs with increased body temperature and decreased pH, allowing for a greater release of O_2 at the peripheral tissues where the P_{O_2} is around 40 mm Hg. This physiologically important mechanism is used during exercise in order to increase O_2 delivery to the working muscle fibers.

The final bottom line of all these processes is the actual content of arterial oxygen, Ca_{O_2}. This can be calculated as follows:

Ca_{O_2} (ml O_2/100 ml blood)

$$= Sa_{O_2} \times 1.34 \times [Hb] \text{ (g/100 ml)}$$

This equation neglects the small amount of oxygen that is physically dissolved in the blood (0.003 ml O_2/100 ml per mm Hg P_{O_2}). Given a normal hemoglobin concentration of 15 g/100 ml and a Pa_{O_2} of 100 mm Hg at sea level, Ca_{O_2} = 97.5 × 1.34 × 15 = 19.6 ml O_2/100 ml. An additional 0.3 ml O_2 would be physically dissolved in the plasma giving a total Ca_{O_2} of approximately 20 ml/100 ml.

The laboratory determination of Ca_{O_2} requires knowledge of hemoglobin concentration and Sa_{O_2}. Sa_{O_2} may be directly obtained from spectrophotometric analysis of blood or derived indirectly from the oxyhemoglobin dissociation curve if P_{O_2}, pH, and body temperature are known. A convenient device for estimating Sa_{O_2} during exercise is the ear or finger oximeter, which approximates Sa_{O_2} from the capillary blood just beneath the skin. This is an important measurement in patients with chronic lung disease, where Sa_{O_2} might significantly decrease during exercise.

It should be clear from the preceding discussion that there are a multitude of factors ranging from the P_{O_2} of inspired air to the hemoglobin concentration that can affect the arterial oxygen content and potentially limit exercise tolerance. These are summarized in Table 2–2. The workup for exercise impairment should include a consideration of these factors. Pulmonary function studies, blood gas analyses, and hematologic studies are all important aspects of the clinical evaluation for suspected disability.

Oxygen Extraction by Skeletal Muscles

The final determinant of $\dot{V}_{O_2}$ max is the capacity of skeletal muscles to extract and

Table 2–2.   Causes of Low Arterial Oxygen Content

I. Reduced ambient O_2 tension ($\downarrow F_{I_{O_2}}$)
  A. High altitude

II. Global alveolar hypoventilation ($\downarrow P_{A_{O_2}}$)
  A. Impaired central respiratory drive
    1. Primary (idiopathic) central alveolar hypoventilation
    2. Pickwickian Syndrome (massive obesity)
    3. Drug induced (barbiturates, morphine)
  B. Neuromuscular diseases affecting respiratory muscles

III. Ventilation–perfusion abnormalities ($\uparrow$ A–a P_{O_2} gradient)
  A. Parenchymal lung diseases
  B. Right-to-left pulmonary or cardiac shunts
  C. Pulmonary embolism

IV. Hematologic abnormalities
  A. Anemia
  B. Abnormal hemoglobins with reduced O_2 affinity
  C. Carbon monoxide exposure

utilize oxygen from the arterial blood. During exercise this is reflected by the arteriovenous O_2 content difference (Ca_{O_2}–$C\bar{v}_{O_2}$). Oxygen extraction by muscle cells is dependent on a number of factors including the intensity of exercise, the capillary density around the muscle fibers, the aerobic enzyme activity within the muscle fiber mitochondria, and the number and size of mitochondria. In healthy individuals at rest, approximately 25% of arterial O_2 is extracted by the muscle fibers with a Ca_{O_2}–$C\bar{v}_{O_2}$ difference of 40 to 50 ml O_2/L; as exercise intensity increases mixed venous O_2 content progressvely falls, and the Ca_{O_2}–$C\bar{v}_{O_2}$ difference widens to 130 to 150 ml O_2/L (Fig. 2–11).

Although the maximal capacity to extract O_2 by skeletal muscles is, to a considerable extent, under genetic control, physical conditioning and deconditioning may significantly modify this capacity. Exercise training studies have shown that in trained muscles adaptive changes occur that include increased density of capillaries around the muscle fibers and increased aerobic enzyme activity in the muscle mitochondria after several months of training.[17] These changes enable the muscle fibers to extract more O_2 per unit of blood flow. As much as 50% of the improvement in $\dot{V}_{O_2}$ max with training is accounted for by peripheral adaptations in the muscles leading to an increased maximal Ca_{O_2}–$C\bar{v}_{O_2}$ difference.[18] In cardiac patients, moreover, where central adaptations within the heart are limited by myocardial damage and left ventricular dysfunction, these peripheral changes within the muscle fibers account for most, if not all, of the increased $\dot{V}_{O_2}$ max with training.[19] This has important implications for cardiac rehabilitation programs, because it implies that patients with major compromises in cardiac function can still improve their functional capacities (i.e., $\dot{V}_{O_2}$ max) with a carefully designed exercise program.

In contrast, decreased physical activity, which occurs with deconditioning or prolonged periods of bed rest, results in a reduction in the oxidative metabolic capacity of skeletal muscles and accounts for much of the decline in $\dot{V}_{O_2}$ max.[17] It is not surprising, therefore, that individuals recovering from an illness involving several weeks or more of bed rest find that usual physical actvities are associated with easy fatigability and weakness. It often takes several months to regain previous levels of conditioning as shown in the classic bed rest study of Saltin.[20]

In addition to deconditioning there are diseases involving skeletal muscles that reduce the ability of muscle fibers to extract and/or utilize O_2, even though the supply of O_2 is more than adequate. These diseases often have a profound effect on exercise tolerance. Primary muscle and neuromuscular diseases causing weakness and inability to exercise include muscular dystrophies (progressive weakness and wasting of muscle fibers), glycogen storage diseases (enzymatic defects in glycogenolysis), periodic paralyses (intermittent attacks of muscle paralysis), and myasthenia gravis (failure at the neuromuscular junction). Decreased mitochondrial O_2 consumption is also a feature of hypothyroidism, a common endocrine abnormality characterized by decreased production of thyroid hormone. Finally, the common electrolyte abnormality of hypokalemia, which is often caused by diuretic therapy, may be associated with muscle weakness and decreased exercise tolerance.

Myocardial Oxygen Supply and Demand

Unlike skeletal muscle, the heart depends almost entirely on aerobic metabolism (oxidative phosphorylation) for its energy requirements. Accordingly, coronary blood flow is exquisitely autoregulated to maintain a balance between myocardial oxygen supply and demand. Myocardial cells efficiently extract 60% to 70% of the oxygen delivered over a wide range of meta-

Table 2–3. Acute and Chronic Adaptations to Exercise

	Acute Response to Exercise	Chronic Adaptation to Exercise Training	Effects of Deconditioning	Causes of Exercise Intolerance
$\dot{V}O_2$	Linear increase to $\dot{V}O_2$ max	Increase in $\dot{V}O_2$ max	Decrease in $\dot{V}O_2$ max	
HR	Linear increase to max HR (220 minus age)	1. No change or possible decrease in max HR 2. Decrease in resting HR and HR response to submaximal exercise	Increase HR response to submaximal workloads	1. Sinus node disease 2. AV node disease 3. Beta-blocking drugs
SV	Increase in early exercise to a plateau	1. Increase in max SV 2. Increase in resting SV and SV response to submaximal exercise	Decrease max SV and SV response to submaximal workloads	1. Valvular heart disease 2. Ischemic heart disease 3. Cardiomyopathy 4. Deconditioning
CaO_2	No change	No change	No change	1. High altitude ($\downarrow$ FIO_2) 2. Hypoventilation ($\downarrow$ PaO_2) 3. Ventilation/perfusion abnormalities ($\uparrow$ A-a$\bigtriangledown$) 4. Hematologic abnormalities
$C\bar{v}O_2$	Progressive fall to minimal value	Decrease in min $C\bar{v}O_2$ with widening of CaO_2–CaO_2 difference	Narrowing of CaO_2–CaO_2 difference due to decreased oxidative enzyme activity in muscle fibers	1. Skeletal muscle disease 2. Neuromuscular disease 3. Systemic diseases affecting oxidative metabolism 4. Deconditioning

AV, atrioventricular; HR, heart rate; SV, stroke volume.

bolic requirements; an increase in oxygen demand by the heart, therefore, can only be met by an increase in myocardial blood flow.

There are three major determinants of myocardial oxygen consumption ($M\dot{V}O_2$): (1) intramyocardial tension (stress); (2) myocardial contractility, and (3) heart rate. Increases in one or more of these factors, as occur during exercise, are normally matched by appropriate increases in coronary blood flow to maintain the supply–demand balance. Recent evidence suggests that autoregulation of coronary blood flow is mediated by the metabolite adenosine, a breakdown product of ATP, which is a potent vasodilator of the coronary vasculature.[21]

According to the Laplace relationship[15] myocardial wall tension (T) is directly proportional to intraventricular radius (r) and pressure (P) and inversely proportional to wall thickness (h), that is, $T = Pr/2h$. Although wall tension cannot be measured directly, the determinants of tension can be studied by various noninvasive and invasive cardiac techniques (Chapter 3).

An indirect measure of $M\dot{V}O_2$ is the heart rate–systolic blood pressure product, commonly known as the double product. Although this readily measured index of $M\dot{V}O_2$ does not take into consideration ventricular volume or myocardial contractility, studies during exercise have demonstrated that it correlates very nicely with directly measured $M\dot{V}O_2$ in healthy subjects.[22] Furthermore, the double product is a useful parameter in the follow-up of patients with coronary artery disease undergoing exercise testing or participating in cardiac rehabilitation programs. Calculating the double product at the onset of exercise-induced angina or ischemic ECG changes (Chapter 5) provides an indirect index of the $M\dot{V}O_2$ threshold above which myocardial ischemia occurs. Changes in this threshold over time, resulting from various medical and/or surgical interventions or occurring naturally with progression of

disease correlate well with the patient's clinical status and coronary angiographic findings.

SUMMARY

This chapter has reviewed anatomic and physiologic concepts of exercise in order to provide a foundation for the subsequent chapters, which deal with more practical aspects of exercise testing, exercise training, and cardiac rehabilitation. The primary focus was on the acute and long-term adaptations to aerobic exercise using the Fick principle to emphasize the close coupling of oxygen uptake, oxygen transport, and oxygen utilization. Table 2–3 summarizes the important points discussed in this chapter, as viewed from the five components of the Fick equation. It is important to remember that many of the causes of exercise intolerance are reversible to some extent with exercise training. In addition, medical management and/or surgical correction of many of these disorders will further enhance the training response.

REFERENCES

1. Guyton, A.C.: Textbook of Medical Physiology. 6th Ed. Philadelphia, W.B. Saunders, 1981.
2. Rushmer, R.F.: Cardiovascular Dynamics. 3rd Ed. Philadelphia, W.B. Saunders, 1970.
3. James, T.N., Sherf, L, Schlant, R.C., and Silverman, M.E.: Anatomy of the heart. In The Heart. Edited by J.W. Hurst. New York, McGraw-Hill, 5th Ed., 1982.
4. DeSanctis, R.W., and Ruskin, J.N.: Disturbances of cardiac rhythm and conduction. In Scientific American Medicine. Edited by E. Rubenstein. New York, Scientific American, 1983.
5. Hutter, A.M.: Ischemic heart disease: Angina pectoris. In Scientific American Medicine. Edited by E. Rubenstein. New York, Scientific American, 1983.
6. Hancock, E.W.: Coronary artery disease—Epidemiology and prevention. In Scientific American Medicine. Edited by E. Rubenstein. New York, Scientific American, 1984.
7. Wasserman, K., Whipp, B.J., and Davis, J.A.: Respiratory physiology of exercise: Metabolism, gas exchange, and ventilatory control. In International Review of Physiology. Respiratory Physiology III. Vol. 23. Edited by J.G. Widdicombe. Baltimore, University Park Press, 1981.

8. Huxley, H.E.: The contraction of muscle. Sci. Am., *19*:319, 1958.
9. Huxley, H.E.: The mechanism of muscle contraction. Science, *164*:1356, 1969.
10. Huxley, A.F.: Muscle contraction. J. Physiol., (Lond.) *243*:1, 1974.
11. Astrand,P., and Rodahl, K.: Textbook of Work Physiology. 2nd Ed. New York, McGraw-Hill, 1977.
12. Komi, P.V., et al.: Skeletal muscle fibers and muscle enzyme activities in monozygous and dizygous twins of both sexes. Acta Physiol. Scand., *100*:385, 1977.
13. Mitchell, J.H., and Blomqvist, G.: Maximal oxygen uptake. N. Engl. J. Med., *284*:1018, 1971.
14. Yeh, M.P., et al.: "Anaerobic threshold": Problems of determination and validation. J. Appl. Physiol., *55*:1178, 1983.
15. Little, R.C.: Physiology of the Heart and Circulation. 3rd Ed. Chicago, Year Book Medical Publishers, 1985.
16. Ellestad, M.H.: Stress Testing: Principles and Practice. 2nd Ed. Philadelphia, F.A. Davis, 1980.
17. Saltin, B., and Rowell, L.B.: Functional adaptations to physical activity and inactivity. Fed. Pro., *39*:1506, 1980.
18. Clausen, J.P.: Effect of physical training on cardiovascular adjustments to exercise in man. Physiol. Rev., *57*:779, 1977.
19. Clausen, J.P.: Circulatory adjustments to dynamic exercise and effects of physical training in normal subjects and in patients with coronary artery disease. Prog. Cardiovasc. Dis., *18*:459, 1976.
20. Saltin, B., et al.: Response to exercise after bed rest and after training. Circulation, *38* (VIII):78, 1968.
21. Berne, R.M.: The role of adenosine in the regulation of coronary blood flow. Circ. Res., *47*:807, 1980.
22. Nelson, R.R. et al.: Hemodynamic predictors of myocardial oxygen consumption during static and dynamic exercise. Circulation, *50*:1179, 1974.

EVALUATION AND EXERCISE PRESCRIPTION

3

CARDIOVASCULAR ASSESSMENT AND TREATMENT

The practice of cardiovascular medicine has undergone remarkable changes in recent years, primarily as a result of technologic advances in diagnostic and therapeutic procedures. There have been both positive and negative consequences to this scientific explosion in cardiology. On the positive side there is now an incredible array of sophisticated diagnostic techniques for quantitating cardiovascular abnormalities to a degree of clarity never before imagined. In addition, new drug therapies and surgical techniques permit earlier and more effective treatments to be administered to patients with heart and vascular diseases. As a result, for the first time in this century, there has been a 30% decline in cardiovascular mortality, which has mostly occurred between 1970 and 1980.[1]

On the negative side, however, these technologic advances have created a severe strain in the nation's health-care budget. A 1982 news report estimated a yearly cost of $39 billion for treating heart disease in this country,[2] and it is likely that current costs are much greater. Most of this expense is related to the practice of high-technology medicine. A second negative consequence of modern scientific cardiology is the dehumanization that inevitably results when the medical focus is predominately on the mechanical aspects of heart disease diagnosis and treatment. This increasing reliance on sophisticated technology has resulted in a loss of some of the more humanistic skills that have traditionally characterized the doctor–patient relationship.

This chapter reviews the process of cardiovascular diagnosis and treatment. Although the focus is on technology, the major objective is to present a logical and comprehensive approach to the management of patients with cardiovascular diseases. The discussion begins with a review of the objectives of the cardiovascular evaluation: What information is needed to successfully manage a patient with suspected or known cardiovascular disease? The next section considers specific methods related to the cardiovascular examination, beginning with the history and physical examination and progressing to more sophisticated and expensive technologies that may be needed to solve certain problems. The chapter concludes with a discussion of cardiovascular therapeutics, emphasizing recent advances in drug and invasive therapies. Throughout this chapter an attempt is made to present a humanistic and cost-effective approach to the workup and treatment of cardiac patients. Specific examples are considered that are most appropriate for health professionals working in cardiac rehabilitation.

OBJECTIVES OF THE CARDIOVASCULAR EVALUATION

The evaluation of a patient with known or suspected cardiovascular disease must be tailored to the specific needs of the patient. Table 3–1 lists the questions that might form the basis for a cardiovascular evaluation. These questions fall into two different categories: (1) questions concerned with the diagnosis of cardiovascular disease and (2) questions related to patient management. The design of an optimal management strategy will certainly be determined, in part, by the specific diagnoses, although prognostic and quality-of-life considerations often contribute significantly to an overall therapeutic plan.

A comprehensive classification system for cardiovascular diagnoses has been developed by the New York Heart Association in their publication *Nomenclature and Criteria for the Diagnosis of Diseases of the Heart and Great Vessels.*[3] This classification scheme subdivides the cardiovascular diagnoses into the five categories listed in Table 3–2.

The *etiologic diagnoses* refer to the causes of heart and blood vessel diseases. Often, this is not known for a particular patient, and the term *idiopathic* is sometimes used to express an unknown etiology. Most of the time, however, a careful evaluation of the patient's clinical status will enable an etiologic diagnosis to be made with a reasonable degree of certainty. Examples of etiologic diagnoses are listed in Table 3–3. By far the most common diagnosis in this country and one that provides the vast majority of patients for cardiac rehabilitation programs is atherosclerotic cardiovascular disease. It should be recognized that patients may have more than one etiologic diagnosis. Furthermore, an etiologic label does not necessarily imply a full understanding of the cause.

The *anatomic diagnoses* are generally more easily determined by the various diagnostic tools discussed in this chapter. Structural abnormalities may involve the chambers of the heart (hypertrophy, enlargement, septal defects, etc.), the cardiac valves (stenosis and insufficiency), the arteries (atherosclerotic lesions, aneurysms), or the veins. Anatomic diagnoses also include specific tumors of the heart, pathologic diagnoses obtained from biopsy specimens, and abnormalities of the pericardium.

The *physiologic diagnoses* refer to abnormalities involving cardiac rhythm and conduction as well as problems of cardiac function and myocardial contractility. Increased pressures in the systemic or pulmonary vascular systems (hypertension) are also classified as physiologic diagnoses.

Cardiac status and *prognostic* considerations are usually made after establishing the etiologic, anatomic, and physiologic diagnoses and after deciding on the most appropriate therapy (Table 3–4). Clinical judgment and experience, knowledge of the natural history and therapy of cardio-

Table 3–1.   Questions For The Cardiovascular Evaluation

1. Is cardiovascular disease present?
2. What is its cause? (etiologic diagnosis)
3. What are the structural abnormalities? (anatomic diagnosis)
4. Are there abnormalities in cardiac function or myocardial contractility?
5. Are there abnormalities in cardiac rhythm or conduction?
6. Is myocardial ischemia present?
7. Is treatment needed?
8. What are the most appropriate therapies?
9. What is the prognosis?
10. How does the cardiovascular disease affect the patient's quality of life?

Table 3–2.   Elements of the Cardiovascular Diagnosis[3]

1. The etiologic diagnosis
2. The anatomic diagnosis
3. The physiologic diagnosis
4. Cardiac status
5. Prognosis

Table 3–3.   Etiologic Cardiovascular Diagnosis (Examples)

Atherosclerotic cardiovascular disease
Congenital heart disease
Rheumatic heart disease
Hypertensive heart disease
Pulmonary heart disease
Infectious heart disease
Idiopathic heart disease (unknown etiology)

Table 3–4. Cardiac Status and Prognosis[3]

Cardiac Status	Prognosis
Uncompromised	Good
Slightly compromised	Good, with therapy
Moderately compromised	Fair, with therapy
Severely compromised	Guarded, despite therapy

vascular diseases, and careful evaluation of the patient's limiting symptoms are all important in making this determination.

One of the real challenges in modern cardiovascular medical practice is knowing how far to go in a particular patient's workup and management. Given the sophistication of diagnostic and therapeutic technologies available today along with the economic incentives for those providing the services, there is an increasing tendency to include costly and often unnecessary procedures in the routine workup of patients with cardiovascular problems. Less and less reliance is given to the information obtained during the history and physical examination in favor of the more quantitative data provided by expensive noninvasive and invasive procedures. Unfortunately, the medical literature does not offer a great deal of insight into the optimal selection of diagnostic tests, although this is discussed to some extent in one recently published textbook on cardiovascular diseases.[4]

One important concept that is relevant to this discussion is the difference between *disease* and *illness*. A disease refers to a specific pathologic process that is taking place within the body that may or may not be causing symptoms. The disease is usually defined by its etiologic, anatomic, and pathophysiologic characteristics that are determined during the physical examination and by various other diagnostic procedures. An illness, on the other hand, is characterized by a constellation of symptoms and findings related to the patient's clinical state of well-being. The complaints experienced by the patient are often heavily influenced by psychosocial determinants

as well as cultural factors, which are best evaluated during doctor–patient interactions. It is this aspect of the cardiovascular evaluation that is neglected when too much emphasis is given to the "hard data" derived from invasive and noninvasive tests. Ideally, the cardiovascular workup as well as the subsequent therapeutic process should be directed toward issues related to both the underlying disease and the resulting illness, if any. This distinction is of particular importance to cardiac rehabilitation programs where the primary goals are directed toward managing the cardiovascular illness rather than the basic disease process.

The methodologies of the cardiovascular examination are reviewed in the next section, beginning with the basic data base of medical history, physical examination, chest radiograph, and electrocardiogram (ECG). This is followed by brief descriptions of the various invasive and noninvasive techniques that are routinely used by cardiovascular specialists.

METHODS OF THE CARDIOVASCULAR EXAMINATION

The Medical History

Probably the most humanistic and cost-effective of all the cardiovascular diagnostic techniques is the medical history. Occasionally, a complete diagnosis and management plan can be determined from the patient history alone. Most often, however, the medical history will provide important clues for making etiologic, anatomic, and physiologic assessments, which are then verified with other diagnostic procedures.

As already discussed, the history may be the only means of evaluating possible psychosocial variables that contribute to the patient's illness. The actual process of obtaining the medical history may also have a therapeutic effect because of the nature of the relationship that develops between the patient and physician during this interaction. Although much of the history may be obtained from self-administered questionnaires or a computer terminal, the physician-administered history is a necessary element in the medical care process.

Table 3–5 lists the components of the medical history that are appropriate for the cardiovascular workup. The actual sequence in which the history is obtained will depend on the particular circumstances of the physician–patient encounter. Often the patient is seeking medical attention because of a specific complaint or an illness that is worrisome. In this situation, the history should begin with a detailed description of the present illness and particular symptomatology. At other times an individual may be undergoing a routine checkup in the absence of any illness. In these situations the history might begin with a review of previous cardiovascular problems, followed by the symptoms review and risk factor assessment. It is important to emphasize that patients who do not *complain* of cardiovascular symptoms may still be experiencing symptoms although perhaps not appreciating their significance.

The differential diagnosis of chest pain symptoms is probably the most frequent diagnostic problem encountered by practicing physicians. The evaluation of chest pain is also of considerable importance to those working in adult fitness, cardiac rehabilitation, and exercise testing laboratories. The medical history is the primary diagnostic tool for this assessment, although additional tests might be needed to confirm a particular diagnosis. Questions dealing with discomfort in the neck, jaw, arms, epigastrium, as well as terms such as burning, numbness, pressure, and difficulty breathing should be included in the history. Table 3–6 lists the possible causes of chest discomfort that need to be considered in the differential diagnosis. Most of these con-

Table 3–5. The Cardiovascular History

History of the present illness

Review of cardiovascular symptoms
  Chest pain or discomfort
  Dyspnea
  Palpitations
  Syncope
  Edema
  Fatigue

Past cardiovascular history
  Rheumatic fever
  Myocardial infarction (MI)
  Cardiovascular surgery
  Congestive heart failure
  Pulmonary embolism
  Bacterial endocarditis
  Cardiovascular therapies

Cardiovascular risk factors
  Cigarette smoking
  Hypertension
  Hypercholesterolemia
  Diabetes mellitus
  Family history of premature coronary disease
  Life-style assessment
    Exercise history
    Diet
    Stress and personality factors

Table 3–6. Causes of Chest Discomfort and its Equivalents

Noncardiovascular conditions
  Chest wall abnormalities
  Esophageal disorders
  Pleural disease
  Gastrointestinal disturbances
  Pulmonary disease
  Psychogenic

Cardiovascular diseases
  Coronary artery disease (CAD)
    Stable angina pectoris
    Unstable angina pectoris
    Variant angina
    Acute myocardial infarction (MI)
    Postmyocardial infarction syndrome (Dressler's)
  Other cardiovascular disorders
    Aortic valve disease
    Hypertrophic cardiomyopathy
    Mitral valve prolapse
    Pericarditis
    Pulmonary hypertension
    Pulmonary infarction
    Dissecting aortic aneurysm

ditions can be diagnosed by a carefully obtained history and physical examination.[5,6] Occasionally, more expensive diagnostic procedures are required to resolve difficult problems. The use of exercise testing in the evaluation of chest pain is discussed in Chapter 5.

The distinction between *typical angina pectoris, atypical angina,* and *nonanginal chest pain* is an important consideration in the evaluation of patients with suspected coronary artery disease. The clinical characteristics of typical angina are listed in Table 3–7. This classic syndrome is almost always due to obstructive coronary atherosclerosis and occurs predictably whenever the myocardial oxygen demands exceed the available supply. Because of this threshold phenomenon, the precipitating factors of exercise and emotional excitement can bring on an anginal attack in a rather reproducible manner. Atypical angina can be defined as a clinical syndrome that is somewhat suggestive of angina pectoris but lacking in one or two of the typical features listed in Table 3–7. These symptoms are also associated with an increased likelihood of obstructive coronary disease but to a lesser extent than typical angina. Finally, nonanginal chest pain refers to symptoms that are very uncharacteristic of angina, lacking in three or more of the classic features described in Table 3–7. These symptoms are not likely to be due to coronary artery disease. Diamond and Forrester[7] have published data for men and women of various ages regarding the probability of underlying coronary disease in typical angina, atypical angina and nonanginal chest pain. These probabilities can be used as pretest probabilities for various noninvasive diagnostic procedures such as exercise testing (Chapter 5).

In patients with typical or atypical anginal symptoms, it is clinically important to further classify the symptoms as *stable* or *unstable.* Stable angina pectoris implies that the symptoms have been present for at least 1 month and that the characteristics of the chest pain, including severity, duration, and precipitating and relieving factors, have not changed during that time. Unstable angina includes recent-onset angina (within 1 month) as well as progressive or accelerating angina in which the symptoms are becoming more severe, lasting longer, more easily provoked and less easily relieved by rest or nitroglycerin. Angina-at-rest associated with transient ST segment elevation is sometimes called *variant* or *Prinzmetal's angina* and is due to coronary artery spasm superimposed on normal or diseased coronary vessels. Patients with unstable anginal syndromes are generally not candidates for exercise testing; they usually are in need of hospitalization for further workup and management.

The other symptoms listed in Table 3–5 may or may not be related to cardiovascular disease. Dyspnea on effort, for example, may be secondary to cardiac or respiratory disorders, or it may be a manifestation of deconditioning. Cardiac dyspnea is usually exertional, although it may occur at night when the patient is lying flat in bed (orthopnea). At times cardiac dyspnea may

Table 3–7. The "Pain" of Typical Angina Pectoris

Quality	Tightness, aching, squeezing, burning, pressing
Location	Substernal, but may also involve left chest, arms, neck, or jaw
Duration	3 to 5 minutes, up to 15 minutes
Precipitating factors	During exertion, emotional upset, cold weather, exertion after meals
Relieving factors	Within 3 to 5 minutes after rest or sublingual nitroglycerin

suddenly wake the patient at night with accompanying feelings of suffocation (paroxsymal nocturnal dyspnea). Cardiac dyspnea symptoms are usually related to interstitial or alveolar pulmonary edema secondary to left ventricular dysfunction or mitral valve disease. Palpitations refer to the subjective awareness of the heart beat and may be the result of disturbances in cardiac rate or rhythm. Syncope or sudden loss of consciousness is frequently secondary to heart disease, although the common faint (vasovagal syncope) needs to be excluded in the differential diagnosis. Edema has many different causes including diseases of the cardiovascular system, liver, and kidneys. Finally, fatigue is almost a universal symptom in patients with a variety of disease and nondisease conditions. The medical history, physical examination, and various noninvasive and invasive laboratory tests may all be needed to resolve difficult diagnostic problems that are manifested by these symptoms.

The Cardiovascular Physical Examination

The physical examination of the cardiovascular system is often the first opportunity to appreciate significant structural or functional abnormalities that may be responsible for limiting symptoms or disability. There are three components to this examination: *inspection, palpation,* and *auscultation.* Each of these modalities requires considerable skill and clinical experience. Unfortunately, there is a tendency today to rely less and less on physical findings in favor of more quantitative information derived from expensive, noninvasive imaging techniques. Although these procedures are sometimes needed to confirm a particular diagnostic impression, many abnormalities of the cardiovascular system can be detected and managed successfully using simple clinical skills.

Inspection

Inspection begins with a general overview of the patient at rest and, if possible,

during activity looking for abnormalities of body habitus, facial appearance and gait. Occasionally, the detection of specific skeletal abnormalities will suggest the presence of underlying congenital heart disease. Examination of the skin may reveal yellow, waxy plaques of xanthelasma around the soft periorbital tissues, which are sometimes associated with hypercholesterolemia and underlying coronary artery disease. Tendon xanthomas, more specific findings of familial hypercholesterolemia, are lumpy, nodular swellings of cholesterol deposits over the Achilles tendons, knees, elbows, or knuckles.

Inspection of the jugular venous pulse in the neck often provides important clues regarding the functional status of the right heart. The right internal jugular pressure and waveform are most suitable for this examination. The patient should be positioned for optimal visualization of venous pulsations just beneath the sternocleidomastoid muscle (30° trunk elevation for normal subjects). In right heart failure or tricuspid valve disease, the jugular venous pressure increases, and greater trunk elevation up to the sitting position may be necessary to see the top of the oscillating venous column. The central venous pressure is estimated by taking the vertical distance from the top of the venous column to the sternal angle of Lewis and adding 5 cm for the distance to the center of the right atrium below the sternal angle. Normal pressure is less than 8 cm of water.

The jugular venous pulse waveform normally consists of a presystolic a wave, which occurs during atrial contraction, and a late systolic v wave, which occurs during atrial filling when the tricuspid valve is closed. Between the a and v waves is the x-descent, which represents atrial relaxation. The y-descent occurs after the v wave and represents early ventricular filling after opening of the tricuspid valve. Large a waves are seen in right ventricular hypertrophy, pulmonary hypertension, and tricuspid stenosis. In tricuspid regurgitation, the v wave becomes prominent with obliteration of the x-descent and fusion with the a wave.

Palpation

During the cardiovascular exam all major arterial pulses including carotid, brachial, radial, femoral, posterior tibial, and pedal pulses should be palpated for patency and waveform characteristics. A grading system ranging from 0 to 3+ is often used to compare pulse intensity, where 0 refers to the complete absence of pulsation, 1+ is diminished pulsation, 2+ is normal pulsation, and 3+ is a large or bounding pulse. Auscultation over the major arteries including the abdominal aorta and its branches should be carried out to detect audible bruits caused by tubulence and usually indicative of partial occlusion from atherosclerosis.

The carotid pulse examination is especially important, since occlusive atherosclerotic disease may lead to catastrophic cerebrovascular accidents if not detected and treated. In addition, the contour of the carotid artery pulsation often provides clues to particular cardiac abnormalities. A low-volume, slowly rising carotid artery waveform (pulsus parvus et tardus) is often the best physical finding for grading the severity of aortic valve stenosis. In contrast, a *bisferiens* pulse has a dynamic, rapid upstroke with two peaks during systole. This abnormal pulse contour is seen in combined aortic regurgitation and stenosis as well as in idiopathic hypertrophic subaortic stenosis.

Palpation of the precordium is an important means of assessing the characteristics of right and left ventricular contraction. Left ventricular size is best appreciated by palpating the apex impulse while the patient is sitting up, leaning forward in held expiration. The center of the point of maximal impulse (PMI) correlates reasonably well with the left heart border. Normally, the PMI is in the fifth intercostal space, midclavicular line. In left ventricular enlargement the PMI is displaced to the left and downward. A sustained, lifting impulse indicates left ventricular hypertrophy usually secondary to aortic stenosis, hypertensive heart disease, or cardiomyopathy. In coronary heart disease (CHD) with an anterior wall aneurysm, there may be an abnormal systolic impulse medial to the apex in the third or fourth intercostal space. Right ventricular hypertrophy is often the cause of a sustained left parasternal lift, which is best appreciated with the palm of the hand placed over the left parasternal region. Heart sounds and murmurs may also be appreciated during palpation, although their definitive characteristics are better determined with auscultation.

Auscultation

The stethoscope was introduced by Laennec in 1826 and quickly became the most important examination tool of the cardiovascular physician. Although in today's fast-moving, high-technology medicine the stethoscope has lost much of its glamour, skillful auscultation of the heart remains one of the most effective diagnostic techniques in medicine.

A systematic approach to cardiac auscultation is necessary to avoid missing significant findings. Table 3–8 summarizes the important aspects of auscultation that are considered in this section. Initially, the patient should be resting comfortably with 30° of trunk elevation in a quiet room. There are four important auscultatory regions of the chest that overlap one another. The aortic areas include the right second intercostal space, the left third intercostal space (Erb's point), and the cardiac apex. The murmur of aortic valvular stenosis may be loudest in any one of these areas. The pulmonic area is primarily confined to the upper left sternal border, while the tricuspid area involves the lower left sternal border. The mitral area is at the cardiac apex and may extend into the left axilla.

Table 3–8.   Auscultation of the Heart

Regions of auscultatory interest
  Aortic areas: right second intercostal space, left
    third intercostal space, and cardiac apex
  Pulmonic area: upper left parasternal region
  Tricuspid area: lower left parasternal region
  Mitral area: cardiac apex and axilla

Heart sounds
  S1: mitral and tricuspid valve closure
  S2: pulmonic and aortic valve closure
  S3: ventricular filling sounds
  S4: decreased ventricular compliance during
    atrial systole
  Ejection click: aortic or pulmonic valve opening
  Midsystolic click: mitral valve prolapse
  Opening snap: opening of mitral valve in mitral
    stenosis

Heart murmurs
  Systolic ejection murmurs
    Functional or innocent flow murmurs
    Aortic stenosis
    Pulmonic stenosis
    Idiopathic hypertrophic subaortic stenosis
    Atypical mitral regurgitation
  Pansystolic or holosystolic murmurs
    Mitral regurgitation
    Tricuspid regurgitation
    Ventricular septal defect
  Late systolic murmurs
    Mitral valve prolapse
  Immediate diastolic decresendo murmurs
    Aortic regurgitation
    Pulmonic regurgitation
  Delayed diastolic murmurs
    Mitral stenosis
    Tricuspid stenosis
  Continuous murmurs (systole and diastole)
    Patent ductus arteriosis
    Arteriovenous fistula

Auscultation should proceed from one area to the next, using both the bell and diaphragm of the stethoscope. The diaphragm, when pressed firmly to the chest wall, selects high-frequency sounds and murmurs. The bell, when held lightly on the chest is best for low frequency murmurs and gallop sounds. Examination of the cardiac apex in the left lateral decubitus position with the bell is optimal for detecting mitral stenosis murmurs and left ventricular gallop sounds. Examination of the right and left parasternal regions with the diaphragm while the patient is sitting up, leaning forward in held expiration is best for detecting early diastolic murmurs of aortic and pulmonary regurgitation.

FIRST HEART SOUND (S1). The first heart sound that initiates ventricular systole has a rather complex origin. The most important component, heard in all areas, is mitral valve closure. Splitting of S1 in the tricuspid area is usually due to tricuspid valve closure, which closely follows mitral closure. In the other areas, however, the second component of a split S1 may be an ejection sound from the aortic or pulmonary valves. S1 is usually loudest at the apex. Increased intensity may be found in patients with short PR intervals, mitral stenosis, and high-output states. Soft S1 sounds are heard in patients with long PR intervals, mitral regurgitation, and low-output states. Variable intensity S1 is usually due to a cardiac arrhythmia such as atrial fibrillation or ventricular tachycardia.

SECOND HEART SOUND (S2). In normal subjects the second heart sound splits physiologically in the pulmonic area. The initial louder component (A2) is due to aortic valve closure; the second and softer component (P2) is due to pulmonic valve closure. With inspiration A2 moves inward, P2 moves outward, and the split widens; during expiration the split narrows until a single sound is heard. Normally P2 is only heard in the pulmonic area. In pulmonary hypertension P2 accentuates and is heard at the apex. Very loud P2 sounds may be palpable in the pulmonic area. Fixed splitting with respiration is heard in atrial septal defects. Increased physiologic splitting is found in conditions where there is a delay in right ventricular ejection (right bundle branch block, pulmonic stenosis). In paradoxic splitting A2 is delayed and follows P2 during expiration. With inspiration the split narrows and becomes single. This is seen when there is a delay in left ventricular ejection as in left bundle branch block, aortic stenosis, or left ventricular failure.

GALLOP SOUNDS (S3, S4). Gallop sounds may originate in either ventricle, although they are most common in the left ventricle. They are best heard with the bell of the stethoscope at the apex. An S3 sound occurs at the peak of rapid ventricular filling in early diastole. It is a normal filling sound in young healthy individuals and may be heard up to age 40. In the dilated, failing ventricle, however, the S3 gallop is a pathologic finding and generally occurs in the setting of sinus tachycardia. An S4 gallop is always an abnormal finding and indicates decreased compliance of the ventricle during atrial systole. It occurs late in diastole just before S1. In coronary artery disease (CAD), an S4 gallop is a common physical finding during ischemia or myocardial infarction (MI). It may be heard immediately after exercise testing in a patient with ischemic ECG findings.

MIDSYSTOLIC CLICKS. These are sounds heard in mid-to-late systole that are due to prolapse of the mitral valve leaflet into the left atrium. A late systolic murmur following the click is indicative of mitral regurgitation. This is a very common, benign developmental abnormality, found especially in young women, and may be associated with resting ST-T wave changes on the ECG and false-positive exercise ECG abnormalities.

SYSTOLIC EJECTION MURMURS. These systolic murmurs begin after S1, end before S2, and have a diamond-shaped configuration. They are harsh, medium-pitched murmurs, which are usually due to turbulent blood flow across the aortic or pulmonic valves. The most common ejection murmur is the benign functional or innocent murmur, which is best heard along the left sternal border in young healthy individuals. These murmurs are generally soft, rather brief in duration and not associated with any cardiac pathology. Murmurs of aortic or pulmonic valve stenosis are usually harsher in quality, and occupy most of systole. In aortic stenosis the murmur radiates into the carotid arteries, although its intensity may be loudest at the mitral area or Erb's point. At times, mitral regurgitation due to papillary muscle dysfunction may be confused with aortic stenosis. Other diagnostic techniques may be necessary to differentiate these two valve lesions.

PANSYSTOLIC MURMURS. These murmurs begin with S1 and usually end with S2. They are most often due to mitral or tricuspid valve regurgitation and have a high-pitched blowing quality. The murmur of mitral regurgitation is best heard at the apex and radiates into the axilla and back. Tricuspid regurgitation is best heard along the lower left sternal border and intensifies with inspiration. It is also associated with giant v waves in the jugular venous pulse. The murmur of ventricular septal defect is loudest along the left sternal border but is more medium pitched and may be associated with a palpable "thrill."

DIASTOLIC MURMURS. Murmurs in diastole are of two types. The immediate, high-pitched decrescendo murmurs of aortic and pulmonic regurgitation are best heard along the right and left sternal borders with the diaphragm. The murmur of mitral stenosis is a delayed, low-pitched diastolic rumbling murmur at the apex, which often begins with an "opening-snap" due to mitral valve opening. Tricuspid stenosis is a similar murmur best heard along the left sternal border, although much less common than mitral stenosis.

An accurate description of a heart murmur includes its intensity (grade 1 to 6), location, timing, configuration, pitch, and duration. In addition, certain maneuvers may be helpful in the differential diagnosis. These include respiratory variations, Valsalva maneuver, exercise, postural changes, pharmacologic agents (amyl nitrite), and postpremature beat changes. Most often the structural abnormality responsible for the murmur and its severity can be adequately assessed with these techniques without the need for more extensive testing.[8]

The Electrocardiogram

The electrical activation of the heart and the derivation of the body surface ECG are discussed in Chapter 2. This secton considers the clinical applications of the ECG to cardiovascular medicine. The ECG may be of value in the detection of anatomic, physiologic, or functional cardiac abnormalities. Because of its low cost, simplicity, and extensive usage over the past 50 years, the ECG continues to be one of the most effective clinical tools in all of medicine. In addition to the resting ECG, which has become an essential diagnostic study in the cardiac workup, there are two special ECG applications that have clinical utility in selected situations: ambulatory electrocardiography and exercise electrocardiography. Because of its importance to cardiac rehabilitation and adult fitness, exercise testing is discussed in considerable detail in Chapter 5.

The most common recording system for resting ECG is the 12-lead ECG, which requires 10 electrodes. Four electrodes are placed on each extremity, and six precordial chest electrodes are placed as follows: V_1, parasternal right fourth intercostal space; V_2, parasternal left fourth intercostal space; V_3 halfway between V_2 and V_4; V_4, left fifth intercostal space, midclavicular line; V_5, anterior axillary line horizontal to V_4; V_6, midaxillary line horizontal to V_5. The 12 leads are divided into six frontal plane bipolar leads and six unipolar chest leads in the horizontal plane. The frontal plane leads are defined as follows: lead I, (−)right arm (RA) versus (+)left arm (LA); lead II, (−)RA versus (+)left leg (LL); lead III, (−)LA versus (+)LL; lead aV_R, (+)RA versus (−)(LA and LL); lead aV_L, (+)LA versus (−)(RA and LL); and lead aV_F, (+)LL versus (−)(RA and LA). The precordial leads are each connected to the central terminal derived from the combination of RA, LA, and LL electrodes, which approximates a zero potential. The right leg electrode is connected to ground.

Method of Interpretation

The optimal interpretation of the 12-lead ECG requires a systematic approach

Table 3–9.   Method of Electrocardiographic Interpretation

Measurements
  Heart rate (atrial and ventricular)
  PR interval (0.12 to 0.20 sec)
  QRS duration (0.06 to 0.10 sec)
  QT interval (heart rate dependent)
  Frontal plane QRS Axis (−30 to +90 degrees)

Rhythm diagnosis

Conduction diagnosis

Waveform description
  P waves (atrial enlargement)
  QRS complexes (ventricular hypertrophy, infarction)
  ST segment (elevation or depression)
  T waves (flattened or inverted)
  U waves (prominent or inverted)

ECG diagnoses
  Within normal limits
  Borderline abnormal
  Abnormal (list diagnoses)

Comparison to previous ECG

in order to avoid missing subtle findings. Table 3–9 describes a logical method for ECG analysis. The terminology and standard format for ECG data presentation are illustrated in Figure 3–1, assuming the standard paper speed of 25 mm/sec. A normal 12-lead ECG is shown in Figure 3–2.

HEART RATE. Usually there is a one-to-one relationship between atrial and ventricular events. If the rhythm is regular the ventricular rate is determined by dividing the RR interval (sec) into 60 to get beats per minute (bpm). For standard paper speeds of 25 mm/sec, it is convenient to remember that atrial or ventricular events occurring one large box apart (0.2 sec) have a rate of 300/min; two boxes (0.4 sec), 150/min; three boxes, 100/min; four boxes, 75/min; five boxes, 60/min; six boxes, 50/min. This provides an easy way to quickly establish approximate heart rates at a glance. In normal sinus rhythm, heart rates below 55 (bpm) are called sinus bradycardia; rates above 100 bpm are called sinus tachycardia; a slight beat-to-beat variation in heart rate with respiration is called sinus arrhythmia.

PR INTERVAL. The PR interval is meas-

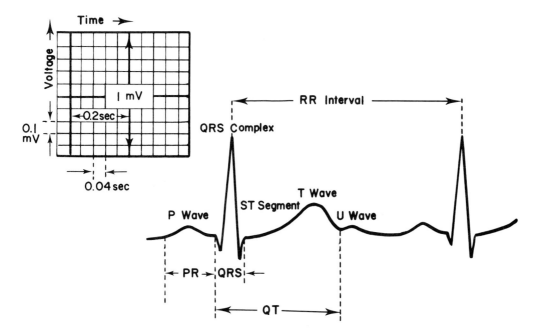

Fig. 3–1. Standard ECG format and terminology. The paper speed is 25 mm/sec and the 1-mV calibration equals 10 mm.

ured from the beginning of the P wave to the onset of the QRS complex. This interval represents the conduction time from the beginning of atrial activation to the beginning of ventricular muscle activation and includes conduction through the atrioventricular (AV) node, bundle of His, and bundle branches. The normal range is from 0.12 sec to 0.20 sec. Short PR intervals may be due to ventricular preexcitation through an AV nodal bypass tract, as seen in the Wolff-Parkinson-White syndrome. In AV junctional rhythms the PR interval may be less than 0.12 sec but the configuration of the P waves suggests retrograde atrial activation (inverted P waves in leads II, III, aV_F). PR intervals longer than 0.20 sec imply conduction delay between atria and ventricles, most often in the AV node. This is called first-degree AV block.

QRS DURATION. This interval represents the ventricular muscle activation time. The normal duration is 0.06 sec to 0.10 sec. Prolonged QRS durations occur when there is intraventricular conduction delay such as seen in bundle branch blocks. Rhythms originating in the ventricles also have wide QRS complexes.

QT INTERVAL. This interval is measured from the beginning of the QRS complex to the end of the T wave and corresponds to the duration of ventricular systole. The upper limits for this measurement are determined by cycle length or heart rate. As an approximate guide, the QT interval is 0.40 sec at a rate of 70 bpm; for each 10 bpm slowing in heart rate, the upper limit increases by 0.02 sec (e.g., for heart rate of 50 bpm, the QT interval should be less than 0.44 sec). For each 10 bpm increment in heart rate above 70 bpm, the upper limit for QT interval decreases by 0.02 sec. These are only approximate limits; tables of normal values are provided in several textbooks of electrocardiography.[9–11] Prolonged QT intervals may be seen in a variety of different clinical circumstances including CHD, central nervous system (CNS) disease, drug therapies (quinidine, procainamide, tricyclic antidepressants), electrolyte abnormalities, and hereditary disorders. Patients with long QT intervals

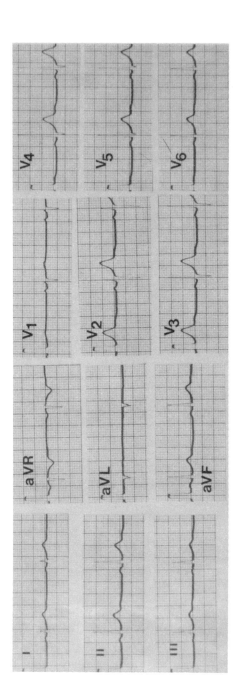

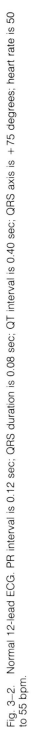

Fig. 3–2.   Normal 12-lead ECG. PR interval is 0.12 sec; QRS duration is 0.08 sec; QT interval is 0.40 sec; QRS axis is + 75 degrees; heart rate is 50 to 55 bpm.

are at increased risk for ventricular arrhythmias, syncope, and sudden death.

FRONTAL PLANE QRS AXIS. This measurement represents the average direction of ventricular activation in the frontal plane. Assuming that the standard leads I, II, and III form an equilateral triangle in the frontal plane (Einthoven's triangle),[9] the axis is determined by vector summation of the individual components of the QRS complex from any two frontal plane leads. Figure 3–3 illustrates the standard lead diagram for plotting the QRS axis. In normal subjects the QRS axis ranges from $+90°$ to $-30°$. An axis to the left of $-30°$ (i.e., more negative) is called left axis deviation. This may result from a conduction block in the left anterior division of the left bundle branch. Right axis deviation refers to an axis to the right (i.e., more positive) than $+90°$. Most often this is due to right ventricular overload conditions.

RHYTHM AND CONDUCTION ANALYSIS. The ECG continues to be the most important tool for assessing disturbances in cardiac rhythm and conduction. Figure 3–4 offers a useful approach to the classification of arrhythmias and conduction abnormalities. Abnormalities of impulse formation should be described in the following terms: (1) site of origin (atria, AV junction, ventricles); (2) rate of occurrence

(normal, slow, fast); (3) regular or irregular; and (4) active (premature) or passive (escape) onset.

The conduction of an electrical event, whether it originates in the sinus node or an abnormal focus, may encounter delays or block anywhere in the conduction system including sinoatrial, intra-atrial, AV junctional, and intraventricular pathways. Conduction delays or block may be either in the antegrade, retrograde, or bilateral directions. Block may be first degree (all impulses conduct but at a slower velocity), second degree (some impulses conduct and some do not), or third degree (no conduction). Second-degree block may be progressive (Wenckebach or Mobitz type I) or nonprogressive (Mobitz type II). Block within the ventricles may involve the right or left bundle branch, the two fascicles of the left bundle, or combinations of pathways.

Figure 3–5 presents an abbreviated atlas of major arrhythmias and conduction disturbances along with a short description of each abnormality. A more thorough discussion of these disorders can be found in a number of excellent textbooks.[9–11]

WAVEFORM DESCRIPTION. Analysis of the individual components of the ECG waveform can provide important clues as to the presence or absence of specific structural abnormalities within the heart. Beginning with the P wave, evidence for right or left atrial enlargement should be sought. Right atrial enlargement is manifest by tall, peaked P waves in leads II, III, and aV_F. Left atrial enlargement causes widening and notching of the frontal plane P-waves. In addition, there is an increase in the terminal negative component of the P wave in lead V1.

Abnormalities of the QRS complex may provide evidence for ventricular hypertrophy. Right ventricular hypertrophy (RVH) causes a rightward shift in the frontal plane QRS axis and increased R wave amplitude in the right precordial leads. Left ventricular hypertrophy (LVH) causes increased

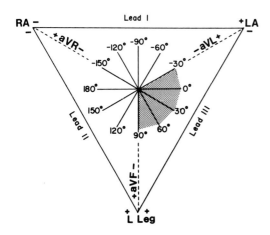

Fig. 3–3. Frontal plane lead diagram for axis determination. The normal range for the QRS axis is shaded.

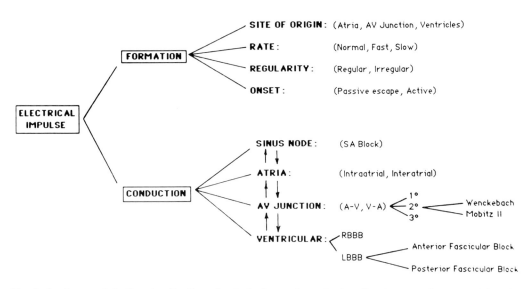

Fig. 3–4. Approach to the classification of arrhythmias and conduction disturbances. Courtesy of Alan E. Lindsay, M.D.

R wave voltage in the left precordial leads and a leftward shift in frontal plane QRS axis. Both RVH and LVH are often accompanied by secondary ST-T wave changes. In leads with tall R waves, the ST segment tends to be depressed with or without inverted T waves. These changes may be the result of subendocardial fibrosis associated with long-standing ventricular hypertrophy.

Electrocardiographic evidence for MI includes abnormalities of the QRS complex, ST segment, and T-waves.[12] The ECG hallmark for MI is the pathologic Q wave, which is defined as a wide (0.04 sec), and/or deep (1/3 QRS amplitude) Q wave. The

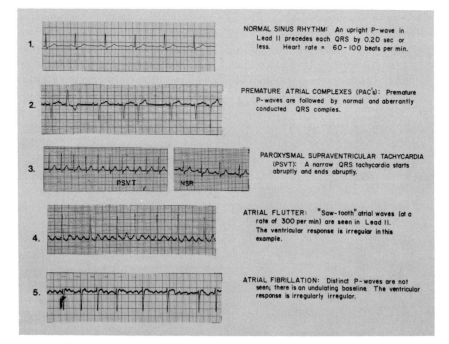

Fig. 3–5. Brief atlas of cardiac arrhythmias and conduction disorders.

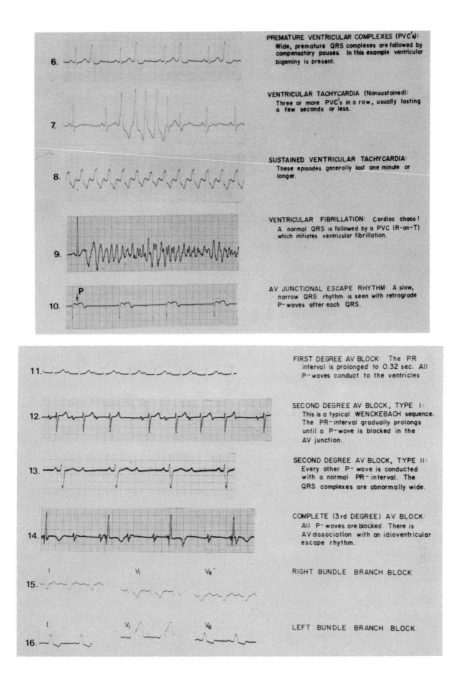

6.

PREMATURE VENTRICULAR COMPLEXES (PVC's):
Wide, premature QRS complexes are followed by
compensatory pauses. In this example ventricular
bigeminy is present.

7.

VENTRICULAR TACHYCARDIA (Nonsustained):
Three or more PVC's in a row, usually lasting
a few seconds or less.

8.

SUSTAINED VENTRICULAR TACHYCARDIA:
These episodes generally last one minute or
longer.

9.

VENTRICULAR FIBRILLATION: Cardiac chaos!
A normal QRS is followed by a PVC (R-on-T)
which initiates ventricular fibrillation.

10.

AV JUNCTIONAL ESCAPE RHYTHM: A slow,
narrow QRS rhythm is seen with retrograde
P-waves after each QRS.

11.

FIRST DEGREE AV BLOCK: The PR
interval is prolonged to 0.32 sec. All
P-waves conduct to the ventricles

12.

SECOND DEGREE AV BLOCK, TYPE I:
This is a typical WENCKEBACH sequence.
The PR-interval gradually prolongs
until a P-wave is blocked in the
AV junction.

13.

SECOND DEGREE AV BLOCK, TYPE II:
Every other P-wave is conducted
with a normal PR-interval. The
QRS complexes are abnormally wide.

14.

COMPLETE (3rd DEGREE) AV BLOCK:
All P-waves are blocked. There is
AV dissociation with an idioventricular
escape rhythm.

15.

RIGHT BUNDLE BRANCH BLOCK

16.

LEFT BUNDLE BRANCH BLOCK

Fig. 3–5 (Continued).

leads exhibiting pathologic Q waves provide evidence for the approximate location of the infarct. Q waves in leads II, III, and aV_F point to an *inferior* wall infarction; Q waves in leads V_1 to V_3 suggest *anterior* wall infarction; Q waves in leads I, aV_L, and/or V_4 to V_6 point to a *lateral* wall infarction. The one infarct location that is not identified by pathologic Q waves is the true posterior infarct, which exhibits tall, wide R-waves in the right precordial leads. These ECG findings represent reciprocal changes from what might be recorded if the ECG leads were in close proximity to the infarcted posterior wall. In acute MI there is ST segment elevation in the leads where pathologic Q waves will develop. As the ST segment elevation subsides, deep T wave inversion develops, which may persist for an indefinite period of time. Persistent ST segment elevation after an infarct has healed is indicative of a ventricular aneurysm. Two ECG examples of MI are illustrated in Figure 3–6. The ECG evidence for myocardial ischemia will be discussed in Chapter 5.

There are many subtle abnormalities in the ECG that can only be appreciated when the ECG data are analyzed within the clinical context of the particular patient being evaluated. This is especially important when interpreting the significance of ST-T wave changes. ST segment depression and T wave inversion may be due to a variety of causes, including electrolyte abnormalities, drugs, myocardial ischemia, ventricular hypertrophy, and neurogenic influences. The interpretation of a particular ST-T wave change is dependent on knowing the patient's clinical status at the

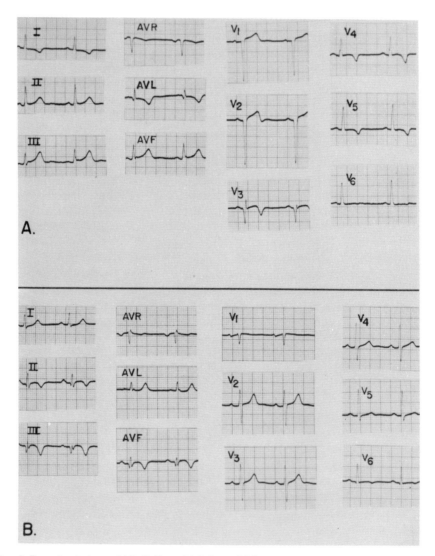

Fig. 3–6.   A, Recent anterior wall MI. B, Recent inferior wall MI.

time the ECG was obtained. The term *nonspecific ST-T wave changes* is used when clinical information is not available or when the specific abnormalities are unclear.

It is also important to compare the patient's most recent ECG with previous ECGs if available. Subtle changes from one ECG to the next may be the only clues to the presence of a new pathologic process.

AMBULATORY ELECTROCARDIOGRAPHY. The ambulatory ECG is an extension of routine ECG testing. This technique is primarily used to detect and quantitate transient arrhythmias and conduction disturbances.[13,14] It is used in the workup of patients complaining of syncope, presyncope, palpitations, and transient neurologic symptoms. It is also an effective tool for following patients with known heart disease who have arrhythmic complications and are on antiarrhythmic medications. Most recently, this technique has been used to detect transient myocardial ischemia in patients suspected of having coronary artery spasm.

The ambulatory ECG usually consists of two leads of continuous ECG data recorded on a small battery-powered tape recorder and carried by the patient for 24 hours. The patient is advised to perform routine activities during the recording period and to keep a diary of all symptoms that have occurred. The tapes are played back at 60 to 120 times real-time and computer processed to quantitate all arrhythmic events. Real-time rhythm strips are made available to the cardiologist for more detailed interpretation. An attempt is made to correlate the specific ECG abnormalities with patient activities and symptoms reported in the diary.

The Chest X-Ray

The chest radiograph completes the four essential tools used in the workup of patients with known or suspected heart disease. Along with the history, physical examination, and resting ECG, the chest radiograph provides important information regarding the state of the cardiovascular system. The standard roentgenographic assessment of the heart consists of four views: posteroanterior, lateral, and right and left anterior obliques. A barium swallow is often included to outline the posterior cardiac structures, which are adjacent to the barium-filled esophagus.

As was discussed for the ECG, a systematic approach to "reading" the chest radiograph is necessary in order to avoid missing subtle abnormalities. In addition, it is important to correlate the abnormal radiographic findings with other clinical information and laboratory data obtained from the patient. The following sequential approach is recommended for complete radiographic analysis: (1) soft tissues and bones of the thorax; (2) pulmonary vasculature and lungs; (3) size and contour of the heart and individual chambers; (4) great vessels and mediastinal structures; (5) abnormal densities and lucencies; (6) pleura and diaphragms. There are a number of excellent texts and review articles discussing various aspects of cardiovascular radiology.[15–17]

Noninvasive Cardiovascular Techniques

Noninvasive diagnostic procedures have revolutionized the study of patients with cardiovascular diseases by providing quantitative and qualitative descriptions of anatomy and physiology to a degree of clarity never before imagined. In general, however, these procedures require expensive, highly sophisticated electronic instrumentation and demand a great deal of expertise from the cardiovascular specialist. Although it is tempting to order these tests in the majority of patients with cardiovascular problems, it is not cost-effective to do so, unless the data are necessary to answer specific questions regarding optimal management. The following noninvasive diagnostic studies are briefly reviewed in this section: (1) echocardiography and doppler techniques, (2) nuclear imaging techniques, (3) positron-emission tomography, and (4) nuclear magnetic resonance.

Echocardiography

This imaging technique involves the transmission of ultrahigh-frequency sound waves into the body in order to detect and image both stationary and moving structures. Short bursts of ultrasound are emitted from a transducer held on the body surface and directed in different directions and tomographic planes. The depth and position of the reflected echos returning from structures within the body are detected by the transducer and electronically amplified to produce either time-motion strip-chart recordings (M-mode) or two-dimensional images in a video format. In recent years computer techniques have been developed to process these two-dimensional images in order to provide quantitative analysis of chamber size, ventricular function, wall motion, and valve areas.

The echocardiographic examination is performed while the patient is supine or in the left lateral decubitus position. Various acoustic windows are chosen for both M-mode and two-dimensional imaging in order to obtain multiple views of the cardiovascular structures. The M-mode images represent an "ice-pick" or unidimensional view of cardiac anatomy. By scanning the M-mode beam in an arc, as illustrated in Figure 3–7, the various cardiac structures from apex to base can be imaged in a time–motion format. The ECG signal is also recorded on the strip chart for timing purposes. Figure 3–7 shows a schematic representation of the M-mode scan from apex to base with the structures labeled.

The two-dimensional or cross-sectional echo evaluation complements the M-mode examination by providing spatial relationships of cardiac anatomy in a video format. Various tomographic cuts of the heart along its long axis and short axis are diagrammed in Figure 3–8. The two-dimen-

sional images are recorded on videotape for subsequent playback and analysis.

Echocardiography has many important clinical applications, which are categorized in Table 3–10.[18] In many instances the echo examination has surpassed the ECG in recognizing chamber enlargement, hypertrophy, and MI. Probably the most obvious and frequent indication for an ultrasound study is the differential diagnosis of heart murmurs.[19] Although the origin of a particular heart murmur can frequently be determined by auscultation, the echo examination provides quantitative information regarding the severity of the valve lesion, its etiology, and the functional consequences. Quantitation of valve areas, chamber size, wall thickness, and ventricular function are all important considerations in determining the need for corrective surgery. Echocardiography is also an important technique for evaluating prosthetic valve function and detecting infective vegetations on diseased or prosthetic valves. Finally, an echo exam is the procedure of choice for recognizing pericardial effusion, tamponade, and atrial myxomas.

In CHD echocardiography may be useful in the identification of high-risk post-MI patients with poor ventricular function.[20,21] In addition the detection of mural thrombus or ventricular aneurysms in these patients may permit more definitive therapies to be administered. Exercise echocardiographic studies are beginning to be reported in the literature as a method for detecting ischemic-induced wall motion abnormalities, which may have prognostic and therapeutic implications.[22]

Echocardiography has proven to be an invaluable asset in the noninvasive evaluation of congenital heart disease, pericardial disease, and cardiomyopathies. In many clinical situations the echo results preclude the need for more expensive and risky cardiac catheterization procedures.

Doppler Echocardiography

The Doppler imaging technique has recently become an important addition to di-

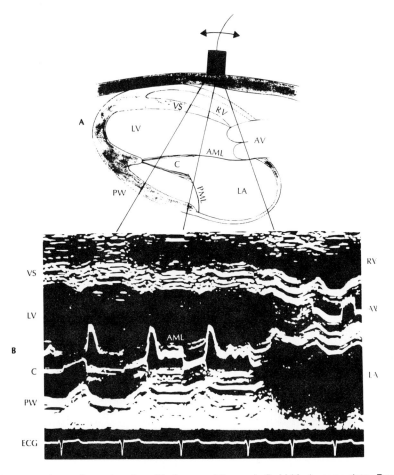

Fig. 3–7.   M-mode echocardiography. *A,* m-Mode scan (diagram). *B,* M-Mode scan data. Reproduced by permission from Nanda, N.C., and Gramiak, R.: Clinical Echocardiography, St. Louis, 1978, The C.V. Mosby Co.

agnostic ultrasound because of its ability to quantitate blood flow velocity in the heart and blood vessels. The Doppler principle is based on the observation that when a sound beam strikes a moving object, the reflected waves have a different frequency from the incident waves, the difference being proportional to the velocity of the moving object.

The two types of Doppler techniques that are currently in use are (1) pulsed Doppler ultrasound and (2) continuous wave Doppler echocardiography.[23] The pulsed Doppler technique permits focusing the ultrasound beam on selected sites in the heart in order to detect blood flow velocity and turbulence in the various car-

diac chambers and great vessels. The localization of heart murmurs and the severity of the valve lesions can be determined with this method. The continuous wave Doppler technique requires a transducer that continuously emits and receives ultrasonic waves. This technique permits an accurate assessment of blood flow velocity in the heart and great vessels similar to an electromagnetic flow meter. This is a useful technique for measuring cardiac output and assessing left ventricular function.

Nuclear Cardiology

The rapid development of radioactive isotope techniques in the 1970s coincided

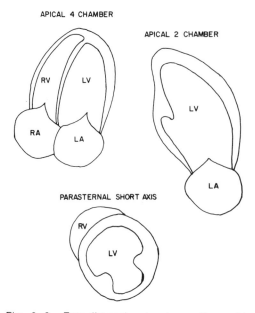

APICAL 4 CHAMBER

APICAL 2 CHAMBER

PARASTERNAL SHORT AXIS

Fig. 3–8. Two-dimensional echocardiographic views. Selzer, A.: Principles and Practice of Clinical Cardiology. 2nd Ed. Philadelphia, W.B. Saunders, 1983.

with the need to improve the recognition of myocardial ischemia and the quantitation of ventricular function as more definitive therapies became available for patients with CHD. Numerous reports in the literature have documented the improved

Table 3–10. Clinical Applications of Echocardiography

Valvular heart disease
  Differential diagnosis of heart murmurs
    Innocent murmur versus organic valvular disease
    Etiology of mitral regurgitation
    Aortic stenosis versus hypertrophic cardiomyopathy
  Prosthetic valve abnormalities
  Detection of valvular vegetations (endocarditis)
  Evaluation of chamber size, ventricular hypertrophy, and ventricular function
Coronary heart disease (CHD)
  Global and segmental wall motion abnormalities
  Ventricular aneurysm detection
  Mural thrombus detection
  Assessment of left ventricular ejection fraction
  Detection of right ventricular infarction
Diagnosis of congenital heart disease
Evaluation of myocardial disease
Evaluation of pericardial diseases

sensitivity and specificity for detecting manifestations of CHD with these techniques.[24] Other nuclear imaging applications to cardiovascular medicine include the detection of right-to-left shunts, the assessment of right ventricular function, and the quantitation of valvular regurgitation.

At present, there are two major nuclear imaging techniques that have clinical utility (1) myocardial perfusion scintigraphy using thallium 201 and (2) radionuclide blood pool ventriculography. Both techniques may be carried out at rest or during exercise testing. The radionuclide images are obtained using a high-sensitivity, high-resolution gamma-ray scintillation camera.[25] Images may be visually analyzed or computer processed for more quantitative and sophisticated analyses. Considerable professional expertise is necessary for reliable interpretations of the data.

MYOCARDIAL PERFUSION IMAGING. Thallium 201 is a radioactive isotope that is an analog of potassium. When injected intravenously in a patient with normal coronary blood flow and myocardial perfusion, there is a rapid accumulation of thallium in an even distribution throughout the myocardium. Ischemic myocardium is initially underperfused and appears as a defect or "cold-spot" surrounded by normally perfused myocardium. If the ischemic abnormality is only transient, as seen during exercise or coronary spasm, there will be a delayed uptake of thallium into the previously ischemic zone with disappearance of the defect. In MI, however, the defect is permanent, since the infarcted myocardium remains underperfused indefinitely. The specific applications of thallium 201 perfusion imaging to exercise testing are discussed in Chapter 5.

RADIONUCLIDE VENTRICULOGRAPHY. This imaging technique is comparable to contrast ventriculography obtained during cardiac catheterization and is used to evaluate ventricular function at rest and during exercise. In patients with CHD the functional consequences of myocardial ischemia or infarction can be assessed by this method in terms of global and segmental wall motion abnormalities. Two methods have been developed for studying ventricular function using technetium 99m bound to red blood cells as the radiotracer. The multigated equilibrium technique uses the ECG signal to control the temporal sequences of images throughout the cardiac cycle. Data are acquired over several hundred cardiac cycles until a sufficient count density is achieved to create a well-defined sequence of images spanning the entire cardiac cycle. The first-pass technique requires a rapid bolus injection of radiotracer, and only the initial pass through the central circulation is analyzed. Both techniques rely on computer processing of angiographic images to compute end-systolic volumes, end-diastolic volumes, and ejection fractions. The use of these radionuclide techniques during supine and upright exercise testing are discussed in Chapter 5.

New Directions in Cardiac Imaging

In recent years there have been a number of new imaging techniques under investigation with a shift in emphasis from morphologic assessment of the cardiovascular system to functional analysis. The two methods that appear to be the most promising are positron-emission tomography (PET) and nuclear magnetic resonance (NMR). Although still considered to be experimental because of cost factors and technical problems, these two procedures will likely have widespread applications in cardiovascular medicine.

POSITRON-EMISSION TOMOGRAPHY. PET is a nuclear imaging technique that involves the use of naturally occurring metabolic substrates labeled with positron-emitting isotopes. Because the radioactive label does not interfere with the biologic behavior of the substrate, the resultant images are dependent on the metabolic pathway used by the particular substrate. There are a variety of different functional studies under investigation.[26] These include (1) blood volume and ventricular function studies using hemoglobin ^{11}CO; (2) oxygen-utilization studies using oxygen 15; (3) myocardial perfusion using rubidium 82 or ammonia ^{13}N; (4) myocardial metabolic studies using palmitate ^{11}C, glucose ^{11}C, or deoxyglucose ^{18}F; and (5) ischemic imaging with pyruvate ^{11}C. All of these radioactive isotopes are rather short-lived and require on site production. Also, considerable expertise is required for data analysis, since in addition to anatomic considerations, interpretation depends on an understanding of the physiologic and metabolic processes of each radioactive substrate.

NUCLEAR MAGNETIC RESONANCE. NMR imaging involves the computer reconstruction of anatomic images resulting from the interaction of large magnetic fields with the hydrogen nuclei (photons) of biologic tissues. Regions of hydrogen nuclei can be localized within the magnetic field to form an analog image of the particular structures being investigated. Electrocardiogram-gated acquisition of NMR data is required for cardiac imaging. The major application of this technique to cardiovascular imaging, thus far, has been in the recognition of ischemic and infarcted myocardium.[27] The characterization of specific tissue abnormalities is related to tissue factors which change the intensity of the magnetic resonance signals. Disease processes altering the magnetic relaxation times of the involved tissue can therefore be imaged by NMR techniques.

Invasive Cardiovascular Diagnostic Procedures

The term *invasive* implies that the body is invaded by the introduction of catheters into the arterial and venous systems and ultimately into the various chambers of the heart and pulmonary arteries. The two major techniques that are used in the evaluation of patients with cardiovascular disease are *cardiac catheterization* and *angiocardiography*. Without a doubt, these procedures have resulted in major advances in diagnostic and therapeutic cardiology over the past 30 years and are now indispensable prerequisites to making many therapeutic decisions. The term invasive also implies an increased risk, considerable expense, and some discomfort to the patient. For these reasons the cost-benefit ratio for each patient needs to be carefully considered before proceeding with catheterization studies. If satisfactory management decisions can be made on the basis of clinical assessment and noninvasive testing, then invasive studies are generally not indicated. If, on the other hand, an operative intervention is being considered, invasive studies are usually necessary to detect and quantitate all the surgically correctable lesions. When invasive studies are planned, it is very important that they be performed in a high-quality, busy, cardiac catheterization laboratory to ensure accurate and reliable results.[28]

Cardiac Catheterization

Patients undergoing catheterization studies are usually admitted to the hospital the day prior to the procedure for a preliminary workup including history, physical exam, ECG and chest radiograph. The catheterizing cardiologist should review the data and determine the specific questions that need to be answered in the catheterization laboratory. If possible, the patient should be hemodynamically stable before studying. The specific catheterization protocol will depend on the particular questions raised during the preliminary workup.

Right heart catheterization, using a percutaneous femoral vein approach or venous cut-down, provides the following observations: (1) pressure measurements in the right atrium, right ventricle, pulmonary arteries, and pulmonary capillary "wedge" position (an indirect reflection of left atrial pressures); (2) pressure gradients across tricuspid and pulmonic valves; (3) cardiac output determination by thermodilution; (4) oxygen contents of the venous blood at different locations in the right heart and pulmonary circulation (calculation of left-to-right shunts).

Left heart catheterization requires either a cut-down on the brachial artery or, more commonly, a percutaneous femoral artery puncture. The following hemodynamic parameters are obtained during this procedure: (1) pressure measurements in the aorta and left ventricle; (2) pressure gradients across the aortic valve; (3) oxygen content of the blood in the left heart and arterial circulation (calculation of right-to-left shunts). When the right heart catheter is in the pulmonary "wedge" position and the left heart catheter is in the left ventricle, a pressure gradient across the mitral valve can be detected to determine the severity of mitral valve stenosis.

In addition to measuring pressures and calculating blood flow, there are two special catheterization procedures that have become clinically useful in recent years: (1) intracardiac electrophysiology studies and (2) endomyocardial biopsy. The electrophysiologic studies involve recording electrical events from different locations in the heart and electrical stimulation of various cardiac chambers to pace or to provoke tachyarrhythmias. One of the earliest applications of these techniques in the 1970s was direct recordings from the bundle of His in patients with known or suspected AV heart block. In this procedure a right heart electrical recording catheter is directed across the tricuspid valve so that the catheter tip lies over the AV junction. Regions of AV block above or below the His bundle recording are easily identified by this method. In patients with the Wolff-Parkinson-White syndrome, direct intracardiac recordings have resulted in accurate localization of the AV nodal bypass tract. These techniques have led to the surgical correction of recurrent paroxysmal supraventricular tachycardias in the Wolff-Parkinson-White syndrome.

The most recent application of invasive electrophysiology is provocative drug testing in patients who are susceptible to life-threatening ventricular arrhythmias. In this procedure sustained ventricular tachycardia is repeatedly provoked by ventricular pacing techniques. Various antiarrhythmic drugs are then administered to determine the optimal drug, drug combination, or dose that will prevent the induction of the arrhythmia.[29] This somewhat complex and risky technique has proven to be extremely useful in certain patients who are at high risk for sudden death. The procedure is only performed in medical centers where there are highly trained personnel using these techniques.

The endomyocardial biopsy technique was initially developed to study the rejection phenomenon in patients who have had cardiac transplants.[30] The technique involves the use of a specially designed biopsy catheter with a forceps handle to manipulate the cutting jaws at the catheter tip.[31] Samples of right and left ventricular endocardium can be obtained for microscopic examination. As investigators gained skill and experience with this procedure, the clinical indications for biopsy increased to include patients with idiopathic cardiomyopathies and suspected myocarditis. In addition the technique has been found to be a useful method of monitoring the cardiotoxic effects of anthracycline chemotherapy. The pathologic diagnosis made from the biopsy samples frequently permits more specific therapies to be administered to patients with severely compromised cardiac function.

Angiocardiography

Most often, angiographic procedures are performed along with right and left heart catheterization studies. These studies involve the selective injection of radiopaque dye into cardiac chambers and blood vessels in order to visualize various segments of the cardiovascular system. The radiographic images are analyzed using cineangiographic techniques or cut-film angiography. Angiography of the right heart is performed to detect certain congenital abnormalities and to evaluate the pulmonary circulation. Abnormalities of the right ventricular outflow tract and pulmonic valve are easily evaluated by this technique. Left ventricular angiography is performed to quantitate the degree of mitral regurgitation and evaluate left ventricular function. Global and segmental abnormalities of left ventricular wall motion can be assessed by this technique. Aortic root angiography is done to evaluate abnormalities of the aortic valve and ascending aorta.

In patients with CAD, the most common invasive diagnostic procedure is the coronary angiogram. In this technique arterial catheters are directed into the right and left coronary arteries in order to selectively visualize different segments of the coronary circulation.[32] Multiple cineangiographic views of each major coronary artery are obtained using hand injections of radiopaque dye. In patients who have had coronary artery bypass surgery, the saphenous vein grafts can also be visualized. Left ventricular angiograms are routinely done in conjunction with coronary studies to evaluate left ventricular function.

The coronary angiogram has become the "gold-standard" method of defining the extent and severity of CAD. Most often this procedure is performed in order to detect surgically correctable lesions or to identify lesions that can be dilated by catheter angioplasty techniques. At times, however, an angiogram may be indicated to evaluate asymptomatic individuals who have abnormal resting ECGs or ischemic ECG responses to exercise. In patients with chest pain being evaluated for heart valve surgery, coronary angiography may identify a subset who need coronary artery surgery at the time of their valve surgery.

The interpretation of coronary angiograms requires a systematic evaluation of each coronary artery. A significant lesion is usually defined as one that occludes at least 70 to 75% of the luminal diameter. The extent of disease is determined by the number of vessels with significant lesions, for example, single-, double-, or triple-vessel disease. A lesion of 50% or greater of the left main coronary artery is considered to be equivalent to double-vessel disease. In addition to the degree of obstruction, the length of the narrowing is also an important determinant of coronary blood flow beyond the lesion. Finally, the location of the lesion in the diseased artery may be an important consideration in determining optimal therapy. Proximal lesions that are not totally obstructing may be relieved by angioplasty procedures without the need for open-heart surgery. Two examples of obstructed coronary arteries seen on angiography are illustrated in Figure 3–9.

CARDIOVASCULAR THERAPEUTICS

The treatment of patients with cardiovascular diseases can be classified as specific therapies, which are directed against particular diseases or manifestations of disease, and nonspecific therapies, which are designed to improve the patient's overall state of well-being. Cardiac rehabilitation and adult fitness, the principal subjects of this book, are primarily nonspecific therapies, although there may be some direct effect in reversing or ameliorating the atherosclerotic process. Therapies can also be categorized as remedial (i.e., directed against an actual disease manifestation), or prophylactic (i.e., aimed at preventing a disease or recurrence of an existing disease). To some extent, exercise therapy is both remedial and prophylactic for patients with CHD, although the major benefits are related to improvements in functional capacity. Finally, therapies may be nonpharmacologic, pharmacologic, or invasive. Nonpharmacologic therapies are directed toward changes in behaviors and life-styles. These are extremely important in the long-term management of patients with CHD. Pharmacologic or drug therapies are directed against specific manifestations and symptoms. Invasive therapies include surgical procedures, angioplasty, and other invasive manipulations of the

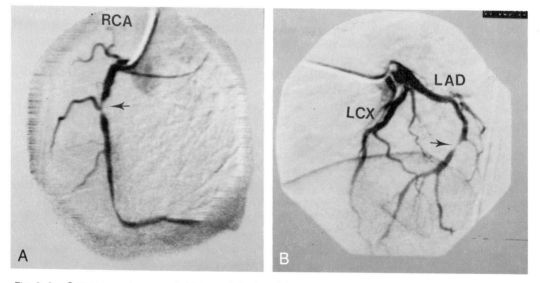

Fig. 3–9. Coronary angiograms. A, High-grade lesion of the proximal right coronary artery (arrow). B, High-grade lesion of the middle segment of the left anterior descending (LAD) coronary artery (arrow). The left circumflex (LCX) artery is also shown.

body. The comprehensive management of cardiovascular diseases often involves many different therapeutic approaches.

A primary consideration in selecting a particular therapy is the cost-benefit ratio. The therapeutic benefits to the patient should clearly outweigh the potential risks, discomforts, and financial obligations. In addition, the objectives of each therapy should be carefully defined prior to its initiation, and periodic follow-up scheduled to evaluate the therapeutic effects. Decisions to modify or discontinue a particular therapy are usually based on cost–benefit issues, which vary from patient to patient.

Nonpharmacologic Management Techniques

Whereas in the past nonpharmacologic therapy consisted primarily of advice given to patients by their physicians regarding diet, exercise, smoking cessation, and other life-style changes, recent advances in the behavioral sciences have led to a more effective and organized approach to patient management. These behavioral techniques are mostly concerned with the elimination of self-destructive behaviors that are associated with an increased risk for atherosclerotic cardiovascular diseases and hypertension. Prevention programs may be primary or secondary, depending on whether the objectives are to prevent the initiation of a new disease process or to prevent recurrences of already existing disease. For atherosclerosis there is suggestive evidence that actual regression of arterial lesions might be possible with these therapies.[33]

In the practice of cardiovascular medicine, nonpharmacologic therapies are often not emphasized to the extent that drug or invasive therapies are. This is not too unexpected, since the main thrust of modern medical training is in the use of pharmacologic and invasive therapies for managing cardiovascular diseases. Physicians are not well trained in the use of be-

havioral techniques, and in general, they do not have the time or inclination to become skilled in administering behavioral therapies. On the positive side, however, is the increasing utilization of behavioral specialists, including psychologists, psychiatrists, social workers, nutritionists, and exercise therapists in the comprehensive management of patients with cardiovascular disease. This is especially evident in cardiac rehabilitation programs where patients interact with a team of behavioral and medical specialists in an effort to modify life-styles, restore health, and optimize function.

Nonpharmacologic therapies may be administered in many different ways. Well-motivated individuals may initiate their own hygienic programs using educational materials obtained from various health agencies or purchased in book stores. Self-administered programs in exercise, weight control, smoking cessation, and stress management are readily available to the general public. The public today is much more enlightened with regard to the pursuit of healthy behaviors than in years past. Physicians are also beginning to recognize the value of these programs in improving the health and well-being of their patients. In addition to self-administered programs for individuals, there are an increasing number of group programs organized by community health agencies or provided in occupational environments where various preventive behaviors and activities are taught. Some of these programs are administered by nonprofessional leaders, while others have professionally trained group facilitators. Finally, in particularly difficult high-risk individuals, there may be a need to utilize counseling services in order to modify various self-destructive behaviors. This is often required for stress-management and modification of type A behavior.

In the following sections the nonpharmacologic approaches for managing hypertension and atherosclerotic diseases are discussed.

Hypertension

Considerable evidence now exists that nonpharmacologic treatments for hypertension are beneficial.[34] These methods of management are particularly effective in patients with borderline or mild hypertension who have yet to begin antihypertensive drug therapy. In addition, nonpharmacologic therapies are also useful as adjuncts to antihypertensive drugs in patients with more severe disease. Three changes in lifestyle are recommended to the majority of hypertensive individuals: (1) dietary modifications, (2) exercise programs, and (3) behavior modification.

Dietary recommendations for hypertensive subjects focus on weight control, sodium restriction, and decreased consumption of saturated fat and cholesterol. For obese hypertensive patients the scientific evidence is convincing that weight loss toward an ideal body weight will result in significant blood pressure lowering.[35,36] Weight reduction techniques include caloric restriction, increased exercise, and behavioral management. In general, all of these methods are necessary for successful long-term weight control. All patients with essential hypertension should be given a moderate sodium-restricted diet to a level of 70 to 90 mEq/day (2 g sodium). If, after several months, there is no significant lowering of blood pressure, continued sodium restriction may no longer be necessary. Saturated fat and cholesterol restriction is recommended because of the increased coronary risk associated with hypertension.

The role of exercise training in managing high blood pressure is less certain, although, if the exercise program is accompanied by substantial reductions in adiposity, there likely will be a blood pressure lowering effect. The specific recommendations for exercise training are discussed in Chapter 6. The many other health benefits of regular exercise make it reasonable to prescribe exercise programs to sedentary hypertensive individuals.

The behavioral techniques that are effective in lowering blood pressure include muscle relaxation and biofeedback. The relaxation response, popularized by Dr. Herbert Benson at Harvard Medical School,[37] involves four essential elements (1) a repetitive mental device (e.g., the word "one" repeated silently with each breath); (2) a passive attitude that disregards distracting thoughts; (3) systematic muscle relaxation, beginning with the feet and progressing up to the face; and (4) a quiet environment. The technique should be practiced for 20 minutes, once or twice daily, at least several hours after a meal. Research studies have indicated fairly substantial long-term blood pressure lowering effects using these methods.[38,39] Other forms of meditation including transcendental meditation, although somewhat more involved than simple relaxation exercises, are also likely to be effective in reducing blood pressure, since they incorporate the same four elements utilized for relaxation.

There are several biofeedback techniques that may be effective in lowering blood pressure. The direct methods provide the subject with feedback such as a light that goes on whenever a specific change in blood pressure occurs as a result of some conscious process. The indirect methods provide feedback to the subject about changes in skin resistance (galvanic skin response) or muscle tension, both of which reflect autonomic arousal and, indirectly, the blood pressure. Biofeedback techniques require long periods of training before significant effects are achieved. Reports in the literature are somewhat conflicting as to the efficacy of these techniques.[40]

Coronary Artery Disease

The nonpharmacologic methods for the prevention of CAD or treating established disease are specifically tailored to the individual's coronary risk factors. The risk factors that can be directly modified or eliminated are hypercholesterolemia, cigarette smoking, hypertension, sedentary life-style, obesity, and type A behavior. Unlike the nonpharmacologic approach to hypertension, however, it is more difficult to prove that risk factor modification has an ameliorating effect on the atherosclerotic process. Nevertheless, the evidence from epidemiologic studies and various intervention trials are sufficiently convincing to warrant an aggressive effort against hypercholesterolemia, cigarette smoking, and hypertension.[41] Furthermore, it is very likely that weight management, exercise training, and modification of type A behavior will have favorable effects on the other risk factors and will also improve the individual's overall sense of well-being.

HYPERCHOLESTEROLEMIA. The evidence relating high blood levels of total cholesterol and low-density lipoprotein cholesterol (LDLC) and low levels of high-denisity lipoprotein cholesterol (HDLC) to coronary risk is indisputable. What is open to question, however, is the effect on the atherosclerotic process of lowering cholesterol levels. The recently completed Lipid Research Clinics Coronary Primary Prevention Trial provided for the first time in a randomized, double-blind study conclusive evidence that cholesterol lowering by diet and the drug cholestyramine resulted in a reduced risk of CHD in men with primary hypercholesterolemia.[42] All participants in that study had an initial cholesterol level of 265 mg/dL or greater. Whether or not dietary management alone of individuals with blood cholesterol levels less than 265 mg/dL will reduce the incidence of coronary disease is still unanswered.

The American Heart Association (AHA) has recently published specific recommendations for treating hypercholesterolemia in adults, based on the position that reductions in elevated blood cholesterol levels in Americans should decrease CHD prevalence.[43] The AHA recommends that the American population at large adopt an eating pattern that would maintain blood total cholesterol levels below 200 mg/dL. A three-phase approach is described in Table 3–11 that involves a progressive reduction in total fat, saturated fatty acids, and cholesterol. Diets should be tailored to meet the needs of the individual.

The treatment of hypertriglyceridemia is somewhat controversial, since the relationship between high blood triglyceride levels and coronary disease is, at best, only minimal, unless there is coexisting hypercholesterolemia.[43] Weight reduction, exercise training, and decreased alcohol consumption are all effective methods of lowering blood triglyceride levels. Reducing saturated fat intake is also recommended.

CIGARETTE SMOKING. The cardiovascular hazards of cigarette smoking are well-known and include MI, angina pectoris, peripheral vascular disease, arrhythmias, and sudden death.[44] It is also known that smoking cessation results in a reduction in coronary mortality and incidence of MI.[45] In addition to cardiovascular effects, cigarette smoking has many other significant health hazards including chronic obstructive lung disease, cancer, peptic ulcer disease, and complications of pregnancy.[46] Of all the known cardiovascular risk factors, it is likely that smoking cessation will have the

Table 3–11. American Heart Association Recommendations for Dietary Management of Hypercholesterolemia[43]

Phase	Recommendations
I	30% total calories as fat ($\frac{1}{3}$ saturated, $\frac{1}{3}$ monounsaturated, $\frac{1}{3}$ polyunsaturated) 55% as carbohydrate (mostly complex) 15% protein Cholesterol intake less than 300 mg/day
II	25% total calories as fat (as above) 60% carbohydrates 15% protein Cholesterol intake 200 to 250 mg/day
III	20% total calories as fat (as above) 65% carbohydrates 15% protein Cholesterol intake 100 to 150 mg/day

greatest impact in lowering the morbidity and mortality from CHD. For this reason, smoking cessation deserves the highest priority among preventive measures for cardiovascular diseases.

There are some cigarette smokers who can abruptly quit smoking on their own or on the recommendations of their physicians. Most individuals who smoke, however, need to use cognitive and behavioral strategies in order to first reduce the number of cigarettes smoked and then quit entirely. Smoking cessation programs may be self-administered, such as the "Freedom From Smoking in Twenty Days" package distributed by the American Lung Association,[47] or they may involve group participation. Cognitive programs require that the smokers think about why they started smoking, what pleasures they derive from smoking, why they want to stop or continue smoking, and then identify individual patterns of smoking habits by keeping daily records. The behavioral methods are then used to change the stimulus-response–reinforcement patterns associated with smoking using a variety of behavioral techniques.[48,49] Substituting other positive health behaviors such as exercise and relaxation techniques are often useful adjuncts to the behavioral methods.

The U.S. Public Health Service has recently released a publication for physicians, "How to Help Your Hypertensive Patients Stop Smoking," which provides a step-by-step cognitive-behavioral approach to smoking cessation.[50] This attractive booklet is designed to encourage physicians to adopt a more structured and effective approach with their patients who smoke.

STRESS MANAGEMENT. One of the big "unknowns" in the risk factor concept of CHD is the role of stress in the initiation and/or aggravation of atherosclerotic disease. Also unclear are the effects of stress management on morbidity and mortality from this disease.

One component of stress reactivity, the type A behavior pattern, has been exten-sively studied and found to be associated with an increased risk of clinical CHD.[51] Type A behavior was initially described by Friedman and Rosenman[52] in 1959 as an emotional syndrome characterized by aggressiveness, competitiveness, an excessive sense of time urgency ("hurry sickness"), and easily aroused hostility. A recent consensus report of a select committee of experts meeting with officials of the National Heart, Lung, and Blood Institute concluded that the type A behavior pattern was a powerful risk factor for coronary disease equal to the relative risk associated with hypertension, cigarette smoking, and hypercholesterolemia.[53] Furthermore, preliminary evidence suggests that behavioral counseling to diminish type A behavior in post-MI patients was associated with a decreased risk of reinfarction and death.[54,55] These data are of particular importance to cardiac rehabilitation programs.

The 1981 Bethesda Conference on the Prevention of Coronary Heart Disease discussed six stress management techniques (Table 3–12) designed to reduce self-destructive behaviors leading to illness and possible cardiovascular disease.[56] Although specifically discussed in relationship to industrial or occupational settings, these techniques are applicable to other clinical settings.

Cognitive Reorganization. This involves the identification of unrewarding, self-defeating behaviors and the substitution of more suitable ones. This may be accomplished in a group therapy environment or by individual counseling.

Assertiveness Training. This is concerned

Table 3–12.   Stress Management Techniques[56]

Cognitive reorganization
Assertiveness training
Relaxation techniques
Time-management strategies
Modification of type A behavior
Environmental restructuring

with learning to express thoughts and feelings in a direct, nonthreatening fashion. Again, this technique is best learned in a group setting using role-playing and problem-solving exercises and developing conflict resolution skills.

Time-Management Strategies. These are designed to reorganize time expenditures and improve work efficiency. These strategies are likely to reduce the stress associated with deadlines and increasing job responsibilities.

Type A Behavior Modification. This technique involves all of the other stress management strategies including relaxation techniques, cognitive restructuring, and restructuring of the environment. Specific details of these techniques are discussed by Friedman et al.[54]

To conclude this discussion of nonpharmacologic therapies in cardiovascular medicine, it is important to emphasize that these methods have a great deal to offer patients in terms of disease prevention, ameliorating illness, and improving quality of life. The underlying principle in all of these techniques is the requirement that the patients assume responsibility for their own health and well-being, a concept that is likely to have considerable impact on the health-care systems of the future. This represents a major shift in emphasis from the patient as a passive recipient of medical care (drugs, surgery, etc.) to an active participant. Motivating patients to assume these new responsibilities may be difficult, unless there is the enthusiastic support of the medical profession and a willingness to refer patients to appropriate programs or counseling services when necessary. Much can be accomplished in the doctor's office[57] and in hospitals[58] using educational materials, counseling by paramedical personnel, and role modeling by health-care professionals.

Cardiovascular Drugs

In the natural history of most cardiovascular diseases, drug therapy frequently becomes necessary to relieve symptoms or other disease manifestations. The various clinical indications for initiating drug therapy are listed in Table 3–13. For each of these indications, there are several different classes of drugs that may be effective, and within each class there are many choices. The factors that lead to the selection of a specific drug for a given patient are many and involve both the science and the art of medicine. Included in the decision-making process are physician experience, desired therapeutic response, ease of administration, side effects, cost, and potential interactions with other drugs. In addition, the pharmaceutical industry may have subtle and not so subtle influences in the selection of specific drugs through the use of clever advertisements, convincing salesmen, exhibits at scientific meetings, and enticing gifts to members of the medical profession.

Antianginal Drugs

Drugs that relieve symptoms of angina pectoris are effective because they restore the balance between coronary blood flow (oxygen supply) and myocardial oxygen demands in ischemic myocardium. The three classes of antianginal drugs that are most applicable to the management of patients with ischemic symptoms are (1) the nitrates, (2) the beta-blockers, and (3) the calcium-channel blockers.

NITRATES The nitrates are the oldest and most commonly prescribed drugs for the treatment of angina pectoris.[59] The primary mechanism of action of these drugs is systemic venodilatation. As a result, the venous return to the right heart is de-

Table 3–13.   Indications for Cardiovascular Drug Therapy

Relief of angina pectoris

Treatment of heart failure

Control of cardiac arrhythmias

Management of hypertension

Antiplatelet and anticoagulant therapy

creased, pulmonary venous return to the left heart is decreased, left ventricular filling pressures are reduced, and myocardial oxygen demands are lowered. Nitrates also have modest arteriolar-dilating effects on the coronary arteries, which may improve coronary blood flow to ischemic myocardium, especially in the setting of coronary spasm.

The two most common forms of nitrate therapy are nitroglycerin and isosorbide dinitrate. Both drugs are available as short-acting (sublingual), intermediate-acting (oral or topical), and long-acting (transdermal patch) preparations. The short-acting drugs take effect within several minutes and may be effective for 15 minutes to several hours. Intermediate-acting drugs are usually effective for 3 to 6 hours; the long-acting topical preparations or transdermal patches may have antianginal effects for 8 to 12 hours.

Headaches are the major side effects of these drugs. In most individuals the headaches will diminish over time, although in some patients the headaches are so severe that continued nitrate therapy becomes impossible. Other side effects include dizziness, light-headedness, and even syncope due to the reduced stroke volume and blood pressure lowering effect of these drugs.

BETA-BLOCKERS. The beta-blocking agents have been used for over 20 years in the treatment of angina pectoris. For most of that time only a single agent, propranolol, was available in this country. In recent years, however, a number of new beta-blockers have been approved for clinical use, and the indications for these drugs have expanded to include hypertension, arrhythmias, MI, and many other clinical conditions.[60]

Beta-blockers work as competitive inhibitors of catecholamine binding at beta-adrenergic receptor sites. In the heart these effects result in decreased myocardial contractility and slowing of the heart rate, both of which reduce the myocardial oxygen requirements. In patients with angina pectoris, these beta-blocking effects result in fewer anginal attacks and increased exercise tolerance.

The available beta-blocking agents differ in terms of their pharmacologic properties. Cardioselective agents (metoprolol, atenolol) have the advantage over nonselective drugs (propranolol, timolol, nadolol) because they minimize unwanted beta-blocking effects on other tissues such as the bronchial tree. In patients with reactive airways disease (chronic bronchitis, asthma) these unwanted effects may aggravate bronchospasm. Another important pharmacologic property differentiating beta-blockers is their lipid solubility. Lipid-soluble drugs (propranolol, metoprolol, timolol) have a relatively short half-life and must be administered two to four times a day. In contrast, the water-soluble agents (atenolol, nadolol) have a long half-life and may be administered once daily.

The major cardiac side effects of these drugs are related to their basic mechanisms of action, bradycardia, and depressed myocardial function. In patients with preexisting left ventricular failure, beta-blockers are relatively contraindicated and must be used with caution. Other important side effects include fatigue, weakness, depression, bronchospasm, decreased libido, and gastrointestinal disturbances.

CALCIUM CHANNEL BLOCKERS. The newest of the antianginal drugs are the calcium channel blocking agents, also known as calcium antagonists. By blocking the entry of ionic calcium into the smooth muscle cells of the arterial walls, these drugs relax smooth muscle and produce vasodilatation.[61] Although initially introduced for the relief of coronary artery spasm, the calcium antagonists are also very effective in relieving angina due to fixed atherosclerotic obstructions.

Three calcium antagonists are currently available in this country for the treatment of all forms of angina: nifedipine, diltiazem, and verapamil. All three drugs are effective in relieving coronary spasm, although they have differing properties on myocardial contractility and cardiac conduction.[62] Verapamil, and diltiazem to a lesser extent, reduce myocardial contractility. Verapamil also slows conduction through the AV node, a property that makes it useful for treating reentrant supraventricular tachycardias. Nifedipine, on the other hand, has peripheral vasodilating effects, which may result in reflex sympathetic stimulation of the heart. In the treatment of angina pectoris, all three drugs work well as single agents or in combination with beta-blockers and nitrates. Side effects are primarily due to excessive vasodilatation, although myocardial depression and bradycardia may also be a problem. In general, the calcium channel blockers are better tolerated than nitrates or beta-blockers.

Antihypertensive Drug Therapy

The major objective in the treatment of hypertension is to reduce cardiovascular morbidity and mortality associated with long-standing elevations in blood pressure. It has been well established that antihypertensive drugs are effective in controlling high blood pressure and prolonging life.[34]

The therapeutic goal is to achieve and maintain diastolic blood pressures below 90 mm Hg and systolic pressures below 140 mm Hg. To accomplish this a "stepped-care" approach has been recommended.[34] Initial therapy should consist of either a beta-blocking agent or a thiazide-type diuretic with increasing dosages, as necessary, to achieve an adequate blood pressure lowering effect. The majority of patients with mild or moderate hypertension will respond to "step 1" drug therapy, especially if nonpharmacologic self-management (weight control, sodium restriction, exercise, relaxation) is also practiced.

If adequate blood pressure control is not achieved on step 1 therapy, the step 2 involves adding a small dose of an adrenergic inhibitor (clonidine, methyldopa, reserpine, prazosin) or a thiazide diuretic (if not already used for step 1). A small percentage of hypertensive patients will require advancing to a third step and rarely to a fourth step. Step 3 requires the addition of a vasodilator such as hydralazine or minoxidil in more resistant cases. Step 4 therapy consists of substituting guanethidine or other adrenergic inhibitors for a step 2 drug. Most patients who require step 3 or step 4 drugs have severe hypertension with evidence for end-organ damage.

At times these patients have to be hospitalized for treatment of hypertensive emergencies, cardiac complications, or CNS catastrophes. Early detection and aggressive management of mild or moderate hypertensive patients using pharmacologic and nonpharmacologic therapies will significantly reduce these serious complications.

Other Cardiovascular Drugs

ANTIARRHYTHMIC DRUGS. The management of patients with cardiac arrhythmias is a complex process that involves a number of important considerations. In the absence of organic heart disease, drug therapy is usually not indicated unless the cardiac rhythm disturbance is associated with disabling or uncomfortable symptoms. Pharmacologic management of the supraventricular arrhythmias such as atrial fibrillation and paroxysmal supraventricular tachycardia may be necessary to control ventricular rate and improve cardiac output, although these arrhythmias are rarely life-threatening.

The most serious indication for antiarrhythmic therapy is in patients with a high risk for sudden death. This is particularly important in patients with CHD who have frequent ventricular arrhythmias. The first year following acute MI in patients with poor ventricular function is associated with a very high risk for sudden death.[63] These patients need careful monitoring for arrhythmic complications.

There are four classes of antiarrhythmic drugs based on electrophysiologic properties.[64] Class I agents include quinidine, procainamide, disopyramide, lidocaine, tocainide, mexiletine, encainide, and flecainide. These drugs appear to act by depressing fast sodium channels, resulting in slowed conduction of electrical impulses within the heart. They also depress phase 4 depolarization of pacemaker cells and decrease automaticity. Class II antiarrhythmic drugs are the beta-blockers. These drugs act primarily by blocking sympathetic nervous system stimulation of the heart. These are the only drugs that have been shown in clinical trials to reduce the incidence of sudden death after acute MI.[65] Class III drugs, including bretylium and amiodarone, prolong cardiac refractory periods and increase the threshold for ventricular fibrillation. Class IV agents are the calcium channel blockers, which were discussed previously for the treatment of angina pectoris. These drugs block the entry of calcium ions into cells of the sinoatrial (SA) and AV nodes (slow channels), resulting in decreased automaticity and slowed conduction.

The antiarrhythmic drug of choice is determined by the pharmacologic and electrophysiologic actions of each drug, the nature of the cardiac arrhythmia, and most often, by the clinical response. In patients at high risk for sudden death, various provocative studies such as exercise testing, ambulatory ECG monitoring and intracardiac electrophysiologic studies may be required to determine the most suitable drug or combination of drugs.

DRUG TREATMENT OF HEART FAILURE. There are three pharmacologic approaches to managing patients with heart failure: (1) inotropic agents to increase myocardial contractility; (2) diuretics to treat fluid overload and reduce ventricular filling (preload); and (3) peripheral vasodilators to reduce the impedance to left ventricular ejection (afterload). The inotropic agents increase myocardial work and oxygen requirements; the afterload- and preload-reducing agents reduce myocardial work and oxygen requirements.

Digitalis preparations, most commonly digoxin, are the oldest and most familiar of the inotropic agents. The primary mechanism of action of these drugs is thought to be the increased availability of calcium ions to the contractile proteins within cardiac muscle cells through the inhibition of membrane sodium-potassium adenosinetriphosphatase (ATPase).[66] This results in increased myocardial contractility. Digitalis also has a heart rate slowing effect and decreases conduction velocity through the AV node. This latter effect is the basis for treating atrial fibrillation with digitalis.

Diuretics promote the excretion of sodium and water from the kidneys and effectively reduce the excess extracellular volume associated with congestive heart failure.[67] These drugs act by interfering with the reabsorption of filtered sodium ions in various segments of the nephron. The thiazide-type diuretics and the loop diuretic furosemide are the most popular drugs for this purpose. The major side effect of these drugs is hypokalemia due to the increased loss of potassium ion in the urine. This can be avoided by the concomitant administration of potassium chloride supplements or the use of potassium-sparing diuretics such as spironolactone or triampterene.

The newest class of drugs for managing chronic heart failure are the vasodilators: hydralazine, prazosin, and captopril. Although originally used for the treatment of hypertension, these drugs have become important additions in the treatment of certain types of heart failure.[68] The decrease in peripheral vascular resistance resulting from vasodilator therapy makes it easier for the left ventricle to contract and deliver an adequate forward stroke volume. This is especially important in patients with aortic or mitral regurgitation where the regurgitant fraction is significantly reduced with vasodilator therapy. The nitrates also have preload- and afterload-reducing properties, which are effective in the management of low-output congestive heart failure.

Invasive Cardiovascular Therapies

The most complex and expensive therapeutic techniques administered to patients with cardiovascular diseases are the invasive procedures. In addition to the many different cardiovascular surgical procedures, the invasive therapies also include artificial pacemakers and other electrophysiologic procedures and percutaneous transluminal coronary angioplasty. By necessity, these techniques require a great deal of technical expertise and experience on the part of the treating physicians and their support personnel. The clinical indications for performing each of these therapeutic procedures have been carefully defined in the medical literature. Patients being considered for a particular procedure usually receive a thorough workup including various noninvasive and invasive tests to determine the need and optimal timing for treatment.

The two invasive therapies most pertinent to patients undergoing cardiac rehabilitation and other forms of exercise therapy are coronary artery bypass grafting (CABG) and percutaneous transluminal coronary angioplasty (PTCA). Because of the importance of these techniques to those working in cardiac exercise programs, a brief discussion of each procedure will be presented.

Coronary Artery Bypass Graft Surgery

Surgical attempts to revascularize ischemic myocardium were totally unsuccessful until direct coronary bypass surgery was introduced in the late 1960s. Within a few years CABG became the most frequently performed cardiac operative procedure in the United States.

The techniques for CABG involve using the patient's greater saphenous vein as a bypass graft between the proximal aorta and the diseased coronary artery distal to the atherosclerotic lesion.[69] As an alternative, the internal mammary artery may be used to provide an artery-to-artery graft, providing the diameter of the internal mammary artery is large enough for adequate blood flow. Internal mammary grafts are technically more complicated and can only be used to bypass lesions of the left anterior descending coronary artery and its diagonal branches.

The indications for coronary artery bypass surgery are continuously evolving as data from prospective randomized therapeutic trials are published. Rahimtoola[70] has critically reviewed the CABG literature up to 1981 in patients with chronic stable angina and reached the following conclusions: (1) CABG prolongs life in comparison to nonsurgical treatment in patients with left main and triple vessel CAD; (2) CABG is generally associated with better symptomatic improvement than medical therapy; (3) operative mortality averages 1% to 2% but varies with age, number of bypassed vessels, and left ventricular function; (4) vein graft occlusion occurs in 10% to 15% of cases; and (5) late survival at 4 years after CABG averages 93%.

In 1983 the results of the Coronary Artery Surgery Study (CASS) were published.[71] This multicenter randomized study of over 3,000 patients was designed to determine the long-term benefits of CABG versus medical therapy in patients with mild angina pectoris and in asymptomatic post-MI patients. There was no significant difference in survival or occurrences of MI between surgically and medically treated patients during an average followup of 5.5 years. Quality of life parameters including relief of symptoms and improved functional capacity were better in the surgically treated group, however.[72] This important study indicates that most patients with mild, stable angina pectoris can be managed conservatively with antianginal medications without the need for coronary angiographic studies or surgery. This is also true for asymptomatic post-MI patients, especially those with good functional capacity. In patients whose symptoms progress in severity or become unstable, more aggressive management may become necessary.

Percutaneous Transluminal Coronary Angioplasty

The most recent and innovative invasive therapy for coronary artery disease is PTCA, introduced by Gruntzig and co-workers in 1977.[73] In this technique the narrowed coronary artery is dilated by a special balloon-tip catheter introduced through a peripheral artery. After the catheter tip is properly positioned within the lumen of the narrowed artery, inflation of the balloon compresses the atherosclerotic lesion. Successful dilation is documented by observing a drop in pressure gradient between the distal lumen of the catheter and the aorta. Repeat coronary angiography also shows reduced lesion size and improved coronary blood flow.

The National Heart, Lung, and Blood Institute (NHLBI) has developed a registry of over 3,000 patients who have had PTCA, documenting the success rate and complications of this procedure.[74] Initial guidelines for PTCA were limited to proximal, single-vessel lesions in patients with stable angina pectoris. As new catheters were designed and techniques improved, the indications for PTCA broadened to include multivessel disease, more distal lesions, unstable angina, and acute MI. The initial success rate for PTCA is 75% to 80% with an approximate 10% restenosis within a year following the procedure.[74] Many patients can undergo repeat PTCA with successful results. Approximately 10% of patients develop acute coronary events during or immediately following the procedure. These include acute MI, pro-longed ischemic pain, coronary artery dissection or embolism. Urgent coronary artery bypass surgery is sometimes necessary to manage these acute complications. The possibility of these complications makes it necessary to have coronary surgical backup in those facilities where PTCA is performed. The mortality rate for PTCA is under 1%. As experience is gained with this technique, the incidence of complications is expected to become negligible.

It is likely that PTCA will have a major impact in the management of patients with CAD. It has already resulted in decreasing the numbers of patients referred for coronary bypass surgery. The procedure is less costly, considerably less invasive, less time-consuming, and associated with less patient morbidity, shorter hospital stays, and earlier return to occupational and recreational activities.

CONCLUSIONS

Although the practice of cardiovascular medicine is rapidly evolving as new technologies and treatments become available, it is not likely that the basic strategy of the cardiovascular workup as presented here will change in the years to come.

Diagnostic procedures should usually proceed from the simple, inexpensive, and qualitative methods to the more complex, expensive, and quantitative methods only if the more sophisticated data are necessary for making optimal management decisions that will significantly affect the clinical status of the patient. Considerable skill is needed by the practicing physician in order to know just how far to go in any given patient's workup. Organizations such as the AHA and the American College of Cardiology are providing valuable guidelines for making cost-effective clinical decisions regarding patient management. It is also likely that the computer will have a significant impact on the practice of medicine by providing patient specific management algorithms in hospitals and doctors' offices.

REFERENCES

1. Levy, R.I., and Moskowitz, J.: Cardiovascular research: Decades of progress, a decade of progress. Science, *217*:121, 1982.
2. Trafford, A.: America's $39 billion heart business. US News and World Report, p. 53, March 15, 1982.
3. The Criteria Committee of the New York Heart Association: Nomenclature and Criteria for Diagnoses of Diseases of the Heart and Great Vessels. 8th Ed., Boston, Little, Brown, 1979.
4. Hurst, J.W.: The approach to the patient: Goals and cardiac appraisal. *In* The Heart. 6th Ed. Edited by J.W. Hurst. New York, McGraw-Hill, 1986.
5. Constant J.: The clinical diagnosis of nonanginal chest pain: The differentiation of angina from nonanginal chest pain by history. Clin. Cardiol., *6*:11, 1983.
6. Levine, H.J.: Difficult problems in the diagnosis of chest pain. Am. Heart J., *100*:108, 1980.
7. Diamond, G.A., and Forrester, J.S.: Analysis of probability as an aid in clinical diagnosis of coronary artery disease. N. Engl. J. Med., *300*:1350, 1979.
8. Crawford, M., and O'Rourke, R.A.: A systematic approach to the bedside differentiation of cardiac murmurs and abnormal sounds. Curr. Probl. Cardiol., *1*:1, 1977.
9. Chow, T.: Electrocardiography in Clinical Practce. Orlando, Fla., Grune & Stratton, 1979.
10. Constant, J.: Learning Electrocardiography. Boston, Little, Brown, 1981.
11. Dubin, D.: Rapid Interpretaiton of EKG's. . . . A Programmed Course. 3rd Ed. Tampa, Fla., Cover Publishing Company, 1974.
12. Schamroth, L.: The Electrocardiology of Coronary Artery Disease. 2nd Ed. Boston, Blackwell Scientific, 1984.
13. Horner, S.L.: Ambulatory Electrocardiography. Applications and Techniques. Philadelphia, J.B. Lippincott, 1983.
14. Winkle, R.A.: Current status of ambulatory electrocardiography. Am. Heart J., *102*:757, 1981.
15. Turner, A.F.: The chest radiograph: a systematic approach to interpretation for the internist. Curr. Probl. Cardiol., *3*:1, 1978.
16. Gedgaudas, E., and Knight, L.: Plain-film diagnosis of heart disease. A physiologic approach. JAMA, *232*:63, 1975.
17. Chen, J.T.T.: The chest roentgenogram. *In* The Heart. 5th Ed. Edited by J.W. Hurst. New York, McGraw-Hill, 1982.
18. Feigenbaum, H.: Echocardiography. 3rd Ed. Philadelphia, Lea & Febiger, 1981.
19. Green, S.F., and Popp, R.L.: Role of echocardiography in diagnosis and management of valvular heart disease. Mod. Concepts Cardiovasc. Dis., *50*:31, 1981.
20. Pandian, N.G., Skorton, D.J., and Kerber, R.E.: Role of echocardiography in myocardial ischemia and infarction. Mod. Concepts Cardiovasc. Dis., *53*:19, 1984.
21. Reeder, G.S., Seward, J.B., and Tajik, A.J.: The role of two-dimensional echocardiography in coronary artery disease. A critical appraisal. Mayo Clin. Proc., *57*:247, 1982.
22. Limacher, M.C., et al.: Detection of coronary artery disease with exercise two-dimensional echocardiography. Circulation, *67*:1211, 1983.
23. Pearlman, A.S., Scoblionko, D.P., and Saal, A.K.: Assessment of valvular heart disease by Doppler echocardiography. Clin. Cardiol., *6*:573, 1983.
24. Okada, R.D., Boucher, C.A., Strauss, H.W., and Pohost, J.M.: Exercise radionuclide imaging approaches to coronary artery disease. Am. J. Cardiol., *46*:1188, 1980.
25. Strauss, H.W., McKusick, K.A., and Bingham, J.B.: Cardiac nuclear imaging: Principles, instrumentation, and pitfalls. Am. J. Cardiol., *46*:1109, 1980.
26. Sobel, B.E., Ter-pogossian, M.M., and Geltman, E.M.: Positron-emission tomography in cardiac evaluation. Hosp. Pract., 93, Nov 1981.
27. Higgins, C.B., et al.: Imaging by nuclear magnetic resonance in patients with chronic ischemic heart disease. Circulation, *69*:523, 1984.
28. Report of the Inter-Society Commission for Heart Disease Resources: Catheterization-angiographic laboratories. Circulation, *53*:A1, 1976.
29. Mason, J.W., and Winkle, R.A.: Electrode catheter arrhythmia induction in the selection and assessment of antiarrhythmic drug therapy for recurrent ventricular tachycardia. Circulation, *58*:971, 1978.
30. O'Connell, J.B., Subramarian, R., Robinson, J.A., and Scanlon, P.J.: Endomyocardial biopsy: Techniques and applications in heart diseases of unknown cause. Heart Transplant., *3*:132, 1984.
31. Mason, J.W.: Techniques for right and left ventricular endomyocardial biopsy. Am. J. Cardiol., *41*:887, 1978.
32. Conti, C.R.: Coronary arteriography. Circulation, *55*:227, 1977.
33. Hammond, H.K.: Regression of atherosclerosis: A review. J. Cardiac Rehab., *3*:347, 1983.
34. The Joint National Committee on Detection, Evaluation and Treatment of High Blood Pressure. The 1984 report of the Joint National Committee on Detection, Evaluation, and Treatment of High Blood Pressure. Arch. Intern. Med., *144*:1045, 1984.
35. Reisin, E., et al.: Effect of weight loss without salt restriction on the reduction of blood pressure in overweight hypertension patients. N. Engl. J. Med., *298*:1, 1978.
36. Gillum, R.F., et al.: Nonpharmacologic therapy of hypertension: The independent effects of weight reduction and sodium restriction in overweight borderline hypertensive patients. Am. Heart. J., *105*:128, 1983.
37. Benson, H.: Systemic hypertension and the relaxation response. N. Engl. J. Med., *296*:1152, 1977.
38. Agras, W.S.: Behavioral approaches to the treatment of essential hypertension. Int. J. Obes., *3*:173, 1981.
39. Agras, W.S.: Relaxation therapy in hypertension. Hosp. Pract., 129, May 1983.

40. Pickering, T.G.: Nonpharmacologic methods of treatment of hypertension: Promising but unproved. Cardiovasc. Rev. Rep., *3*:82, 1982.

41. Kannel, W.B., et al.: Optimal resources for primary prevention of atherosclerotic diseases. Circulation, *70*:157A, 1984.

42. Lipid Research Clinics Program: The Lipid Research Clinics coronary primary prevention trial results: I. Reduction in incidence of coronary heart disease. JAMA, *251*:351, 1984.

43. AHA Special Report: Recommendations for treatment of hyperlipidemia in adults: A joint statement of the Nutrition Committee and the Council on Arteriosclerosis. Circulation, *69*:1065A, 1984.

44. Kannel, W.B.: Update on the role of cigarette smoking in coronary artery disease. Am. Heart J., *101*:319, 1981.

45. Gordon, T., Kannel, W.B., McGee, D., and Dawber, T.R.: Death and coronary attacks in men who give up cigarette smoking. A report from the Framingham Study. Lancet, *2*:1345, 1974.

46. Holbrook J.H.: Tobacco and health. CA, *27*:343, 1977.

47. Freedom From Smoking in Twenty Days. American Lung Association, New York, 1986.

48. Danaher, B.G., and Lichtenstein, E.: Become an Ex-smoker. Englewood Cliffs, N.J., Prentice-Hall, 1977.

49. Pomerleau, D.E., and Pomerleau, C.S.: Break the Smoking Habit. Champaign, Ill., Research Press, 1977.

50. The Physician's Guide: How to Help Your Hypertensive Patients Stop Smoking. US Department of Health and Human Servces, National Institutes of Health, NIH Publication No. 83-1271, April 1983.

51. Rosenman, R.H., et al.: Coronary heart disease in the Western Collaborative Group Study: Final follow-up experience of 8½ years. JAMA, *233*:872, 1975.

52. Friedman, M., and Rosenman, R.H.: Association of specific overt behavior pattern with blood and cardiovascular findings. JAMA, *169*:1286, 1959.

53. The Review Panel on Coronary-Prone Behavior and Coronary Heart Disease: Coronary-prone behavior and coronary heart disease: A critical review. Circulation, *63*:1199, 1981.

54. Friedman, M., et al.: Feasibility of altering type A behavior pattern after myocardial infarction. Recurrent coronary prevention project: Methods, baseline results, and preliminary findings. Circulation, *66*:83, 1981.

55. Friedman, M., et al.: Alteration of type A behavior and reduction in cardiac recurrences in post myocardial infarction patients. Am. Heart J., *108*:237, 1984.

56. Eliot, R.S., et al.: Task force 3: The physician in the work setting. Am. J. Cardiol., *47*:751, 1981.

57. Reeves, T.J., et al.: Task force 2: The physician in the office (adult medicine). Am. J. Cardiol., *47*:747, 1981.

58. Gillespie, L., et al.: Task force 4: The physician in the hospital. Am. J. Cardiol., *47*:766, 1981.

59. Abrams, J.: Nitroglycerine and long-acting nitrates in clinical practice. Am. J. Med., *76* (Suppl. 6A):85, 1983.

60. Conolly, M.E. Kersting, F., and Dollery, C.T.: The clinical pharmacology of beta-adrenoceptor-blocking drugs. Prog. Cardiovasc. Dis., *19*:203, 1976.

61. Braunwald, E.: Mechanism of action of calcium-channel blocking agents. N. Engl. J. Med., *307*:1618, 1982.

62. Mitchell, L.B., Schoreder, J.S., and Mason, J.W.: Comparative clinical electrophysiologic effects of diltiazem, verapamil and nifedipine: A review. Am. J. Cardiol., *49*:629, 1982.

63. Epstein, S.E., Palmeri, S.T., and Patterson, R.E.: Evaluation of patients after acute myocardial infarction. N. Engl. J. Med., *307*:1487, 1982.

64. Winkle, R.A.: Cardiac Arrhythmias. Current Diagnosis and Practical Management. Reading, Mass., Addison-Wesley, 1983.

65. May, G.S., et al.: Secondary prevention after myocardial infarction: A review of long-term trials. Prog. Cardiovasc. Dis., *24*:331, 1982.

66. Noble, D.: Mechanism of action of therapeutic levels of cardiac glycosides. Cardiovasc. Res., *14*:495, 1980.

67. Earley, L.E.: Diuretics. N. Engl. J. Med., *276*:966, 1967.

68. Chatterjee, K., and Parmley, W.W.: The role of vasodilator therapy in heart failure. Prog. Cardiovasc. Dis., *19*:301, 1977.

69. Jones, E.L., and Hatcher, C.R.: Techniques for surgical treatment of atherosclerotic coronary artery disease and its complications. *In* The Heart, 5th Ed. Edited by J.W. Hurst. New York, McGraw-Hill, 1982.

70. Rahimtoola, S.H.: Coronary bypass surgery for chronic angina—1981. Circulation, *65*:225, 1982.

71. CASS Principal Investigators and Their Associates: Coronary Artery Surgery Study (CASS): A randomized trial of coronary artery bypass surgery. Survival data. Circulation, *68*:939, 1983.

72. CASS Principal Investigators and Their Associates: Coronary Artery Surgery Study (CASS): A randomized trial of coronary artery bypass surgery. Quality of life in patients randomly assigned to treatment groups. Circulation, *68*:951, 1983.

73. Gruntzig, A.: Transluminal dilatation of coronary artery stenosis. Lancet, *1*:263, 1978.

74. Kent, K.M., Mullin, S.M., and Rassamani, E.R. (eds.): Proceedings of the National Heart, Lung, and Blood Institute Workshop on the Outcome of Percutaneous Transluminal Coronary Angioplasty. Am. J. Cardiol., *53*:1C-146C, 1984.

4

SCREENING FOR EXERCISE PROGRAMS

This chapter describes various assessment techniques that are generally recommended for most adults, including high-risk adults and cardiac patients, prior to their initiating exercise programs. It may be somewhat unrealistic to expect that most individuals will have immediate access to facilities where these tests can be conducted. Nevertheless, the dramatically increased public awareness and interest in healthy life-styles has resulted in a growing "wellness" industry, which is now providing a variety of evaluative services related to cardiovascular risk assessment and exercise testing. Many of these services are available in physicians' offices, hospitals, and health clubs. Fitness and risk factor evaluations are also provided by some state and local health agencies. It is likely that the number of these facilities and services will continue to expand in the next several years to accommodate the growing public interest in healthy life-styles.

All patients with known cardiovascular, pulmonary, or metabolic diseases should undergo a careful medical examination including exercise electrocardiogram (ECG) testing before starting an aerobic exercise program. There are a number of reasons why screening tests are also recommended for some apparently healthy individuals prior to beginning exercise. Identification of persons at risk for exercise-related cardiovascular complications is the primary

concern among health professionals working in this area. A second purpose of the screening evaluation is to identify adverse life-styles or behaviors that might be susceptible to modification during the exercise training program. Many of these behaviors also increase the risk for developing cardiovascular disease. Third, the assessment may include an orthopedic evaluation to detect existing or potential musculoskeletal problems that might be aggravated by certain exercise activities or require special training considerations. Finally, the evaluation establishes a baseline for those parameters likely to change with training and provides a more objective means for quantifying the degree of improvement.

This chapter considers the use of ques-

Table 4–1.   Screening for Exercise Programs

1.   Health history and life-style questionnaires
2.   Physical assessment techniques
    Height and weight
    Body composition
       Hydrostatic weighing
       Skinfold measurements
       Electrical impedance plethysmography
       Ideal body weight
    Blood pressure
    Muscle strength, endurance, and
      flexibility
    Submaximal exercise testing for fitness
      evaluation
    Pulmonary function screening tests
3.   Laboratory assessment
    Blood lipids
    Blood glucose
    Complete blood count (CBC)

tionnaires and simple assessment techniques that can be administered by allied health personnel. Discussions of exercise ECG testing and other physician-administered procedures are found in Chapters 3 and 5. Table 4–1 outlines the major topics discussed here.

HEALTH HISTORY AND LIFE-STYLE QUESTIONNAIRES

Self-administered questionnaires have a number of advantages over interview techniques for obtaining medical history and life-style information. They can be completed prior to the individual's fitness evaluation, thereby saving valuable professional time during the assessment. The data base obtained using questionnaires is generally more comprehensive than that obtained by an interviewer. Also, much of the data can be standardized and collected in a computer-usable format to facilitate computerized data management. This provides an important data base for performing follow-up studies and answering research questions. Table 4–2 lists the categories of data that are of interest in screening individuals for exercise and other health-enhancing programs. The completed questionnaires should be re-

Table 4–2.   Questionnaire Data for Fitness Evaluations

Medical history
Past history of:
Cardiovascular disease
Pulmonary disease
Neuromuscular problems
Orthopedic problems
Surgery
Current symptoms
Current medications
Life-style information
Smoking history
Nutrition and weight history
Exercise habits
Substance abuse
Psychosocial information
Personality classification (type A/B)
Analysis of life stressors
Family history

viewed by a health professional and, if necessary, further details obtained by interviewing the client. An example of a comprehensive questionnaire developed for cardiovascular risk assessment is shown in Figure 4–1.

PHYSICAL ASSESSMENT TECHNIQUES

In the evaluation of candidates for adult fitness and cardiac rehabilitation programs, there are several important physical measurements that should be obtained by allied health personnel. These include (1) weight and height, (2) body composition, (3) blood pressure, (4) muscle strength and endurance, (5) submaximal exercise testing, and (6) pulmonary function screening tests. Although these procedures are rather easy to understand, they must be performed carefully by experienced personnel. Often the simplest techniques are carried out most carelessly.

Weight and Height

Accurate weight and height measurements are desirable for utilizing the height–weight charts developed by the Metropolitan Life Insurance Company (see Tables 15–3 and 15–4).[1] Although these optimal weights are sometimes inaccurate in subjects with increased lean body mass, such as athletes with considerable skeletal muscle tissue, they provide useful guidelines for the average person. If possible the same scale should be used each time the subject is weighed. The zero position should be checked before each weighing, and the scale should be recalibrated periodically. Subjects should be weighed without shoes and with a minimal of clothing. For height measurements the subject should stand without shoes with the back to the measuring device, feet together, and arms relaxed at the sides. With the eyes directed straight ahead, the measuring square is adjusted to rest lightly on the

THE FITNESS INSTITUTE

AT LDS HOSPITAL

Health Assessment Questionnaire

— THIS INFORMATION WILL BE KEPT CONFIDENTIAL —

(Please Print)

General Information

NAME: _____ SEX: _____
(LAST)   (FIRST)   (M.I.)

DATE OF BIRTH: _____ AGE: _____
(MONTH)   (DAY)   (YEAR)

SOCIAL SECURITY NUMBER: _____ ____ _____

HOME ADDRESS: _____

_____
(CITY)   (STATE)   (ZIP CODE)

TELEPHONE: HOME _____ - _____ - _____ BUSINESS: _____ - _____ - _____
(AREA CODE)   (AREA CODE)

MARITAL STATUS: ☐ Single ☐ Married ☐ Divorced ☐ Widowed ☐ Separated

RACE: ☐ Caucasian ☐ Black ☐ Oriental ☐ Spanish American ☐ Other _____

EDUCATION (Check highest level attained): ☐ Grade School ☐ Jr. High ☐ High School
                                           ☐ College ☐ Graduate School

OCCUPATION: _____

PERSONAL PHYSICIAN: _____
(NAME)

_____
(ADDRESS)

_____
(CITY)   (STATE)   (ZIP CODE)

YES NO
☐   ☐   Would you like a copy of your report sent to your physician?

FILE NO. _____

Date: _____ / _____ / _____
(MO)   (DAY)   (YEAR)

Fig. 4–1. Cardiovascular risk assessment questionnaire. The Fitness Institute, LDS Hospital, Salt Lake City, Utah.

Insurance Information

Health Insurance: _____

Policy Number: _____

Group Number: _____

Name of Policy Holder: _____

Employer: _____

Work Address: _____

What is/are your reason(s) for coming to The Fitness Institute?

☐ A complete fitness evaluation.

☐ Physician referral for an exercise test.

☐ Cardiopulmonary Rehabilitation Program.

☐ School for Weight Management.

☐ Underwater weighing test for determination of percent of body fat.

☐ Other (please explain): _____

Personal Health History

(Check the box if your answer is **yes.** Leave others blank.)

☐ Has a doctor ever told you your blood pressure was too high?

☐ Are you currently taking medications for high blood pressure?

☐ Have you ever had a stroke? When ? _____ (year)

☐ Has a doctor ever said that you had heart trouble?

☐ Have you ever had chest discomfort brought on by exercise and relieved by rest?

☐ Have you had a heart attack? How many ? _____ Date(s):_____

☐ Have you had a coronary angiogram? Date: _____

☐ Have you had open heart surgery? Date: _____

☐ Do you have irregular heart beats from time to time?

☐ Do you often have difficulty breathing?

Fig. 4–1 (continued).

☐ Do you get short of breath before anyone else?

☐ Do you ever get short of breath when sitting or sleeping?

☐ Have you ever been told your cholesterol was high?

☐ Do you have a chronic, recurring or morning cough?

☐ Have you ever coughed up blood?

☐ Do you tire easily during everyday activities?

☐ Do you have swollen, stiff or painful joints?

☐ Have you ever had muscle, bone or joint illnesses or injuries (including your back) in the past?

Describe: _____

_____

_____

☐ Do you have any muscle, bone or joint problems (including your back) that affect you now?

Describe: _____

_____

_____

☐ Have you been under the care of a physician for any orthopedic or neuromuscular problems?

Describe: _____

_____

_____

Fig. 4–1 (continued).

Do you currently or have you ever had any of the following: (indicate the year)

_____ anemia

_____ pneumonia

_____ kidney trouble

_____ urinary tract problems or infections

_____ rheumatic fever

_____ heart murmur

_____ venereal disease

_____ jaundice or hepatitis

_____ liver disease

_____ mumps

_____ asthma

_____ dizziness or fainting spells

_____ hemorrhoids

_____ malaria

_____ thyroid disease

_____ measles

_____ scarlet fever

_____ mononucleosis

_____ emphysema

_____ hernia

_____ polio

_____ bronchitis

_____ varicose veins or phlebitis

_____ diverticulitis

_____ hives

_____ nervous exhaustion

_____ joint or bone abnormalities

_____ cancer

_____ any nervous or emotional problem

_____ typhoid

_____ chickenpox

_____ diabetes or abnormal blood sugar test

Other: _____

_____

_____

List any medications you are currently taking:

_____

_____

_____

List any vitamin or dietary supplements you are currently taking:

_____

_____

_____

Fig. 4–1 (continued).

<u>Hospitalizations and Tests</u>

List previous hospitalizations for surgical procedures or medical problems:

Year   **Reason for Admission**

_____   _____

_____   _____

_____   _____

_____   _____

_____   _____

_____   _____

Indicate previous tests and year performed:

Tests	**Year**
☐ upper GI X-ray	_____
☐ lower GI X-ray	_____
☐ gallbladder X-ray	_____
☐ proctoscopic exam	_____
☐ chest X-ray	_____
☐ TB skin test	_____
☐ allergy tests	_____
☐ complete physical examination	___/___ Mo Yr
☐ electrocardiogram	___/___
☐ chest X-ray	___/___
☐ exercise electro-cardiogram (stress test)	___/___

Fig. 4–1 (continued).

Personal Habits

Smoking History

( ) Have you ever smoked cigarettes, cigars or pipe?   **(If not, skip to next section)**

( ) Do you smoke at present? When did you quit: _____ (year) Years smoked:_____

( ) Smoke cigarettes? Packs per day: _____

( ) Smoke cigars? Cigars per day: _____

( ) Smoke pipe? Pipefuls per day: _____

( ) Would you like to quit smoking?

Nutrition History

What do you consider a good weight for yourself? _____ pounds

What is the most you ever weighed (excluding pregnancy)? _____ lbs, at age: _____ Yrs.

Weight now: _____ lbs. One year ago: _____ lbs. At age 21: _____ lbs.

How do you feel about your current weight? ( ) very satisfied ( ) satisfied ( ) not concerned
     ( ) dissatisfied ( )very dissatisfied

Number of meals you usually eat per day: _____

Number of times per week you usually eat: _____ breakfast _____ snacks _____ beef
     _____ pork _____ fish _____ fowl _____ desserts _____ fried foods

Number of eggs you usually eat per week: _____ **(Do not count those used in cooking)**

Number of servings (cups, glasses, containers) per week you usually consume of:
     _____ homogenized (whole) milk _____ skim (non-fat) milk
     _____ two percent fat milk _____ buttermilk

Do you ever drink alcoholic beverages? ( ) yes ( ) no
     If yes, what is the approximate intake of these beverages?
          beer: ( ) none   ( ) occasional   ( ) often: _____ drinks per week
          wine: ( ) none   ( ) occasional   ( ) often: _____ drinks per week
          liquor: ( ) none   ( ) occasional   ( ) often: _____ drinks per week

Do you use: ( ) salt   ( ) salt substitute   ( ) none

Do you salt your food at the table?   ( ) no   ( ) lightly   ( ) moderately   ( ) heavily

Do you add salt in cooking?   ( ) no   ( ) lightly   ( ) moderately   ( ) heavily

Do you drink coffee? ( ) yes ( ) no   ( ) regular   ( ) decaffeinated

How many cups per day do you average? _____

Do you drink tea?   ( ) yes   ( ) no   ( ) herbal   Cups/glasses per day _____

Do you place specific emphasis on high fiber in your diet? ( ) yes ( ) no

Do you usually eat a filling breakfast? ( ) yes ( ) no

Fig. 4–1 (continued).

Have any of your blood relatives had:

    ( ) heart attack under age 60?   relation: _____

    ( ) stroke under age 60?   relation: _____

    ( ) diabetes?   relation: _____

    ( ) high blood pressure?   relation: _____

    ( ) elevated cholesterol?   relation: _____

    ( ) obesity? (20 or more lbs. overweight)   relation: _____

    ( ) sudden death?   relation: _____

    ( ) cancer? (type or location)   relation: _____

    _____

    ( ) epilepsy?   relation: _____

    ( ) asthma?   relation: _____

    ( ) bleeding disorders?   relation: _____

General Health Status

How would you evaluate your health status over the past 6 months?

    ( ) same   ( ) better   ( ) somewhat worse   ( ) significantly worse

Do you presently feel that you are in good health?

    ( ) not at all   ( ) much less than average   ( ) less than average   ( ) average

    ( ) better than average health   ( ) outstanding health

How many hours of sleep do you usually get a night?

    _____ hours

Do you wear seat belts when riding in or driving motor vehicles?

    ( ) no   ( ) sometimes   ( ) usually   ( ) always

Explain any other medical problem not covered in this questionnaire.

_____

_____

_____

_____

_____

_____

_____

_____

Fig. 4–1 (continued).

Are you interested in a weight control program? ( ) yes   ( ) no   ( ) presently involved

    If yes, to what extent do you feel your weight affects your daily activity?

       ( ) no affect   ( ) some affect   ( ) often interferes   ( ) very interfering

    How much weight would you like to lose? _____ lbs.

Exercise History

Are you currently involved in a regular exercise program? ( ) yes   ( ) no

Do you regularly walk or run one or more miles continuously? ( ) yes   ( ) no

    If yes, average number of miles per day: _____ miles. Days per week: _____ days.

    What is your average time per mile? _____ min.   ( ) Don't know

What other regular exercise activities are you involved in? ( ) none

    ( ) golf   ( ) bowling   ( ) tennis   ( ) handball   ( ) soccer

    ( ) basketball   ( ) volleyball   ( ) racquetball   ( ) squash   ( ) cycling

    ( ) swimming   ( ) other: _____

How many days per week do you exercise? _____ Minutes per day? _____

How much physical exertion (sufficient to produce perspiration) is required in your job?

    ( ) none   ( ) very little   ( ) moderate   ( ) heavy

Are you interested in getting into a regular exercise program? ( ) yes   ( ) no

    If yes, what activity or activities would you prefer in a program for yourself?

       ( ) walking and/or running   ( ) bicycling   ( ) swimming   ( ) other: _____

Family History

Father: ☐ alive   current age: _____ current health problems: _____

       ☐ deceased   age at death: _____ cause of death: _____

Mother: ☐ alive   current age: _____ current health problems: _____

       ☐ deceased   age at death: _____ cause of death: _____

Brothers: number   living: _____ age(s): _____ current health problems: _____

       number deceased: _____ age at death: _____ cause of death: _____

Sisters: number   living: _____ age(s): _____ current health problems: _____

       number deceased: _____ age at death: _____ cause of death: _____

Children: number   living: _____ age(s): _____ current health problems: _____

       number deceased: _____ age at death: _____ cause of death: _____

Fig. 4–1 (continued).

scalp, and measurements are recorded to the nearest ¼ inch or 0.5 cm.

Body Composition

Although the standard height–weight tables for small, medium, and large frame size provide reasonable approximations of the normal weight range for many people, there is considerable interest among health professionals, as well as the general public, in quantifying the relative composition of body weight in terms of percent body fat and lean body mass. The emphasis in today's culture on leanness, fitness, and high-fashion clothing, together with preconceived notions of obesity as defined by standard height–weight tables, often results in obsession in some larger sized individuals about losing excessive amounts of weight. For many, being "overweight" is not necessarily "over-fat." Body composition analysis offers a more realistic determination of ideal body weight because the techniques quantitate the percent body fat relative to total weight. Problems of both underweight and overweight can be more objectively analyzed by these techniques.

There are several indirect techniques for assessing body composition that are used in clinical practice. These include (1) hydrostatic (underwater) weighing, (2) skinfold measurements, and most recently, (3) electrical impedance plethysmography. Each of these methods has advantages and disadvantages in terms of accuracy, cost, convenience, and subject distress. The following sections briefly consider these procedures. Readers interested in a comprehensive review of the science of body composition analysis should consult a recently published symposium sponsored by the American College of Sports Medicine.[2]

HYDROSTATIC WEIGHING. The hydrostatic weighing technique (Fig. 4–2) is a method for determining body density (Db) using Archimedes' principle.[3] This principle states that the loss of weight of an object when submerged in water is equal to the weight of the water displaced by the object. From the weight of the displaced water (Mw) and the known density of water (Dw) at specific temperatures (Table 4–3), the volume of displaced water (Vw) can be computed as follows:

$$Vw = \frac{Mw}{Dw}$$

Since water is not compressible, the volume of displaced water (Vw) is equal to the volume of the submerged object or person (Vb). If the weight of the person in air is Mb, the density of the person (Db) is easily computed:

$$Db = \frac{Mb}{Vb}$$

In actual practice the underwater weight consists of two components: the measured weight in water *plus* the weight of water displaced by air in the lungs, airways, and gastrointestinal system. Many laboratories have the subject expire two-thirds vital capacity, using a spirometer, leaving the remaining one-third vital capacity plus residual volume in the lungs before completely submerging under water. Residual volume can be estimated from prediction equations based on age, sex, and height,[4,5] or it can be directly measured using the helium-dilution or nitrogen washout techniques.[4] The prediction equations for men and women follow:

Men: Residual Volume (L)

$$= 0.0216H + 0.207A - 2.840$$

Women: Residual Volume (L)

$$= 0.0197H + 0.201A - 2.421$$

where H is the height (cm) and A is age (years). For most clinical applications estimated residual volumes are adequate. Using this information body density is actually computed from the following equation:

$$Db = \frac{Mb}{\dfrac{(Mb - Mw)}{Dw}} - (RV + 100 \text{ ml})$$

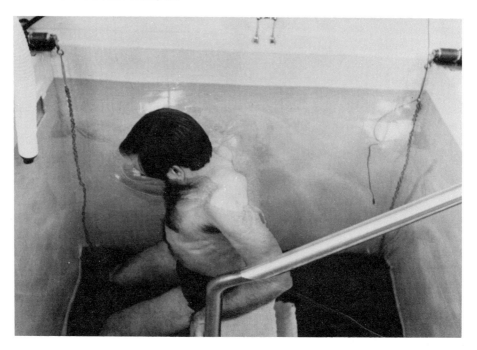

Fig. 4–2.   Hydrostatic weighing technique. The Fitness Institute, LDS Hospital, Salt Lake City, Utah.

where RV is the air remaining in the respiratory system (residual volume plus one-third vital capacity), and 100 ml is the estimated volume of air in the gastrointestinal system. Some laboratories have the subject exhale maximally before submerging. In this situation only the residual volume remains in the lungs.

While the calculation of body density is relatively straightforward, involving few assumptions and fairly simple measure-

ments, the estimation of percent body fat from body density is based on equations derived from the careful dissection of relatively few fresh human cadavers. The general assumption in deriving these equations is that the densities of adipose tissue and fat-free lean body mass as measured in these few studies are constant for all individuals and across all population groups. This is probably not a very realistic assumption. Nevertheless, a number of equations for predicting percent body fat from body density have been developed. The equation of Brozek et al.:[6]

$$\% \text{ Body Fat} = \frac{457}{Db} - 414$$

and that of Siri:[7]

$$\% \text{ Body Fat} = \frac{495}{Db} - 450$$

are in common clinical usage. Both of these equations provide similar results for adult individuals under age 50. For older adults, youth, and children, the equations may overestimate the body fat content because

Table 4–3.   Density of Water at Various Temperatures

Temperature (C)	Density
30°	0.99568
31°	0.99537
32°	0.99506
33°	0.99473
34°	0.99440
35°	0.99406
36°	0.99372
37°	0.99336
38°	0.99299
39°	0.99260

Modified from West, R.C. (ed.): Handbook of Chemistry and Physics. 50th Ed. Cleveland, The Chemical Rubber Co, 1969.

the fat-free body density is lower in these populations.[8] In addition, the equations are probably most valid only in subjects ranging from 10% to 30% body fat. Other sources of error using hydrostatic weighing techniques have been discussed by Pollock et al.[9]

SKINFOLD MEASUREMENTS. The estimation of body density from skinfold measurements is based on the assumption that there is a valid mathematic relationship between subcutaneous fat and body density. Over the years, many prediction equations have been proposed for body density based on the sum of various skinfolds. Most recently, generalized equations have been developed for men and women that take into consideration age, sex, and the curvilinear relationships between body density and skinfold thickness.[10] These equations for predicting body density from skinfolds generally correlate well with hydrostatically determined body density, providing that experienced personnel perform the measurements. The advantages of skinfold measurements over hydrostatic weighing are that they require little time, use inexpensive equipment, require minimal space, and need minimal patient cooperation.

Skinfolds are measured with calipers (e.g., Harpenden Skinfold Calipers, British Indicators, Ltd.) calibrated in divisions of 2 mm, although readings are interpreted to the nearest millimeter. Skinfold measurements should be obtained by the same individual each time, if possible, in order to reduce interindividual variation. A fold of skin and subcutaneous tissue is picked up between the thumb and forefinger of the left hand and lifted firmly away from the underlying muscle. The fold should be held between the fingers when the measurement is being made. The calipers are applied to the fold 1 cm below the finger, such that pressure on the fold at the point measured is exerted by the calipers' face only and not by the fingers. The calipers are applied to the skinfold by removing the fingers from the trigger lever. The value

registered on the calipers sometimes decreases as one watches the pointer of the dial. This decrease can usually be stopped by taking a firmer pinch with the left hand. If it continues, the reading must be taken immediately after application of the spring pressure.

A variety of sites for skinfold measurements in men and women have been recommended by various authors using different regression models for predicting body density. The generalized equations developed by Jackson and Pollock[10] seem to minimize the large prediction errors found at the extremes of the body density distribution. Equations based on age, sex, and the sum of three skinfolds are reasonably accurate for most clinical purposes. In women Jackson and Pollock[11] recommend the following three sites for skinfold measurements (Fig. 4–3):

(A) Triceps: a vertical fold on the posterior aspect of the upper arm, halfway between the acromion and olecranon processes. The arm should be extended and relaxed.

(B) Suprailium: a diagonal fold above the iliac crest in the anterior axillary line along lines of Linn.

(C) Thigh: a vertical fold on the anterior aspect of the thigh half way between the knee and the hip.

Using the sum of these three skinfolds and age, body density can be estimated from the regression equation.[10] The percent body fat is then computed using the formula of Siri:[7] $\% \text{ Fat} = \dfrac{495}{Db} - 450$. Table 4–4, from Jackson and Pollock,[11] provides the percent body fat for women using these equations.

In men, Jackson and Pollock[11] recommend the following three sites for skinfold measurements (Fig. 4–4):

(A) Chest: a diagonal fold one half the distance between the anterior axillary line at the axilla and the nipple.

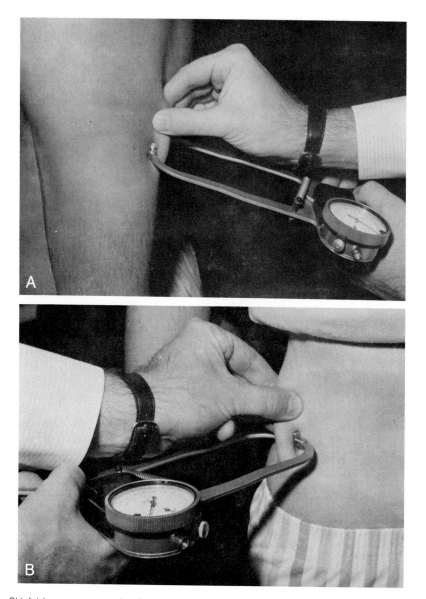

Fig. 4–3. Skinfold measurement sites for women. *(A)* Triceps. *(B)* Suprailium.

(B) Abdominal: a vertical fold 2 cm lateral to the umbilicus.

(C) Thigh: (same procedure as that for women, see Fig. 4–3C)

Again, body density is determined from the sum of these three skinfolds and age using the generalized prediction equations.[10] Table 4–5, reprinted from Jackson and Pollock[11] provides the percent body fat for men using age, sum of skinfolds, and the equations previously described.

Other sites for skinfold measurements should be considered under special circumstances. For some individuals, the thigh or chest skinfold may be particularly difficult to obtain. Substituting sites in the axilla or subscapular region and using different regression equations would provide an acceptable alternative for estimating body density.[9]

ELECTRICAL IMPEDANCE PLETHYSMOG-RAPHY. The most recent development in

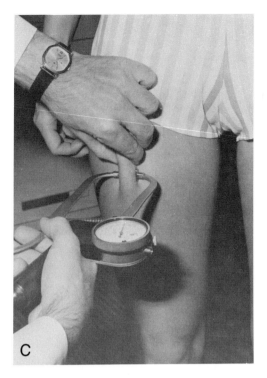

C

Fig. 4–3 (continued).   (C) Thigh.

body composition analysis is the technique of impedance plethysmography. This relatively simple method is based on the concept that fat-free body mass, because of its high water content, is more highly conductive to electrical current than is adipose tissue. The method involves the introduction of low amperage alternating current through two electrodes attached to distal skin sites on the wrist and ankle and recording the resistance in ohms from two additional electrodes on the limbs. The actual procedure is easy to perform and takes only 4 to 5 minutes. One battery-operated, portable impedance analyzer for body composition studies is commercially available (RJL Systems, 9930 Whittier, Detroit, MI, Model BIA-103) and costs approximately $5,000.

At this time there are still very few published data on the accuracy of the impedance technique. A study by Lukaski et al.[12] compared the impedance measurements with hydrostatic weighing in 37 healthy men, with a mean age of 30 years, and found a good correlation between the two techniques. It is likely that more studies will be published in the coming years attempting to validate this potentially useful method of body composition analysis. Until then, however, hydrostatic weighing, in spite of its limitations, will remain the "gold-standard" clinical technique for determining percent body fat.

IDEAL BODY WEIGHT. There is a wide range of normal values in men and women for the "optimal" body fat content. Lohman[8] suggests that, for men, a 10% to 22% body fat content is satisfactory for health maintenance; for women, 20% to 32% is considered within the normal range. It should be emphasized that these rather wide ranges offer considerable flexibility to individuals desiring to be in the normal body weight range. Some people might prefer to be at the lower end of these ranges for psychological or athletic reasons. In fact, competitive endurance athletes may find a significant improvement in performance when their body fat content is far below the recommended range for healthy men and women. The ideal body fat content for various athletic activities has not been scientifically established.

Once the percent body fat has been determined, the desired weight at a particular body fat content can be calculated according to the following formula:[9]

Desired Weight

$$= \frac{\text{Weight} - (\text{Weight} \times [\% \text{ fat}/100])}{1 - x}$$

where x is the desired percent fat expressed as a decimal. It is suggested that each individual be given a range of optimal weights, based on the normal range of body fat content and the individual's particular needs.

Blood Pressure

Hypertension, an often silent disease until major cardiovascular or renal compli-

Table 4–4.   Percent Body Fat for Women Using the Sum of Triceps, Suprailium, and Thigh Skinfolds

Sum of Skinfolds (mm)	Age (years)								
	<22	23–27	28–32	33–37	38–42	43–47	48–52	53–57	>57
23–25	9.7	9.9	10.2	10.4	10.7	10.9	11.2	11.4	11.7
26–28	11.0	11.2	11.5	11.7	12.0	12.3	12.5	12.7	13.0
29–31	12.3	12.5	12.8	13.0	13.3	13.5	13.8	14.0	14.3
32–34	13.6	13.8	14.0	14.3	14.5	14.8	15.0	15.3	15.5
35–37	14.8	15.0	15.3	15.5	15.8	16.0	16.3	16.5	16.8
38–40	16.0	16.3	16.5	16.7	17.0	17.2	17.5	17.7	18.0
41–43	17.2	17.4	17.7	17.9	18.2	18.4	18.7	18.9	19.2
44–46	18.3	18.6	18.8	19.1	19.3	19.6	19.8	20.1	20.3
47–49	19.5	19.7	20.0	20.2	20.5	20.7	21.0	21.2	21.5
50–52	20.6	20.8	21.1	21.3	21.6	21.8	22.1	22.3	22.6
53–55	21.7	21.9	22.1	22.4	22.6	22.9	23.1	23.4	23.6
56–58	22.7	23.0	23.2	23.4	23.7	23.9	24.2	24.4	24.7
59–61	23.7	24.0	24.2	24.5	24.7	25.0	25.2	25.5	25.7
62–64	24.7	25.0	25.2	25.5	25.7	26.0	26.4	26.7	26.9
65–67	25.7	25.9	26.2	26.4	26.7	26.9	27.2	27.4	27.7
68–70	26.6	26.9	27.1	27.4	27.7	27.9	28.1	28.4	28.6
71–73	27.5	27.8	28.0	28.3	28.5	28.8	29.0	29.3	29.5
74–76	28.4	28.7	28.9	29.2	29.4	29.7	29.9	30.2	30.4
77–79	29.3	29.5	29.8	30.0	30.3	30.5	30.8	31.0	31.2
80–82	30.1	30.4	30.6	30.9	31.1	31.4	31.6	31.9	32.1
83–85	30.9	31.2	31.4	31.7	31.9	32.2	32.4	32.7	32.9
86–88	31.7	32.0	32.2	32.5	32.7	32.9	33.2	33.4	33.7
89–91	32.5	32.7	33.0	33.2	33.5	33.7	33.9	34.2	34.4
92–94	33.2	33.4	33.7	33.9	34.2	34.4	34.7	34.9	35.2
95–97	33.9	34.1	34.4	34.6	34.9	35.1	35.4	35.6	35.9
98–100	34.6	34.8	35.1	35.3	35.5	35.8	36.0	36.3	36.5
101–103	35.3	35.4	35.7	35.9	36.2	36.4	36.7	36.9	37.2
104–106	35.8	36.1	36.3	36.6	36.8	37.1	37.3	37.5	37.8
107–109	36.4	36.7	36.9	37.1	37.4	37.6	37.9	38.1	38.4
110–112	37.0	37.2	37.5	37.7	38.0	38.2	38.5	38.7	38.9
113–115	37.5	37.8	38.0	38.2	38.5	38.7	39.0	39.2	39.5
116–118	38.0	38.3	38.5	38.8	39.0	39.3	39.5	39.7	40.0
119–121	38.5	38.7	39.0	39.2	39.5	39.7	40.0	40.2	40.5
122–124	39.0	39.2	39.4	39.7	39.9	40.2	40.4	40.7	40.9
125–127	39.4	39.6	39.9	40.1	40.4	40.6	40.9	41.1	41.4
128–130	39.8	40.0	40.3	40.5	40.8	41.0	41.3	41.5	41.8

From Jackson, A.S., and Pollock, M.L.: Practical assessment of body composition. Phys. Sportsmed., 13:76, 1985. (Reprinted by permission of the Physician and Sportsmedicine, a McGraw-Hill publication.)

cations appear, is one of the most common and potentially deadly afflictions of adult individuals in our society. Blood pressure screening, therefore, should be an important aspect in the evaluation of candidates for exercise programs.

Proper technique is essential for obtaining accurate blood pressure measurements. The subject should be resting comfortably in a chair with the arm bared. Rolled-up sleeves should be avoided, since upper arm contriction might affect the validity of the reading. Cuff size is also important and has been standardized by the American Heart Association (AHA).[13] For each cuff size the proper range should be marked on the inside of the cuff so that when the cuff is wrapped around the arm, the index line at the end of the cuff falls within that range. If the index line falls outside the range for that sized cuff, a smaller or larger cuff should be used for that subject. Each testing facility should own standard-sized, large-sized, and pediatric cuffs. Finally, a well-maintained mercury sphygmomanometer or a properly calibrated aneroid manometer should be used for obtaining the blood pressure measurements.

Before taking the subject's pressure, the

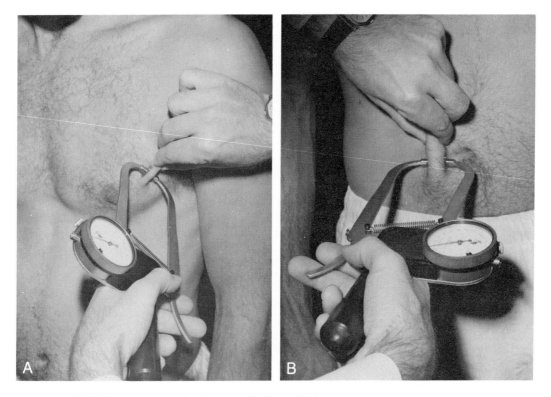

Fig. 4–4.   Skinfold measurement sites for men. *(A)* Chest. *(B)* Abdomen.

peak systolic pressure should be estimated by inflating the cuff to a pressure that obliterates the distal radial pulse. The diaphragm of the stethoscope is then positioned over the brachial artery and the cuff inflated approximately 30 mm Hg above the estimated systolic pressure. The cuff is then slowly deflated 2 mm Hg/s until the first Korotkov sounds are audible. The *systolic blood pressure* is defined as the pressure at which the Korotkov sounds are heard for two consecutive beats. As the cuff continues to deflate slowly, the *diastolic blood pressure* is defined as the point when the Korotkov sounds completely disappear (phase V). The average of two or more blood pressure readings should be used to determine the subject's initial measurement.[14]

The 1984 Report of the Joint National Committee on Detection, Evaluation, and Treatment of High Blood Pressure[14] provides up to date guidelines and recommendations for hypertension screening and management. Table 4–6 summarizes the current classification of systolic and diastolic hypertension and provides recommendations for follow-up. It is important to provide individuals with their actual numerical blood pressure values and also give them the appropriate guidelines for follow-up as defined in Table 4–6. Recommendations for managing hypertension in competitive athletes have recently been published by Walther and Tifft.[15]

Muscle Strength, Endurance, and Flexibility

Muscle function tests range from simple field tests to very elaborate laboratory evaluations using expensive muscle testing equipment. These latter tests are generally used by research exercise physiologists, health professionals working with competitive athletes, or medical specialists study-

Table 4–5.   Percent Body Fat for Men Using the Sum of Chest, Abdomen, and Thigh Skinfolds

Sum of Skinfolds (mm)	Age (years)								
	<22	23–27	28–32	33–37	38–42	43–47	48–52	53–57	>57
8–10	1.3	1.8	2.3	2.9	3.4	3.9	4.5	5.0	5.5
11–13	2.2	2.8	3.3	3.9	4.4	4.9	5.5	6.0	6.5
14–16	3.2	3.8	4.3	4.8	5.4	5.9	6.4	7.0	7.5
17–19	4.2	4.7	5.3	5.8	6.3	6.9	7.4	8.0	8.5
20–22	5.1	5.7	6.2	6.8	7.3	7.9	8.4	8.9	9.5
23–25	6.1	6.6	7.2	7.7	8.3	8.8	9.4	9.9	10.5
26–28	7.0	7.6	8.1	8.7	9.2	9.8	10.3	10.9	11.4
29–31	8.0	8.5	9.1	9.6	10.2	10.7	11.3	11.8	12.4
32–34	8.9	9.4	10.0	10.5	11.1	11.6	12.2	12.8	13.3
35–37	9.8	10.4	10.9	11.5	12.0	12.6	13.1	13.7	14.3
38–40	10.7	11.3	11.8	12.4	12.9	13.5	14.1	14.6	15.2
41–43	11.6	12.2	12.7	13.3	13.8	14.4	15.0	15.5	16.1
44–46	12.5	13.1	13.6	14.2	14.7	15.3	15.9	16.4	17.0
47–49	13.4	13.9	14.5	15.1	15.6	16.2	16.8	17.3	17.9
50–52	14.3	14.8	15.4	15.9	16.5	17.1	17.6	18.2	18.8
53–55	15.1	15.7	16.2	16.8	17.4	17.9	18.5	19.1	19.7
56–58	16.0	16.5	17.1	17.7	18.2	18.8	19.4	20.0	20.5
59–61	16.9	17.4	17.9	18.5	19.1	19.7	20.2	20.8	21.4
62–64	17.6	18.2	18.8	19.4	19.9	20.5	21.1	21.7	22.2
65–67	18.5	19.0	19.6	20.2	20.8	21.3	21.9	22.5	23.1
68–70	19.3	19.9	20.4	21.0	21.6	22.2	22.7	23.3	23.9
71–73	20.1	20.7	21.2	21.8	22.4	23.0	23.6	24.1	24.7
74–76	20.9	21.5	22.0	22.6	23.2	23.8	24.4	25.0	25.5
77–79	21.7	22.2	22.8	23.4	24.0	24.6	25.2	25.8	26.3
80–82	22.4	23.0	23.6	24.2	24.8	25.4	25.9	26.5	27.1
83–85	23.2	23.8	24.4	25.0	25.5	26.1	26.7	27.3	27.9
86–88	24.0	24.5	25.1	25.7	26.3	26.9	27.5	28.1	28.7
89–91	24.7	25.3	25.9	26.5	27.1	27.6	28.2	28.8	29.4
92–94	25.4	26.0	26.6	27.2	27.8	28.4	29.0	29.6	30.2
95–97	26.1	26.7	27.3	27.9	28.5	29.1	29.7	30.3	30.9
98–100	26.9	27.4	28.0	28.6	29.2	29.8	30.4	31.0	31.6
101–103	27.5	28.1	28.7	29.3	29.9	30.5	31.1	31.7	32.3
104–106	28.2	28.8	29.4	30.0	30.6	31.2	31.8	32.4	33.0
107–109	28.9	29.5	30.1	30.7	31.3	31.9	32.5	33.1	33.7
110–112	29.6	30.2	30.8	31.4	32.0	32.6	33.2	33.8	34.4
113–115	30.2	30.8	31.4	32.0	32.6	33.2	33.8	34.5	35.1
116–118	30.9	31.5	32.1	32.7	33.3	33.9	34.5	35.1	35.7
119–121	31.5	32.1	32.7	33.3	33.9	34.5	35.1	35.7	36.4
122–124	32.1	32.7	33.3	33.9	34.5	35.1	35.8	36.4	37.0
125–127	32.7	33.3	33.9	34.5	35.1	35.8	36.4	37.0	37.6

From Jackson, A.S., and Pollock, M.L.: Practical assessment of body composition. Phys. Sportsmed., 13:76, 1985. (Reprinted by permission of the Physician and Sportsmedicine, a McGraw-Hill publication.)

ing neuromuscular and orthopedic disorders. For the purpose of screening subjects for exercise programs, simple field tests are usually adequate. Readers interested in more sophisticated testing procedures should consult several recently published books by Baumgartner and Jackson,[16] Wilmore,[17] and Berger.[18]

MUSCLE STRENGTH. A battery of tests involving major muscle groups is suggested for evaluating muscle strength. Table 4–7, published by Pollock et al.,[9] lists normal reference values for men and women for several muscle-strength tests based on the one-repetition maximal test. Each test consists of a series of trials designed to determine the maximal weight that can be lifted only once before fatigue. If only one test is selected, Pollock et al.[9] recommend the one-repetition maximal bench press, since this test most closely correlates with total dynamic strength.

Muscle strength of the hand and forearm can be tested using a handgrip dyna-

Table 4–6. Classification of Blood Pressure and Recommended Follow-up Criteria

Range (mm Hg)	Category	Recommended Follow-up
Diastolic		
<85	Normal blood pressure	Recheck within 2 years
85–89	High normal blood pressure	Recheck within 1 year
90–104	Mild hypertension	Confirm within 2 months
105–114	Moderate hypertension	Evaluate or refer promptly (within 2 weeks)
>114	Severe hypertension	Evaluate or refer immediately
Systolic (diastolic <90)		
<140	Normal blood pressure	Recheck within 2 years
140–159	Borderline isolated systolic hypertension	
140–199		Confirm within 2 months
>159	Isolated systolic hypertension	
>199		Evaluate or refer promptly (within 2 weeks)

Modified from The 1984 Report of the Joint National Committee on Detection, Evaluation, and Treatment of High Blood Pressure. Arch. Intern. Med., *144*:1045, 1984.

Table 4–7. Normal Reference Values for Strength Testing Based on the One-Repetition Maximal Test

Body Weight (lb)	Bench Press (lb)		Standing Press (lb)		Curl (lb)		Leg Press (lb)	
	Men	Women	Men	Women	Men	Women	Men	Women
80	80	56	53	37	40	28	160	112
100	100	70	67	47	50	35	200	140
120	120	84	80	56	60	42	240	168
140	140	98	93	65	70	49	280	196
160	160	112	197	75	80	56	320	224
180	180	126	120	84	90	63	360	252
200	200	140	133	93	100	70	400	280
220	220	154	147	103	110	77	440	308
240	240	168	160	112	120	84	480	336

From Pollock, M.L., Wilmore, J.H., and Fox, S.M.: Health and Fitness through Physical Activity. New York, Wiley, 1978.

mometer (Harpenden, British Indicators, Ltd., England). After adjusting the grip for the subject's hand size, three attempts at maximal grip strength should be made with each hand, alternatively. The highest figure (in kilograms) is used for the final score. Table 4–8 illustrates a rating scale for men and women.

MUSCLE ENDURANCE. The testing of muscle endurance is somewhat controver-

Table 4–8. Hand Grip Strength Test

Score	Men	Women
Excellent	65 or above	42 or above
Good	56–63	37–41
Average	44–55	30–36
Fair	36–43	24–29
Poor	30–35	19–23

sial, since many of the recommended field tests are biased by variations in muscle strength. In order to standardize for these differences among individuals, Pollock et al.[9] suggest using a fixed percentage of 70% of the maximal muscle strength for testing endurance; that is, determining the maximal number of repetitions that can be carried out by a particular group of muscles at 70% maximal strength. Unfortunately, normal reference values for these tests are not yet available. Norms for more standard endurance tests, such as push-up and sit-up tests, have been published.[9]

MUSCLE FLEXIBILITY. Accurate tests of muscle flexibility require quantifying the range of motion of the different joints. One useful screening test is the sit-and-reach test, which is used to assess the flexibility of the lower back and posterior thigh muscles. In this test a calibrated flexibility testing bench (e.g., Health Accessories, Seattle, Wash.) is used as illustrated in Figure 4–5. The subject assumes the sitting position with the knees fully extended, feet together, and soles touching the seat of the bench. On command, the arms are extended and the fingers pointed as the subject reaches forward maximally, pushing a slider along the calibrated back of the bench. Scoring for this test is illustrated in Table 4–9.

Submaximal Exercise Testing for Fitness Evaluation

Submaximal exercise testing to estimate maximal aerobic capacity ($\dot{V}O_2$ max) is a poor substitute for maximal testing, although it may be useful in asymptomatic, low-risk subjects for whom a more costly maximal diagnostic test is not needed. These tests can also be administered in the field by allied health professionals without ECG monitoring or physician supervision and, as a result, are reasonably inexpensive.

A number of submaximal exercise test protocols have been developed for assessing cardiovascular fitness. The prediction of maximal $\dot{V}O_2$ from submaximal heart rates and work loads is possible because of the near linear relationship between exercise heart rate and $\dot{V}O_2$, and between $\dot{V}O_2$ and work load.[19] It should be noted, however, that there are many limitations to the prediction of $\dot{V}O_2$ max from submaximal testing protocols, and at best, these tests provide only approximate measures of cardiovascular fitness.

A stationary bicycle ergometer is the preferred method for submaximal testing, since it is inexpensive, reasonably portable, and the work load can be quantitated in watts or kilopond-meter (kpm)/min. A nomogram for the prediction of maximal $\dot{V}O_2$ from heart rate and bicycle work load has been developed by Astrand[20] and is illustrated in Figure 4–6. To predict maximal $\dot{V}O_2$ (L/min), a straight line is drawn from the steady-state heart rate to the $\dot{V}O_2$ equivalent of the work load achieved. The intersection of that line with the $\dot{V}O_2$ max scale is the predicted $\dot{V}O_2$ max. For subjects

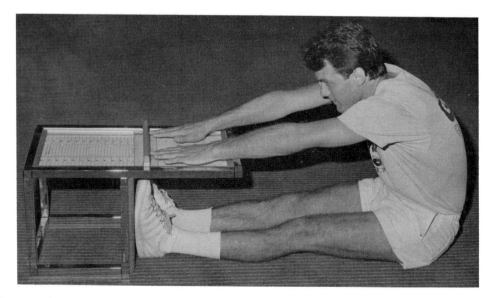

Fig. 4–5. Sit-and-reach test for muscle flexibility.

Table 4–9.   Sit and Reach Test (inches)

Excellent	+7 or above
Good	+4 to +6
Average	−1 to +3
Fair	−3 to −2
Poor	−4 or less

over 35 years of age, Astrand[20] recommends multiplying the predicted $\dot{V}O_2$ max obtained from the nomogram by a correction factor (Table 4–10).

Several bicycle testing protocols have been described that utilize the Astrand[20] nomogram. For younger and more physically active subjects, the test described by Astrand and Ryhming[19] provides a reasonably accurate estimate of fitness. In this protocol an initial work load of 50 W (300 kpm/min) for women or 100 W (600 kpm/min) is chosen. If after 6 minutes the heart rate is below 130 bpm, the work load is increased by 50 W, and exercise is continued for another 6 minutes. Increments of 50 W every 6 minutes are continued until a target heart rate of approximately 70% of the predicted maximal heart rate (220 minus age) is reached. Once the target heart rate is obtained, exercise should be continued for several minutes until a steady-state heart rate is achieved for that work load. The maximal $\dot{V}O_2$ can then be estimated from the steady-state heart rate and work load using the Astrand nomogram (Fig. 4–6).

A modification of the Astrand-Ryhming test has been described by Siconolfi et al.[21] that is more applicable to older and less physically active individuals. For men over age 35 and for all women, the initial bicycle workload is 25 W (150 kpm/min). Work load is increased 25 W every 2 minutes until a target heart rate of 70% maximal predicted heart rate is achieved. Exercise is then continued at that work load until a steady-state heart rate has been maintained for at least 2 minutes. For men under the age of 35, the initial workload is 50 W. Work load is then increased by 50 W every 2 minutes until the exercise heart rate is

over 60% maximal predicted heart rate and then by 25 W every 2 minutes until heart rate reaches the target rate of 70% predicted maximal. Exercise is continued until steady-state heart rates are maintained, defined as a change in heart rate of less than 5 bpm over 2 consecutive minutes. $\dot{V}O_2$ max (L/min) is then estimated from the steady-state heart rate and the final work load using the Astrand nomogram.

In the study by Siconolfi et al.,[21] the modified Astrand-Ryhming test,[19] previously described, was validated against directly measured $\dot{V}O_2$ max in 50 subjects from 20 to 70 years of age. The data from these subjects were used to derive equations for predicting $\dot{V}O_2$ max by multiple regression analysis. For males the following equation was derived:

$$\gamma = 0.348 \, (x) - 0.035 \, (age) + 3.011$$

where γ is the $\dot{V}O_2$ max (L/min), x is the $\dot{V}O_2$ max obtained from the Astrand nomogram (not corrected for age), and age is in years ($R = 0.86$, standard error of estimate $= 0.359$ L/min). For women the equation was as follows:

$$\gamma = 0.302 \, (x) - 0.019 \, (age) + 1.593$$

where γ and x are as defined previously ($R = 0.97$, standard error of estimate $= 0.199$ L/min). Using these equations $\dot{V}O_2$ max was predicted in a second group of 63 subjects with no significant differences found between directly measured $\dot{V}O_2$ max and $\dot{V}O_2$ max estimated from regression equations. The overall correlation (R) between measured and estimated $\dot{V}O_2$ max for the 63 subjects was 0.94 with a standard error of 0.248 L/min. Furthermore, in this study the $\dot{V}O_2$ max estimated from the above equations was a better predictor of the directly measured $\dot{V}O_2$ max than the $\dot{V}O_2$ max obtained from the Astrand nomogram.

It seems reasonable, from these data, to recommend the modified Astrand-Ryhming protocol described by Siconolfi et al.[21] and the preceding equations to predict $\dot{V}O_2$ max in sedentary, asymptomatic low-risk

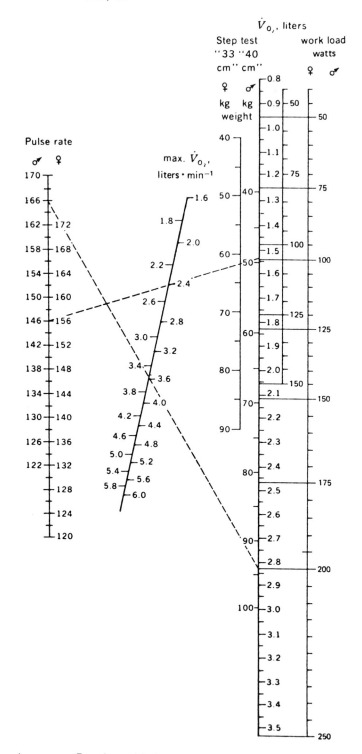

Fig. 4–6.   Astrand nomogram. From Astrand, I.: Aerobic work capacity in men and women with special reference to age. Acta Physiol. Scand., *49*(Suppl. 169): 1960.

Table 4–10.   Correction Factor for $\dot{V}O_2$ Max Prediction in Subjects Over Age 35[20]

Age	Factor
35	0.87
40	0.83
45	0.78
50	0.75
55	0.71
60	0.68
65	0.65

individuals. It should be emphasized, however, that the Astrand nomogram is not valid in individuals taking a variety of medications that affect the heart rate response to exercise (beta-blockers, sympathomimetic agents, some calcium channel blockers). For these people as well as for older, more high-risk, and/or symptomatic individuals, the maximal exercise test protocols that involve ECG monitoring and physician supervision are recommended. These are described in Chapter 5.

Pulmonary Function Screening Tests

Routine spirometry is a useful procedure that is easily performed by allied health personnel. The tests may provide the initial evidence for early cardiopulmonary disorders. Individuals complaining of unexplained dyspnea on exertion are especially good candidates for pulmonary function studies, since this common symptom may only reflect deconditioning in some subjects but, in others, may also be a manifestation of serious heart or lung disease. The two spirometric parameters of particular interest are the forced vital capacity (FVC) and the forced expiratory volume in one second (FEV_1). Minimal standards for spirometers and the interpretation of spirometric tracings have been published.[22]

Figure 4–7 illustrates the spirometric lung volumes. The FVC is defined as the maximal volume of air that can be forcefully exhaled following a maximal inhalation. The subject's FVC should be compared to the published normal reference values based on age, sex, and height.[4] Restrictive lung diseases, characterized by stiff lungs, have reduced lung volumes including the FVC. Obstructive lung diseases, on the other hand, are characterized by increased airways resistance on expiration and a reduction in FEV_1. Normally, the FEV_1 is about 80% of the FVC. In obstructive lung diseases, such as asthma, chronic bronchitis, and emphysema, the FEV_1 is less than 75% of the FVC.

Adequate spirometric tracings for analysis require careful attention to details. The following steps published by the Intermountain Thoracic Society[4] are recommended:

1. Have the patient seated comfortably upright.
2. Loosen all tight clothing including underclothing (belt, girdle, brassiere, etc.).
3. Remove dentures if present.
4. Explain carefully and fully what is to be done prior to starting, demonstrating each phase of the test.
5. Put mouthpiece in patient's mouth, between and beyond the teeth, and be sure no leaks are present.
6. Occlude the patient's nose with a nose clip.
7. Then instruct patient to slowly but maximally exhale, observing both the patient and the tracing.
8. When the expiration is maximal (residual volume has been reached), then instruct the patient to breathe in as deeply as possible (to total lung capacity).
9. When patient reaches full inspiration, change chart speed to the fast speed (at least 30 mm/sec) and when attained:
   a. Vigorously encourage the patient to blow out the air as rapidly as possible by loudly commanding "blow." (You should be embarrassed by the commotion you must make.)
   b. Urge patient to keep exhaling, "blow-blow," until the breath is

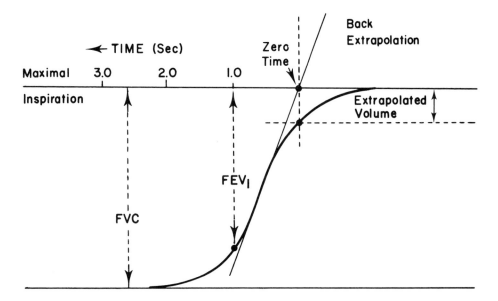

Fig. 4–7.   Measurement of spirometric tracing to determine FEV₁.

completed as evidenced by a constant level on the kymograph (straight horizontal line—not due to breath holding).

c. If the spirogram does not become horizontal, the technician should not terminate the study but should encourage the patient to continue until he or she is unable to go on. Caution: hypoxemic patients may become distressed and, in such instances, the study should be terminated prematurely.

d. At the point where expiration has been assessed to be complete, instruct the patient to maximally and rapidly inhale back to the point of maximal inspiration. Command patient to "suck it in."

10. Disconnect patient, remove nose clips, let patient relax, and flush out the spirometer.

11. Repeat study until three acceptable tracings are obtained. Acceptability will be determined by the technician's observation that the subject understood the instructions and performed the test with a smooth continuous ex-halation, with apparent maximal effort, with a good start, and without:

a. Coughing.

b. A Valsalva maneuver (glottis closure).

c. An early termination of expiration. (In a normal patient, this would be before completion of the breath; in an obstructed patient this would be assumed to have taken place if the expiration time was less than 5 seconds.)

d. A leak.

e. An obstructed mouthpiece (for example, obstruction due to the tongue being placed in front of the mouthpiece or false teeth falling in front of the mouthpiece).

f. An unsatisfactory start of expiration, characterized by excessive hesitation or false starts. Unsatisfactory starts prevent accurate back extrapolation and determination of time zero. To achieve accurate time zero, the extrapolated volume on the spirogram should be less than 10% of the FVC or 100 ml, whichever is greater.

g. An excessive variability among the three acceptable curves. The FVC and FEV_1 of the two best of the three acceptable curves should not vary by more than 5% of reading or 100 ml, whichever is greater.

13. Record the technician's assessment of patient performance and cooperation (good, fair, poor) with respect to lung function. A maximal effort may be misleading if the patient pits one group of muscles against another. If flow from the mouth is limited by pitting one group of respiratory muscles against another, the value of the spirogram as an indicator of mechanical properties of the lung is reduced.

(From Clinical Pulmonary Function Testing. A Manual of Uniform Laboratory Procedures. 2nd Ed. Salt Lake City, Utah, Intermountain Thoracic Society, 1984.)

Once the spirometric tracings have been obtained, the one spirogram representing the subject's best effort should be used for performing all calculations. This should be the tracing with the largest absolute sum of the FEV_1 plus the FVC.[4] Figure 4–7 illustrates a sample spirogram with the measurements. For the purposes of calculating the FEV_1, zero time is determined by back extrapolation. As seen in Figure 4–7, a line is drawn along the steepest slope and extended back to intersect the maximal inspiratory level. If the "extrapolated volume" (Fig. 4–7) is more than 10% of the FVC or 100 ml, the tracing is considered suboptimal.[4]

The FVC and FEV_1 should be expressed in liters to two decimal places, and the ratio FEV_1/FVC, to one decimal place. For convenience a transparent spirometric ruler can be used over the tracings to convert the chart displacement in millimeters to volumes. The measured volumes in ambient temperature, pressure, saturated should then be converted to body temperature, pressure, saturated by multiplying the volumes times a conversion factor based on room temperature and barometric pressures.[4] The final volumes should be compared to normal reference values based on age, sex, and height.[4] Abnormalities should be categorized as mild, moderate, or severe, using published criteria.[4]

LABORATORY ASSESSMENT

The only blood tests that might be considered to be routine in screening subjects for adult fitness programs and cardiac rehabilitation are the blood lipids. Some evaluation centers might also include a fasting blood glucose to screen for diabetes mellitus and a complete blood count to screen for anemia. The technique of venipuncture is easily learned by allied health personnel, and venous blood samples are readily obtained from most individuals.

Blood Lipids

The blood lipids have become extremely important laboratory measurements in recent years because of the following observations: (1) atherosclerosis continues to be our nation's number one cause of death and disability;[23] (2) the risk of atherosclerosis, in general, and specifically coronary heart disease (CHD) appears to be directly proportional to the blood levels of total cholesterol (TC) and low-density lipoprotein cholesterol (LDLC) and inversely proportional to the level of high-density lipoprotein cholesterol (HDLC);[24,25] (3) blood cholesterol and LDLC levels are influenced in a major way by dietary saturated fat and cholesterol intake;[26,27] and (4) recent scientific evidence strongly suggests that lowering blood cholesterol levels by diet and drug therapy significantly reduces the incidence of CHD in hypercholesterolemic subjects.[28] Since the main objective of adult fitness and cardiac rehabilitation programs is to improve the cardiovascular health and well-being of participants, it seems reasonable to include lipid screening in the initial evaluation of applicants to these programs.

The most cost-effective initial lipid screening test is the TC level, which can be measured any time, fasting or not. If the TC is lower than 200 mg/dl, no further testing is necessary, and subjects with these low values do not need to be particularly concerned about their diets. Those with cholesterol levels above 200 mg/dl should have a fasting lipid screen, which includes TC, HDLC, and triglycerides.[29] The remaining lipids can be easily calculated from these values. The very low-density lipoprotein cholesterol (VLDLC) is estimated by dividing the triglycerides by 5, providing that the triglycerides are below 500 mg/dl. The important LDLC is obtained by subtracting the sum of the HDLC and VLDLC from the TC.

Individuals who have LDLC levels above 200 mg/dl are considered to be at high risk for coronary atherosclerosis and should be aggressively managed by their physicians. In those with LDLC values between 100 and 200 mg/dl, calculating the LDLC/HDLC ratio might identify a high-risk subset (ratio above 3:1) who might benefit from dietary therapy. Hypertriglyceridemia (triglycerides greater than 150 mg/dl) is a common lipid abnormality that usually occurs as a secondary disorder associated with obesity, diabetes mellitus, or excessive alcohol intake. In these conditions the risk for atherosclerosis is more related to the primary metabolic abnormality than to the hypertriglyceridemia per se. Complete guidelines for managing the hyperlipidemias have been published.[29,30]

Blood Glucose

The fasting blood glucose determination is a crude screening test for diabetes mellitus that is not very sensitive unless the fasting glucose is over 150 mg/dl. In asymptomatic subjects over age 40 as well as obese individuals over age 30, it is recommended that a yearly blood glucose be obtained 2 hours after a large breakfast. If the blood glucose value is less than 120 mg/dl, diabetes is essentially ruled out.[31]

CONCLUSIONS

Although the physician-administered medical history, physical examination, and maximal exercise stress test are all important in screening individuals at high risk for cardiovascular disease as well as those with already existing disease, techniques that are usually carried out by allied health professionals are important as well. Not all of these screening tests are necessary for adult fitness or cardiac rehabilitation programs, but they are very likely to improve the overall quality of those programs by providing more comprehensive and individualized data from which to develop the exercise prescriptions.

REFERENCES

1. Metropolitan Life Insurance Company: Four Steps to Weight Control. New York, Metropolitan Life Insurance, 1969.
2. Lohman, T.G., et al.: Symposium on body composition. Med. Sci. Sports Exerc., 16:578, 1984.
3. McArdle, W.D., Katch, F.I., and Katch, V.L.: Exercise Physiology. Philadelphia, Lea & Febiger, 1981.
4. Clinical Pulmonary Function Testing. A Manual of Uniform Laboratory Procedures. 2nd Ed. Salt Lake City, Utah, Intermountain Thoracic Society, 1984.
5. Crapo, R.O.: Lung volumes in healthy nonsmoking adults. Bull. Eur. Physiopathol. Respir., 18:419, 1982.
6. Brozek, J., et al.: Densitometric analysis of body composition: review of some quantitative assumptions. Ann. N.Y. Acad. Sci., 110:113, 1963.
7. Siri, W.E.: Body composition from fluid spaces and density: Analysis of methods and techniques for measuring body composition. Washington, D.C., National Academy of Sciences National Research Council, 1961.
8. Lohman, T.G.: Body composition methodology in sports medicine. Phys. Sports Med., 10:47, 1982.
9. Pollock, M.L., Wilmore, J.H., and Fox, S.M.: Exercise in Health and Disease. Evaluation and Prescription for Prevention and Rehabilitation. Philadelphia, W.B. Saunders, 1984.
10. Jackson, A.S., and Pollock, M.L.: Steps toward the development of generalized equations for

predicting body composition in adults. Can. J. Appl. Sports Sci., 7:187, 1982.

11. Jackson, A.S., and Pollock, M.L.: Practical assessment of body composition. Phys. Sports Med., 13:76, 1985.

12. Lukaski, H.C., et al.: Assessment of fat-free mass using bioelectric impedance measurements of the human body. Am. J. Clin. Nutr., 41:810, 1985.

13. Kirkendall, W.M., et al.: AHA Committee Report: Recommendations of Human Blood Pressure Determination by Sphygmomanometers. Circulation, 62:1146A, 1980.

14. The 1984 Report of the Joint National Committee on Detection, Evaluation, and Treatment of High Blood Pressure. Arch. Intern. Med., 144:1045, 1984.

15. Walther, R.J., and Tifft, C.P.: High blood pressure in the competitive athlete: guidelines and recommendations. Phys. Sports Med., 13:93, 1985.

16. Baumgartner, J.A., and Jackson, A.S.: Measurement and Evaluation in Physical Education. 2nd Ed. Dubuque, Ia., William C. Brown, 1982.

17. Wilmore, J.H.: Training for Sport and Activity—The Physiological Basis of the Conditioning Process. 2nd Ed. Boston, Allyn & Bacon, 1982.

18. Berger, R.A.: Applied Exercise Physiology. Philadelphia, Lea & Febiger, 1982.

19. Astrand, P.O., and Ryhming, I.: A nomogram for calculation of aerobic capacity (physical fitness) from pulse rate during submaximal work. J. Appl. Physiol., 7:218, 1954.

20. Astrand, I.: Aerobic work capacity in men and women with special reference to age. Acta Physiol. Scand., 49(suppl 169):1, 1960.

21. Siconolfi, S.F., et al.: Assessing $\dot{V}O_2$ max in epidemiologic studies: Modification of the Astrand-Ryhming test. Med. Sci. Sports Exerc., 14:355, 1982.

22. Gardner, R.M., et al.: ATS statement—Snowbird workshop on standardization of spirometry. Am. Rev. Respir. Dis., 119:831, 1979.

23. Heart Facts 1984. Dallas, American Heart Association, 1983.

24. Kannel, W.B., Castelli, W.P., and Gordon, T.: Cholesterol in the prediction of atherosclerotic diseases. New perspectives based on the Framingham Study. Ann. Intern. Med., 90:85, 1979.

25. Kannel, W.B., and Schatzkin, A.: Risk factor analysis. Prog. Cardiovasc. Dis., 26:309, 1983.

26. Levy, R.I., Rifkind, B.M., Dennis, B.H. (eds.): Nutrition, Lipids, and Coronary Heart Disease: A Global View. New York, Raven Press, 1979.

27. Shekelle, R.B., et al.: Diet, serum cholesterol and death from coronary heart disease: The Western Electric Study. N. Engl. J. Med., 304:65, 1981.

28. The Lipid Research Clinics Coronary Primary Prevention Trial Results. I. Reduction in incidence of coronary heart disease. Lipid Research Clinic Program. JAMA, 251:351, 1984.

29. Brown, W.V., Goldberg, I.J., and Ginsberg, H.N.: Treatment of common lipoprotein disorders. Prog. Cardiovasc. Dis., 27:1, 1984.

30. AHA Special Report: Recommendations for treatment of hyperlipidemia in adults. Circulation, 69:1065A, 1984.

31. Classification and diagnosis of diabetes mellitus and other categories of glucose intolerance. National Diabetes Data Group. Diabetes, 28:1039, 1979.

5

CLINICAL EXERCISE TESTING: METHODOLOGY, INTERPRETATION, AND APPLICATIONS

Exercise testing has become an important assessment tool in the evaluation of individuals participating in adult fitness and cardiac rehabilitation programs. In addition there are many other applications of this technique in the practice of cardiovascular and pulmonary medicine. This chapter reviews clinical applications of exercise testing that are of interest to personnel working in adult fitness facilities, cardiac rehabilitation centers, and exercise testing laboratories.

Table 5–1 lists the topics that are considered in this chapter. Although exercise testing procedures vary somewhat from laboratory to laboratory, depending on needs, personnel, equipment, and particular schools of training, the underlying principles in each of these areas of discussion are reasonably standardized within the exercise testing community.

Like many other areas of scientific investigation, principles of exercise testing are in a continuous process of evolution. New ideas, concepts, equipment, and data that challenge existing methods of practice appear frequently in the literature. Many of these will ultimately be modified or rejected in favor of more traditional methods; some, however, will significantly improve certain aspects of the exercise test. Although change and new ideas are important for the growth of an investigative tool, the cost–benefit issues of each new technology should be carefully resolved before its widespread adoption.

CLINICAL INDICATIONS FOR EXERCISE TESTING

The appropriate use of exercise testing in clinical practice requires a careful consideration of the possible applications of this technique in various clinical situations. Certainly, there are many questions regarding the presence of cardiovascular abnormalities that can be resolved without exercise testing, using information derived from the history, physical examination, chest radiograph, and resting electrocardiogram (ECG) (Chapter 3). There may also be a tendency in some exercise facilities to recommend routine exercise testing prior to initiating a fitness program in individuals who are clearly not at risk for cardiovascular disease. In these situations the occasional abnormal response may lead to even more costly and unnecessary medical testing to exclude the presence of disease.

Table 5–1. Exercise Testing: Indications, Methodology, and Applications

1. Clinical indications for exercise testing
    Diagnostic indications for exercise testing
    Evaluations of cardiovascular functional
        capacity
    Contraindications to exercise testing
2. Exercise test methodologies
    Choice of exercise device
    ECG lead systems
    Electrodes and skin preparations
    Exercise test protocols
    Procedures before exercise
    Procedures during exercise
    Exercise test end points
    Procedures after exercise
    Complications of exercise testing
3. Exercise electrocardiography
    Electrophysiology of myocardial ischemia
    ECG manifestations of myocardial ischemia
    Conduction disturbances during exercise testing
    Exercise test arrhythmias
4. Clinical judgment in exercise testing
    Exercise test accuracy
5. Application of Bayes' theorem to exercise testing
6. Diagnostic exercise testing
    Screening of asymptomatic individuals
    Differential diagnosis of chest pain
    Evaluation of syncope and palpitations
7. Advances in diagnostic testing
    Computer processing of the exercise ECG
    Multivariate analysis of exercise test data
    Quantitative ST segment analyses
    Precordial and body surface ECG mapping
    Cardiokymography
    Radionuclide stress testing
8. Identification of high-risk and low-risk patients
    Risk assessment in asymptomatic populations
    Evaluating the severity of CAD
    Exercise testing after MI
9. Evaluation of cardiovascular functional capacity
    Measurement of maximal oxygen uptake
    Classification of physical fitness
    Functional capacity of patients with cardiac
        disease
    Adult fitness evaluations

CAD, coronary artery disease; ECG, electrocardiogram; MI, myocardial infarction.

There are essentially two broad indications for exercise testing: (1) *diagnostic* and (2) *functional*. Diagnostic testing is performed primarily to resolve questions regarding the presence or absence of myocardial ischemia, usually secondary to coronary atherosclerosis. Functional testing, on the other hand, is used to evaluate physical working capacity and often considers questions that are independent of the presence or absence of heart disease. In most clinical situations, however, both diagnostic and functional information contribute to the overall interpretation of the test results.

Diagnostic Indications
for Exercise Testing

The detection of myocardial ischemia in the adult population continues to be a major challenge to the medical profession, since coronary heart disease (CHD) is still the leading cause of death and disability in our society.[1] Statistics from the Framingham heart disease study[2] indicate that myocardial infarction (MI) and sudden cardiac death are frequently the first clinical manifestations of coronary disease.[2] The challenge, therefore, is to detect myocardial ischemia earlier in the natural history of coronary disease in order to prevent the more serious complications of advanced disease. As discussed later, the exercise test is by no means free of diagnostic errors and is only of practical value in certain subsets of the population (Table 5–2).

There is a wide range of opinion regarding the testing of asymptomatic individuals for exercise-induced myocardial ischemia. With the recent increased public interest in wellness and exercise, and the somewhat cautious recommendations of professional organizations such as the American Heart Association (AHA) and the American College of Sports Medicine (ACSM), there is a tendency to overuse the physician-supervised maximal exercise test in screening for early CHD. Nevertheless, it is clear that there is a population of high-

Table 5–2. Diagnostic Indications for Exercise Testing

Asymptomatic, middle-aged individuals with strongly positive coronary risk factors
Differential diagnosis of chest discomfort
Asymptomatic postmyocardial infarction patients
Evaluation of syncope and palpitations

risk asymptomatic individuals, mostly men over the ages of 40 to 45 years with significant coronary risk factors who are at increased risk of developing symptomatic CHD. These people are candidates for diagnostic exercise testing, especially if they are interested in modifying their sedentary life-styles.

Symptoms of chest discomfort are among the most frequent reasons for seeking medical attention. As discussed in Chapter 3, the physician can often determine whether or not the symptoms represent angina pectoris from the patient's description of the discomfort. Chest pain descriptors such as quality of discomfort, location, duration, predictability, and precipitating and relieving factors will usually enable the symptoms to be classified as typical angina pectoris or nonanginal chest pain. At times, however, the symptoms will only be suggestive of ischemic heart disease. Exercise testing is often very helpful in resolving this issue.

The use of exercise testing to detect myocardial ischemia in post-MI patients is an important consideration just prior to hospital discharge or shortly after discharge. The identification of ischemic ECG abnormalities in those patients is usually indicative of multivessel coronary artery disease (CAD) and suggests an increased risk for reinfarction and mortality in the first year following the acute MI.[3] The absence of ischemic ECG abnormalities, on the other hand, coupled with a reasonable exercise tolerance and blood pressure response, identifies a very low-risk subgroup of patients who are able to return to productive life-styles soon after discharge.[4]

Exercise testing can also be used to evaluate the cause or mechanisms of sudden loss of consciousness (syncope) and palpitations, especially when it is suspected that exertional activities are among the precipitating factors of these symptoms. Exercise testing is often used in conjunction with ambulatory ECG monitoring in the diagnostic workup of these patients.

Evaluation of Cardiovascular Functional Capacity

The second major clinical purpose of exercise testing is assessing the functional cardiovascular and/or respiratory status in a variety of clinical situations (Table 5–3). Questions regarding the need for further diagnostic studies, therapeutic decisions, and prognosis can often be resolved by evaluating functional capacities in the exercise laboratory. For many patients with heart disease, the knowledge of an adequate functional capacity is a major factor in their psychological well-being and productivity.

In coronary disease functional exercise testing often provides information needed for optimal management (Table 5–4). Information derived from functional testing is used to determine the type of physical

Table 5–3. Exercise Testing for Functional Assessments

Functional assessments in patients with cardiovascular diseases
    Coronary heart disease
    Valvular disease
    Cardiomyopathy
    Congenital heart disease
    Peripheral vascular disease

Evaluation of patients with respiratory disease
Assessment of patients with known or suspected disabilities
Assessment for exercise training programs

Table 5–4. Functional Exercise Testing in Coronary Heart Disease

Quantitation of physical working capacity for occupational and leisure time activities
    Stable anginal pectoris
    After myocardial infarction
    After coronary artery bypass surgery
    After coronary angioplasty

Prognostic stratification of patients into high-risk and low-risk subgroups

Therapeutic considerations
    Evaluating the need for surgery
    Selection of optimal therapy
    Assessing the effects of therapy

Cardiac rehabilitation
    Design of initial exercise prescription
    Determining rate of exercise progression

activities that can be safely engaged in during work and recreation. In general, patients feel reassured knowing their particular exercise limitations.

Identification of high-risk subsets of coronary patients has recently been emphasized in the literature, since many new technologies and therapies are now available that significantly improve long-term outlook. In fact, the study and treatment of high-risk patients have so preoccupied the medical community that insufficient attention has been given to the recognition of low-risk patients, who probably represent the majority of the coronary disease population. Changing economic forces in medicine will likely result in more emphasis on low-risk patients, since these patients can be encouraged to lead productive life-styles without the need for costly diagnostic and treatment procedures. Of all the uses of exercise testing discussed in this chapter, the identification of low-risk coronary patients is likely to be the most cost-effective.

The decision to treat or not to treat and the choice of therapy are frequently determined by the patient's functional capacity and exertional symptoms. Coronary patients with good functional capacity and minimal symptoms during exercise are usually not candidates for surgical therapy. The multiplicity of drugs available today for the treatment of angina, arrhythmias, and heart failure requires careful assessment of the functional consequences of various therapies in order to optimize dosages and types of drugs needed to manage particular problems.

Exercise testing for cardiac rehabilitation is, of course, an important prerequisite for the successful management of most patients with chronic CAD. The design of exercise programs and the rate at which patients progress in their rehabilitation will depend on the exercise test results. This is further discussed in Chapters 12 to 14.

There are many indications for exercise testing in evaluating patients with other forms of cardiovascular and pulmonary disease. Decisions regarding the need for cardiac catheterization studies, the choice and regulation of various drug therapies, and optimal timing of operative interventions can all be enhanced by evaluation of functional capacity. Exercise testing is often required in the assessment of disability claims involving a variety of conditions associated with work intolerance. An objective evaluation of functional capacity helps in determining the extent to which an individual is able to perform physically demanding tasks. Furthermore, the extent of impairment involving the cardiovascular, respiratory, and musculoskeletal systems can often be determined and recommendations given for appropriate rehabilitation.

Finally, functional testing is frequently recommended in high-risk adults prior to initiating a fitness program. The results of the exercise test are taken into consideration in structuring a safe and effective exercise program.

Contraindications to Exercise Testing

Although there are many indications for exercise testing in clinical practice, the test is not without potential risk or discomfort to the patient. Each patient, therefore, should be assessed prior to testing to determine if the benefits of testing clearly outweigh the possible risks, and that the test results will contribute to patient management. Most of the contraindications listed in Table 5–5 are relative, since there may be occasions when low-level exercise testing is conducted under careful supervision to answer specific questions needed for optimal management. Certainly, a number of the noncardiac contraindications listed in Table 5–5 can usually be resolved prior to exercise testing, or testing may not even be appropriate under some circumstances. Common sense is usually sufficient to resolve these issues.

Table 5–5.   Contraindications to Exercise Testing

Unstable or severe cardiovascular disorders
  1. Recent, acute myocardial infarction
  2. Unstable angina pectoris
  3. Uncontrolled cardiac arrhythmias
  4. Severe congestive heart failure
  5. Severe aortic stenosis
  6. Active myocarditis, pericarditis, or endocarditis
  7. Dissecting aortic aneurysm
  8. Recent systemic or pulmonary emboli
  9. Systolic blood pressure >200 mm Hg, or diastolic blood pressure >120 mm Hg
  10. Acute thrombophlebitis

Noncardiovascular conditions
  1. Active infections
  2. Severe emotional distress
  3. Uncontrolled metabolic disease such as thyrotoxicosis, myxedema, diabetes, etc.
  4. Neuromuscular, musculoskeletal, and arthritic conditions that preclude exercise
  5. Other systemic illnesses that would make exercise difficult

EXERCISE TEST METHODOLOGIES

Table 5–1 lists the methodologic aspects of exercise testing that are discussed in this section. It is important to realize that procedures vary from laboratory to laboratory without necessarily affecting the quality of testing. Every attempt is made in this review to be consistent with standards developed by the AHA[5] and the ACSM.[6]

Choice of Exercise Device

The stationary bicycle ergometer and the motor-driven treadmill are the two most common modalities for clinical exercise testing. Each has advantages and disadvantages, and many laboratories have the flexibility of using either device, depending on the particular needs of the patient. In North America the treadmill is more popular, primarily because individuals in our society are better able to achieve high work loads on the treadmill. Treadmill protocols are more flexible than bicycle protocols, since speed and grade may be varied independently to increase the work load. Unlike the bicycle, the treadmill test is not patient dependent, and, therefore, it is more reproducible. In addition, work loads are more accurately measured on the treadmill than on the bicycle, where pedaling frequency is an important determinant of the total work.

The bicycle, on the other hand, is less costly, requires less space, and is more portable, less likely to break down, and less noisy. At high work loads on the bicycle, it is easier to obtain good ECG data free of motion artifact. Blood pressures are also more easily measured on the bicycle. Some patients may be less anxious on the bicycle, since they are more in control of their exercise efforts. For individuals who have difficulty walking because of age, debilitating illnesses, or orthopedic problems, the bicycle ergometer may be the only method of assessing exercise tolerance. The bicycle may also be positioned for supine leg exercise during cardiac catheterization or nuclear imaging studies. Finally, arm crank ergometry may be conducted with these devices to assess the cardiovascular effects of upper extremity exercise.[7,8] This may be particularly useful in coronary disease patients who do physically demanding upper extremity work.

Regardless of which exercise device is used for testing, it is important to understand the methods for calibrating the work load. The treadmill varies its workload by changing speed (mph) and elevation (percent grade). The accuracy of the speed meter is checked by placing a visible marker on the treadmill belt and counting the number of belt revolutions in one minute. The belt speed is calculated using the following formula:

$$S = \frac{C \times R}{1,056}$$

where S is speed in mph, C is the belt circumference measured in inches, and R is the number of belt revolutions in 1 minute. If the calulated speed is not the same as that indicated by the speed meter, the meter should be adjusted as described in the "owner's manual" for that particular treadmill.

The percent grade of the treadmill is calculated by measuring the vertical heights from the floor to the treadmill belt at two different points. If the horizontal difference between the two points on the floor is x, and the difference in vertical heights at the two points is y, then the percent grade is $y/x \times 100$. If the elevation meter on the treadmill is different from the calculated grade, the meter should be adjusted accordingly.

Calibrating the bicycle ergometer is more complicated and depends on whether the ergometer is mechanically braked or electrically braked. Methods for calibration have been described in the literature[9] as well as in the manuals for each type of ergometer.

Electrocardiographic Lead Systems

One area of exercise testing that is not well standardized is the choice of an ECG lead system. There are a number of reasons for this, not the least of which is that the ideal lead system has yet to be defined. Chaitman and Hanson[10] reviewed the literature on lead systems up to 1981 without reaching any definite conclusions as to which particular system or individual leads are best for identifying myocardial ischemia. It is clear, however, that multiple leads are becoming increasingly popular in today's exercise testing laboratories.

By far the most popular of the multiple-lead systems is the modified 12-lead system first described by Mason and Likar in 1966[11] and illustrated in Figure 5–1. Although originally the arm electrodes were placed below the clavicles just medial to the deltoid muscles, there is less motion artifact when these electrodes are placed directly over the clavicles in the midclavicular lines. The leg electrodes are positioned in the anterior axillary lines, halfway between the costal margins and the iliac crests; the six chest electrodes are in their usual positions as in the standard resting ECG (Chapter 3). The Mason–Likar modification results

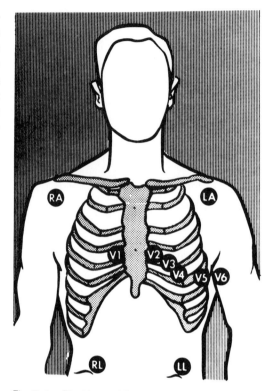

Fig. 5–1.   The Mason–Likar modified 12-lead system. From Koppes, G., McKiernan, T., Bassan, M., and Froelicher, V.F.: Treadmill exercise testing. Part 1. Edited by W.P. Harvey and S.M. Fox. Curr. Probl. Cardiol., 7:26, 1977. © 1977, Year Book Medical Publishers. Reproduced with permission.

in some changes in the configuration of the ECG waveform from the standard ECG, which may interfere, in some cases, with recognition of old inferior wall MI.[10]

Bipolar ECG leads have the advantages of being simpler, requiring less time to set up, and being less costly and generally less noisy in terms of artifact.[12–15] Several commonly used bipolar lead sites are illustrated in Figure 5–2. Most of these leads use the V_5 chest position for the positive pole and somewhat resemble standard lead V_5, but with larger QRS voltages. It has been suggested that these leads are more sensitive to ST segment changes due to myocardial ischemia than standard leads.

Chaitman et al.[16] advocate combining several of the bipolar leads with the Mason–Likar system into a 15-lead system to

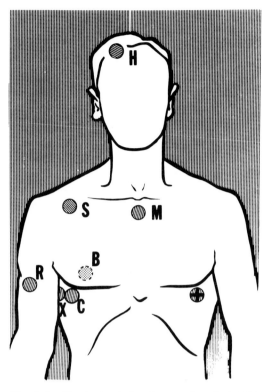

Fig. 5–2. Bipolar lead sites for exercise electrocardiography. The positive pole is located in the V_5 chest position. From Froelicher, V.F., et al.: A comparison of two bipolar exercise ECG leads to V_5. Chest, 70:611, 1976.

optimally detect ischemic ECG changes in high-risk symptomatic patients. In addition they feel that this lead system facilitates the detection of multivessel disease. It is not yet possible, however, to define the ideal combination of leads for testing low-risk, asymptomatic individuals, since an increase in the number of leads may also increase the false-positive error in this population.

Electrodes and Skin Preparation

The ECG detection of myocardial ischemia during progressive exercise becomes more difficult with increasing heart rates. Unless special attention is given to electrodes and skin preparation, the deteriorating signal/noise ratio with increasing exercise will preclude obtaining adequate ECG data for interpretation. Motion arti-

fact accounts for most of the electrical noise that is superimposed on the ECG signal during exercise. Although considerable bioengineering efforts have been implemented to reduce unwanted artifact using expensive computer processing techniques, the simplest and most effective method is still careful preparation of the patient prior to testing.

The patient should be supine while electrodes are being placed in order to ensure accurate location of the electrode sites. Male patients will often need to be shaved around the electrode sites before skin preparation. The patient should be informed of this prior to shaving in order to avoid unnecessary distress. One should also explain that there likely will be some minimal chest wall irritation for several weeks following the test as the hair regrows. The actual electrode sites will depend on the particular lead system. Sites over large muscles should be avoided in order to minimize artifact due to myoelectric potentials.

Tam and Webster[17] have studied the possible causes of motion artifact by measuring potential drops at the electrode/paste interface and the skin/paste interface, concluding that the latter was the major source of artifact. They also showed how skin abrasion to remove the superficial horny layer of epidermis (stratum corneum) could significantly lower the electrical impedance across the skin/paste interface and improve the signal/noise ratio. Skin abrasion can best be accomplished using an abrading paste rubbed over the electrode sites. Alternatively, one can also use fine-grain sandpaper or a dull dental burr. Special care is needed to avoid abrading into the superficial capillaries immediately below the stratum corneum. It is usually a good idea to clean the sites with alcohol or acetone prior to electrode application.

Many excellent exercise test electrodes are now available that are specially designed to minimize motion artifact. Most of these electrodes incorporate a recessed silver–silver chloride disk adjacent to a sponge soaked with electrolyte solution, which forms a low-resistance interface between electrode disk and skin. An adhesive pad surrounds the disk and holds it to the skin. In some individuals who sweat excessively during exercise, the adhesive does not hold, and it may be necessary to wrap the electrodes to the chest and abdomen with an Ace bandage or use an elastic vest. It is generally not necessary to check the impedance across each electrode–skin interface with an ohm meter to verify that the impedance is less than 5,000 ohms. Tapping each electrode while observing the oscilloscopic ECG signal for noise will usually identify bad electrodes needing replacement. This is most often due to drying out of the electrolyte sponge in the electrode. Finally, it is important to make sure that the electrode wires are not pulling on the electrodes when the patient is sitting or standing, since deformation of the skin can cause spurious shifts in ECG baseline.

Exercise Test Protocols

Most clinical indications for exercise testing require an incremental protocol beginning at a low work load and progressing to higher work loads until either a predetermined end point is reached (submaximal protocols) or until signs or symptoms develop that preclude further exercise (sign- or symptom-limited protocols). If the limiting symptoms are reflective of the subject's functional capacity, the test is called *maximal*. Steady-state or constant work-load protocols are sometimes used in the evaluation of suspected pulmonary disorders, but they are not commonly used in clinical cardiovascular testing.

The progressive work-load protocols may be *intermittent*, with periods of rest alternating with increasing work loads, or *continuous*, where the work load increases in a series of stages without intermittent rest periods. Although the intermittent protocols may enable the subjects to reach

higher maximal work loads, they are not practical for routine clinical testing because of the long time required to complete the protocol.

It is important that exercise test personnel have a working knowledge of different protocols in order to have the flexibility to accommodate different patient populations. In any particular patient, a protocol should be chosen that best answers the clinical questions being asked with minimal risk to the patient. Serial testing in a given patient should usually follow the same protocol to enable comparisons to be made over time. For maximal testing, standardized protocols are preferred, since comparisons can be made between patients, and normal reference values for different age groups have been published in the literature.

Protocols for Bicycle Testing

Before beginning exercise the seat height and handle bar should be adjusted for patient comfort and efficiency of pedaling. The seat height should be set so that there is only minimal (5°) flexion at the knee when the foot is at its lowest position on the pedal. Pedaling frequency should be 50 to 60 rpm in order to achieve valid work loads; this can be monitored with a metronome or an rpm meter.

The optimal bicycle protocol is one that matches the duration of exercise to the subject's functional capacity. Buchfuhrer et al.[18] have shown that exercise tests that are either of short duration (less than 8 minutes) with large incremental steps or of long duration (greater than 17 minutes) with small incremental steps are associated with lower measures of functional capacity ($\dot{V}O_2$ max) than tests of 8 to 17 minutes' duration. They recommend, for both bicycle and treadmill testing, that the work-rate increment be selected to bring the subject to maximal effort in 10 ± 2 minutes. This implies that subjects be assessed prior to testing to estimate their functional ability to exercise in order to determine the optimal incremental work rate. Each subject should be questioned about habitual physical activity and classified as active or inactive, depending on whether or not they exercise 3 or more days a week for at least 15 to 30 minutes a day. Body weight should also be taken into consideration, since larger individuals may have a performance advantage on the bicycle due to large leg muscles.

Exercise should begin with the subject pedaling against minimal resistance for 1 minute as a warm-up. Thereafter the work rate can be increased in increments of 15 watts (~90 kpm/min) to 25 watts (~150 kpm/min) each minute, depending on the subject's heart rate response, aiming for a test duration of 10 ± 2 min. Extremely sedentary subjects or individuals with cardiopulmonary disorders may require even smaller increments.

Protocols for Treadmill Exercise

A number of continuous incremental treadmill protocols have achieved popularity in the United States and elsewhere. Many of these have been evaluated and compared in the literature, with data published relating work rate and time to the subject's oxygen uptake.[19–23] Protocols vary in terms of percent grade, speed, duration, and size of increments between stages. Five commonly used protocols are illustrated in Table 5–6.

The Bruce protocol is probably the most popular of treadmill protocols, owing in part to the many important contributions to exercise testing made by Dr. Robert Bruce at the University of Washington.[19] In this protocol both speed and grade are increased every 3 minutes in rather large increments. An optional warm-up (stage 1/2) period may or may not be needed. The primary advantage of this protocol is the relatively short duration needed for most subjects to reach maximal effort. In some people this is a disadvantage, because the large increments may be too great to accurately assess functional capacity. In addition, subjects who exercise beyond stage III may have to run on the treadmill to keep up, making "clean" ECG recordings and blood pressure measurements more difficult.

The Balke protocol[20] is a much smoother and more slowly progressive protocol, where the speed remains constant at 3.3 mph and the grade increases by 1% every minute (except for the first increment of 2%). Only selected stages are illustrated in Table 5–6. This protocol was developed primarily to assess physical fitness in reasonably healthy military personnel and not for cardiovascular screening. Its major disadvantage for healthy individuals is its duration; for older and more diseased populations, the 3.3-mph speed may be too great. There have been a number of modifications of this protocol to improve its applicability to clinical testing. Speeds of 2.0 mph or 3.0 mph are often utilized.

At the US Air Force School of Aerospace Medicine (USAFSAM) a modification of the Balke protocol has been designed for Air Force personnel.[21] This protocol is clinically more practical for screening the apparently healthy population because of the reduced time to maximal effort. Like the Balke protocol, subjects walk at a constant speed of 3.3 mph, but with 5%-grade increments every 3 minutes. The oxygen uptake values established for the Balke protocol apply quite nicely to those measured at the end of each USAFSAM protocol stage.[21] Similar blood pressure and heart rate responses have also been observed.

In the Ellestad protocol,[22] the speed increases progressively from 1.7 to 6.0 mph with no change in the grade (10%) until stage 5, when the grade increases to 15%. Like the Bruce test this protocol may require running in the higher stages, with the disadvantage of increased motion artifact and difficulty in obtaining accurate blood pressures. Short-statured individuals are at

Table 5–6.　Treadmill Exercise Protocols in Clinical Practice

Protocol	Stage	Grade (%)	Speed (mph)	Total Time (min)	O₂ Uptake (ml/kg/min)	METs
Bruce[19]	(1/2)	5	1.5	3	11	3
	I	10	1.7	6	17	4
	II	12	2.5	9	25	7
	III	14	3.4	12	35	10
	IV	16	4.2	15	47	13
	V	18	5.0	18	56	16
Balke[20]	1	0	3.3	1		
	3	3	3.3	3	17	4
	6	6	3.3	6	21	6
	9	9	3.3	9	26	7
	12	12	3.3	12	31	9
	15	15	3.3	15	36	10
	18	18	3.3	18	41	12
USAFSAM[21]	I	0	3.3	3	14	4
	II	5	3.3	6	21	6
	III	10	3.3	9	28	8
	IV	15	3.3	12	36	10
	V	20	3.3	15	46	13
	VI	25	3.3	18	52	15
Ellestad[22]	1	10	1.7	3	17	4
	2	10	3.0	5	25	7
	3	10	4.0	7	33	9
	4	10	5.0	10	45	12
	5	15	5.0	12	51	14
	6	15	5.0	15	56	17
Modified Naughton[24]	1	0	2.0	3	7.0	2
	2	3.5	2.0	6	10.5	3
	3	7.0	2.0	9	14.0	4
	4	10.5	2.0	12	17.5	5
	5	14.0	2.0	15	21.0	6
	6	17.5	2.0	18	24.5	7
	7	12.5	3.0	21	28.0	8
	8	15.0	3.0	24	31.5	9
	9	17.5	3.0	27	35.0	10

MET, metabolic equivalent.

a distinct disadvantage, since they must begin running at a lower stage of exercise.

Finally, the modified Naughton protocol was developed to assess the cardiovascular status of post-MI patients before hospital discharge or shortly after discharge.[23,24] This particular protocol has also been used extensively in recent years to identify high-risk and low-risk patients after acute MI. In this protocol the speed remains 2 mph for the first six stages while the grade increases by 3.5% every 3 minutes; the speed then increases to 3 mph for the remaining stages with 2.5% increments in grade. The work load increases in increments of 1 metabolic equivalent (MET) (3.5 ml O₂/kg/min). This protocol is also very useful in evaluating patients with depressed ventricular function due to severe valvular heart disease or cardiomyopathy.

It should be emphasized that the MET levels of the different protocols assume that a steady state has been reached for each particular work load. This requirement is not always satisfied in some protocols, especially at high work loads.

Procedures Before Exercise

The preparation of a patient for exercise testing begins with an explanation of the purpose for the test and the various procedures that will be conducted during the test. Every effort should be made to familiarize the patient with the test procedures and relieve any anxieties or concerns. The specific instructions prior to testing will vary from one laboratory to another. In general, patients should be advised not to eat, smoke, or consume alcoholic drinks for 2 to 3 hours before testing. Comfortable clothes and walking shoes should be worn or brought to the laboratory. Women are advised to wear a loose-fitting blouse that buttons in front, along with shorts or slacks. A snug-fitting bra is usually recommended to secure the breasts and minimize electrical interference while exercising.

Informed consent implies that the patient is aware of the potential benefits and occasional risks of the test and consents to be tested. Most often this is accomplished by having the patient read and sign a consent form after all questions have been answered to the patient's satisfaction. Sample consent forms have been published by the AHA[5] and the ACSM.[6] Each exercise testing laboratory should design a consent form that is compatible with state and local laws governing consent as well as the hospital or other institutional review board (Fig. 5–3). It is unlikely that signed consent will offer any legal protection to a laboratory where an exercise complication is the result of negligence or improper procedures.

Patient Interview and Examination

If the patient is being tested for a known or suspected cardiovascular problem, a brief physician evaluation is necessary to rule out any contraindications to testing and to gather information that will facilitate interpreting the test results. In some laboratories a preliminary history and review of cardiovascular risk factors are obtained by the exercise test technologist as the patient is being prepared for the test. Alternatively, a self-administered questionnaire may be completed by the patient prior to testing. If the patient has a history of chest discomfort, the symptoms should be reviewed by the physician and classified as typical angina pectoris, atypical angina, or nonanginal chest pain.[25–27]

A brief cardiovascular examination should be performed with special attention given to heart murmurs and gallops. Severe aortic stenosis is a contraindication to testing. This is recognized by a harsh systolic heart murmur at the base with delayed and diminished carotid arterial pulses. Findings of mitral valve prolapse, including a midsystolic click with or without a late systolic murmur, are also important to recognize, since this common condition may be associated with resting ST-T wave changes and false-positive exercise tests.

ECG Data Collection

The resting 12-lead ECG should be reviewed by the supervising physician prior to testing. Although uncommon, ECG findings of acute MI have been observed in patients referred for evaluation of chest pain. These patients need intensive coronary care not exercise testing. Diagnostic ECG stress testing may not be feasible in the setting of left bundle branch block or other resting ECG abnormalities associated with marked ST-T wave changes. These individuals might be better evaluated with radionuclide techniques.

The resting ECG should be obtained in the supine and standing positions. In addition some laboratories routinely hyperventilate all patients prior to testing to look for ST-T wave changes that may mimic myocardial ischemia during exercise. However, if there are no ST-T wave changes from supine to standing position, it is unlikely that hyperventilation will cause significant changes. For these reasons it may only be useful to hyperventilate those individuals (mostly women) who have labile, positional ST-T wave changes. Hyperventilation-induced changes do not preclude the possibility of true ischemic ECG changes during exercise.

THE FITNESS INSTITUTE'S EXERCISE TEST CONSENT FORM

NAME: _____DATE: _____

AGE: _____SEX: _____PHYSICIAN: _____

INFORMED CONSENT: In order to evaluate the functional performance and capacity of the heart, lungs, and blood vessels, each individual consents, voluntarily, to perform an exercise test. Before being tested, she/he is questioned and examined by a physician, and has an electrocardiogram recorded (to show whether or not testing should proceed), after which he/she walks on a treadmill, with speed and incline increased every three minutes, until the limits of fatigue, breathlessness, chest pain, and/or other symptoms are of such severity that he/she should stop the effort. Blood pressure and electrocardiogram are monitored while he/she is exercising. In some instances expired air will be collected and oxygen uptake determined.

RISKS of testing including occasional changes in the rhythm of the heart beats and the possibility of excessive changes in blood pressure. There is a remote chance of fainting and even a more remote chance of a heart attack. Professional supervision protects against injury, by providing appropriate precautionary measures, and in the unlikely event that these precautions are insufficient, emergency hospital treatment is available.

BENEFITS of testing include quantitative assessment of working capacity and critical appraisal of the disorders or diseases that impair capacity, the knowledge of which facilitates better treatment and more accurate prognosis for future cardiac events.

Both the right to withdraw from the test at any time with impunity and the right to withhold confidential information from nonmedical persons (such as employers and insurance agents) without consent are assured. The welfare of each person will be protected.

In addition to participating in this exercise test, each person permits his/her name to be registered for future follow-up studies.

CONSENT:

Having read the information statement above and had the opportunity to ask questions, I hereby willingly consent to be tested.

DATE: _____SIGNED: _____

TIME: _____WITNESS: _____

Fig. 5–3.   Consent form for exercise testing.

Blood Pressure Measurements

Blood pressures should be obtained at rest in the supine and standing positions and during each stage of exercise. Some practice is necessary to accurately measure exercise blood pressures, especially during treadmill testing where ambient noise and patient movement often interfere with the measurements. Automated blood pressure recording devices have been designed for exercise testing and may offer significant advantages over manually obtained measurements. One such device, using a microphone pickup of Korotkoff's sounds and ECG-assisted microprocessing of unwanted noise, has been favorably evaluated in the literature.[28,29] Disadvantages of these devices are that they are expensive, take longer to measure the blood pressure (30 to 45 seconds), and may be uncomfortable for the patient because of the slow deflation time.

Procedures During Exercise

During exercise the patient should be carefully observed and periodic assessments made of symptoms, ECG data, blood pressure, and any untoward physical signs. Continuous observation of ECG rhythm and waveform on the oscilloscope is essential, both during and after exercise. Most modern exercise ECG monitors have delay capabilities (memory) to obtain hard copy rhythm strips of arrhythmic events noted on the oscilloscope. Samples of the ECG for waveform analysis should be obtained at the end of each stage.

Chest pain during exercise is an important observation, especially if the patient is being evaluated for suspected or known coronary disease. Careful observation of the patient, the ECG, and blood pressure will usually enable the patient's symptoms to be classified as anginal or nonanginal chest pain. It may not be necessary to stop the test at the onset of chest pain, if the intensity of pain is mild, if the patient's blood pressure is stable or rising, and if the ECG does not show significant ST-T wave changes. Indications for terminating the test include (1) increased pain intensity (3 + out of 4 +), (2) failure of systolic blood pressure to rise or a fall in blood pressure, (3) marked ST segment depression or any abnormal ST segment elevation.

Exercise Test End Points

The decision to stop an exercise test is sometimes determined by the patient (limiting symptoms), sometimes by the physician (abnormal findings), and sometimes by the protocol (submaximal end points). A list of these various end points is given in Table 5–7.

The patient's request to stop should al-

Table 5–7.   Exercise Test End Points

Patient-determined end points
Patient wants to stop
Significant chest discomfort
Marked fatigue
Severe dyspnea
Other limiting symptoms (dizziness, leg cramps, joint discomfort, etc.)
Physician-determined end points
Patient does not look good (ataxia, confusion, pallor, cyanosis, etc.)
ECG end points
Marked ST depression or elevation
Bundle branch or AV nodal heart block
Ventricular tachycardia or fibrillation
Increasing frequency of PVCs, couplets, etc.
Uncontrolled supraventricular arrhythmias
Reduction in systolic blood pressure and/or heart rate with increasing work loads
Systolic blood pressure >250 mm Hg or diastolic blood pressure >120 mm Hg
Equipment failure
Protocol-determined end points
Heart rate determined
Work load determined

AV, atrioventricular; ECG, electrocardiogram; PVCs, premature ventricular complexes.

ways be a serious consideration for terminating the test. At times, however, when the patient seems poorly motivated and is clearly in no distress, the supervising physician may encourage the patient to continue exercising until more limiting signs or symptoms are noted. In general, when doing a diagnostic test, if the patient fails to achieve 90% of predicted maximal heart rate (220 minus age) without chest pain or ECG manifestations of ischemia, the test is considered inadequate to rule out ischemic heart disease. For this reason it is sometimes important to urge the patient to continue exercising until a more appropriate heart rate response is achieved (assuming the patient is not taking heart-rate-slowing drugs). Patients who are not accustomed to exercise may misinterpret their symptoms as limiting when, in fact, they are clearly submaximal. Careful preparation of the patient before testing and kind encouragement during testing will often improve the exercise response.

Physician-determined end points may be absolute or relative, depending on the particular circumstances. Clinical judgment, experience, and knowing the patient being tested are all important factors in safely completing the exercise test. Rate-dependent bundle branch block, for example, may not always be an indication to terminate a test, especially if this is a previously recognized phenomenon and not related to myocardial ischemia.

The protocol-determined end points are related to the submaximal protocols designed for low-level exercise testing. The predischarge exercise test after acute MI may be terminated when the patient's heart rate reaches 70% of predicted maximal heart rate or when the work load reaches 5 METs.

Procedures After Exercise

After a brief cool-down period, while the patient is still standing on the treadmill or sitting on the bicycle, the ECG should be recorded. Patients on the treadmill should hold on to the rails, because venous pooling may cause light-headedness. If the test is a diagnostic test and if significant ECG abnormalities did not develop during exercise, the patient should return to the supine position during the recovery period. The increased venous return that occurs when supine may aggravate borderline ischemic myocardium because of increased end-diastolic pressure and result in diagnostic ECG changes. For patients who develop significant ischemic ECG changes during exercise, however, it may be preferable to sit during the recovery period, because the supine position may increase the risk of ventricular arrhythmias. Regardless of patient position, the ECG should be recorded every 2 to 3 minutes until the waveform is back to the control configuration.

During recovery the patient should be examined for new gallops or murmurs resulting from myocardial dysfunction. An S-4 gallop may be indicative of decreased compliance associated with myocardial ischemia. A new systolic murmur at the apex is usually due to papillary muscle dysfunction. These are usually transient findings associated with reversible myocardial ischemia.

Exercise Test Data Forms

Figure 5–4 is an example of a two-page exercise test report form, which is a modification of a form published by Koppes et al.[30] The form attempts to capture all the clinically important information needed for interpreting the exercise test results. The first page of the form asks for clinical data, cardiovascular risk factors, reasons for testing, description of the resting ECG, and exercise test data for each stage of exercise and recovery. The second page asks for physical findings before and after exercise, reasons for stopping, specific ECG abnormalities, prognostic indicators, and interpretive statements. This form is most applicable to diagnostic exercise testing of patients with known or suspected heart disease. Other forms may be more appropriate for functional testing where more physiologic parameters need to be assessed.

Complications of Exercise Testing

Although rare, exercise testing may be associated with untoward events. In a recent survey of the exercise testing community, Stuart and Ellestad[31] collected data on over 500,000 exercise tests and determined that, for each 10,000 tests, there were approximately 3.5 MIs, 4.8 serious arrhythmias, and 0.5 deaths. Table 5–8 lists the requirements for minimizing exercise test complications. Periodic inservice training should be given to the exercise testing staff to review emergency treatment procedures, so that any potentially serious or life-threatening complications can be recognized early and effectively managed.

EXERCISE ELECTROCARDIOGRAPHY

Electrophysiology of Myocardial Ischemia

Although the ECG has great utility in the recognition of myocardial ischemia, the

INTERMOUNTAIN HEALTH CARE, INC.
A community hospital system serving the Intermountain West

CARDIOLOGY DIVISION
LDS HOSPITAL
325 8th Ave., S.L.C., Utah (801) 350-1185

REPORT OF
TREADMILL EXERCISE TEST
(PAGE ONE)

PATIENT IDENTIFICATION	
Hospital No.	
Name:	
Address	
PVT MD:	Phone:

SEND REPORT TO

TREADMILL NO.	AGE	SEX	WT. (KG.)	HT. (CM)

☐ INPATIENT
☐ OUTPATIENT

DATE (MO., DAY, YR.)	24 HR. TIME

PREVIOUS TEST   NO.
☐ NO ☐ YES, LAST:

HOURS SINCE
LAST MEAL
LAST CIGARETTE

MEDICATIONS
☐ DIGITALIS   ☐ NITRATES
☐ BETA-BLOCKER   ☐ QUINIDINE/PRONESTYL
☐ DIURETIC   ☐ OTHER

CARDIAC RISK FACTORS

HISTORY OF HYPERTENSION
☐ YES ☐ NO ☐ SUSP

NOW ELEVATED
☐ YES ☐ NO

ON TREATMENT
☐ YES ☐ NO

CIGARETTE SMOKING
☐ NO ☐ PAST ONLY ☐ YES

NO. YEARS AGO QUIT | PACK-YEARS | PACKS/DAY

CHOLESTEROL LEVEL ☐ Not Known
☐ NORMAL ☐ HIGH:

FAMILY HISTORY PREMATURE ASHD ☐

ACTIVITY STATUS
☐ Sedentary   ☐ Active Recreation
☐ Recent Bed Rest ☐ Active Occupation ☐ Athlete

OTHER RISK FACTORS

RESTING ECG   DESCRIBE
☐ NORMAL ☐ ABNORMAL

CLINICAL REASONS FOR TEST

EVALUATION OF ATYPICAL SENSATION OR PAIN POSSIBLY DUE TO ASCVD (Explain)
☐

EVALUATION OF ANGINA: ONSET:
☐ TYPICAL   ☐ ATYPICAL   ☐ UNSTABLE

ARRHYTHMIA EVALUATION   ☐ SUSPECT ONLY
☐ PVDs   ☐ SVT   ☐ OTHER:

OTHER HEART DISEASE
☐ VALVULAR: ☐ OTHER:
☐ MITRAL PROLAPSE ☐ CONGENITAL

EVALUATION POST AMI   TIME SINCE LAST INFARCT:
☐   WEEKS   MONTHS   YEARS

CORONARY ANGIOGRAM: DATE

SCREENING ASYMPTOMATIC INDIVIDUAL
☐

☐ FUNCTIONAL CAPACITY EVALUATION
☐ EXERCISE PRESCRIPTION

CORONARY BYPASS SURGERY (DATE AND TYPE)

☐ OTHER

STAGE	MPH/ GRADE	METS	MIN/SEC IN STAGE	HR (AT END OF STAGE)	BP	DESCRIBE: CHEST PAIN/ARRHYTHMIAL/ST CHANGES/LEADS
Supine	3.5 cc O_2/Kg/Min = 1 MET					
HV For 30 Sec	(BASAL)					
Stand						
1/4	1.7 /0%	2				
1/2	1.7 /5%	3				
I	1.7/10%	4				
II	2.5/12%	7				
III	3.4/14%	10				
IV	4.2/16%	14				
V	5.0/18%	16				
						PREDICTED MAX HEART RATE 220- = /Min.
Immed	MAX SBP (_____) X					
1 min.	MAX HR (_____) =					
3 min.	.... x 10³					
5 min.	$\dot{V}O2$ MAX { est. =					
7 min.	{ mxed. =					
...... min.						

CARDIOLOGY 18-78

Fig. 5–4.   Data form for diagnostic exercise testing. The Fitness Institute, LDS Hospital, Salt Lake City, Utah. Modified from Koppes, G., McKiernan, T., Bassan, M., and Froelicher, V.F.: Treadmill exercise testing. Part 1. Curr. Probl. Cardiol., 7:34, 1977.

INTERMOUNTAIN HEALTH CARE, INC.
A community hospital system serving the intermountain West
CARDIOLOGY DIVISION
LDS HOSPITAL
325 8th Ave., S.L.C., Utah (801) 350-1185

REPORT OF
TREADMILL EXERCISE TEST
(PAGE TWO)

PATIENT IDENTIFICATION

PROBABILITY OF CAD	☐ Unlikely	☐ Probable	EXPLAIN		
PRIOR TO TEST = %	☐ Possible	☐ Very Probable			

PHYSICAL	PRE	S3	☐ YES ☐ NO	S4	☐ YES ☐ NO	MURMUR ☐ YES ☐ NO	TYPE
EXAM	POST	S3	☐ YES ☐ NO	S4	☐ YES ☐ NO	SIGNS/SYMPTOMS CHF ☐	MURMUR ☐ YES ☐ NO TYPE

REASONS FOR STOPPING 1. Primary 2. Secondary 3. Tertiary	CHEST PAIN	DYSPNEA	FATIGUE/WEAKNESS	CLAUDI-CATION	GENERAL APPEARANCE	CNS SYMPTOMS
	HYPER-TENSION	HYPO-TENTION	ST CHANGES	ARRHYTHMIA	TECHNICAL PROBLEM	PHYSICAL DISABILITY
	POOR PATIENT COOPERATION	LEG FATIGUE	OTHER:			

ECG RESPONSE	ARRHYTHMIA	NO	FEW PVD's	FREQ PVD's	VT	FREQ PADs	SVT
		OTHER	EXPLAIN:				
	CONDUCTION	NORMAL EXPLAIN:	LBBB	RBBB	BLOCK	AXIS SHIFT	
	ST SEGMENT	NORMAL EXPLAIN:	BORDERLINE	DEPRESSION	ELEVATE	NORMALIZE	
	T & U WAVES	NORMAL EXPLAIN:	T-INVERSION	TALL T	U-INVERSION	PROMINENT U	

PATIENT RESPONSE	MAX HR ☐NL ☐HI ☐LO	SYSTOLIC BP ☐NL ☐HI ☐FALL	FUNCTIONAL CAPACITY ☐EXCELLENT ☐NORMAL ☐LOW	FAI = % ☐ VERY LOW
	ANGINA ☐ YES ☐ NO	ATYPICAL PAIN ☐ YES ☐ NO	CHF SIGNS ☐ YES ☐ NO	OTHER COMPLICATIONS ☐ YES ☐ NO	MAXIMAL EFFORT ☐ YES ☐ NO

PROG-NOSTIC INDI-CATORS	ONSET ST-DEPRESSION STAGE: HR=	MAX ST-DEPRESSION MM LEADS:	MAX EXERCISE STAGE: HR=	POST-EXERCISE DURATION OF ST DEPRESSION min,	ANGINA ONSET HR=
	OTHER				

INTERPRETATION

NORMAL MAXIMAL TEST	COMMENTS	
NORMAL SUBMAXIMAL TEST	% MAX HR = %	COMMENTS
BORDERLINE ABNORMAL	EXPLAIN	
ABNORMAL ST DEPRESSION	LOW RISK / HIGH RISK	EXPLAIN
ABNORMAL ST ELEVATION	COMMENTS	
OTHER ABNORMALITIES	EXPLAIN	

NEW PROBABILITY OF CAD AFTER TEST = %	COMMENTS:

Interpreted By: _____ Date _____

Approved By: _____ Date _____

CARDIOLOGY 1A-78

Fig. 5–4 (continued).

Table 5–8.   Minimizing the Risks of Exercise Testing

1. Trained personnel (testing, treatment, CPR)
2. Physician attendance during testing
3. Continuous ECG monitoring during and after exercise
4. Pretest history and physical exam
5. Resting ECG evaluation
6. Patient awareness of signs and symptoms
7. Emergency resuscitation equipment and drugs
8. Terminate test at appropriate time
9. No shower until cool-down

CPR, cardiopulmonary resuscitation; ECG, electrocardiogram

underlying cellular electrophysiologic events that are responsible for the ECG abnormalities are only partially understood. Nevertheless, in preparation for a discussion on exercise ECGs, it is useful to review the pathophysiology of myocardial ischemia and the mechanisms responsible for ischemic ECG changes.

Myocardial ischemia is that process resulting from an imbalance between myocardial oxygen supply and demand such that the myocardial cells are deprived of oxygen. Most often, as in the setting of fixed coronary atherosclerotic lesions, an increased myocardial oxygen demand is brought on by exercise or some other stress, and the coronary blood supply becomes inadequate to meet the increased requirements. What follows is a sequence of events, initially reversible, that have mechanical, metabolic, and electrophysiologic consequences. The mechanical consequences are due to the inability of hypoxic myocardial cells to contract and are recognized clinically as segmental wall motion abnormalities or decreased left ventricular ejection fraction. The metabolic consequence is the production of lactate by hypoxic cells, which can be detected during cardiac catheterization with blood samples from the coronary sinus. The electrophysiologic consequences are responsible for the ischemic ECG changes.

Figure 5–5 illustrates the relationship between the intracellular action potential of a ventricular muscle cell and the surface ECG. The QRS complex represents the sequence of ventricular muscle activation and occurs during phase 0 of the action potentials. The ST segment reflects phase 2 of repolarization, and the T wave occurs during phase 3. In this diagram the U wave and the P wave are drawn as superimposed waveforms, since they are independent of ventricular muscle depolarization and repolarization. It is important to note that the resting membrane potential, phase 4, is responsible for the TQ segment of the ECG. As will be seen, the TQ segment has a major role to play in the ECG manifestations of myocardial ischemia. The following discussion on the derivation of ischemic ECG abnormalities is based on several recent reviews and research studies.[32–36]

In the setting of myocardial ischemia, the intracellular action potential becomes markedly altered. Several changes occur within seconds of oxygen deprivation that affect the shape and the duration of the action potential. The most specific change seems to be a decrease in the resting membrane potential, or phase 4, resulting from a partial failure of the membrane sodium–potassium pump and accumulation of potassium in the extracellular space.[34] The second change is a decrease in action potential duration and amplitude due to more rapid repolarization during phases 2 and 3.

The ECG alterations in myocardial ischemia are determined by the relationship between the body surface ECG leads and the location of the ischemic myocardium in the ventricles. In the setting of exercise-induced ischemia, the left ventricular subendocardium is most vulnerable. Figure 5–6 illustrates the relationship between ischemic subendocardial action potentials and the ECG.

Figure 5–6A depicts a normal segment of the ventricular wall simplified into endocardial and epicardial cell regions. An action potential from each region is diagrammed, along with a representative ECG

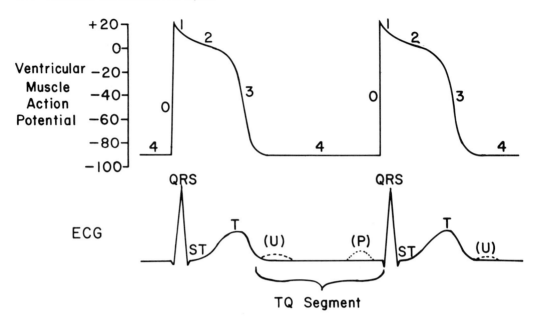

Fig. 5–5.   Relationship between intracellular action potential of ventricular muscle (top) and the body surface (bottom). See text.

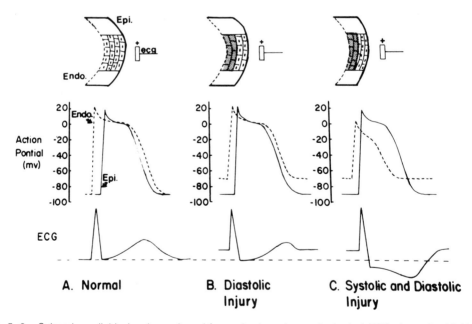

Fig. 5–6.   Subendocardial ischemia as viewed from a body surface unipolar (+) ECG electrode. (A) Normal ECG before ischemia. (B) Diastolic current of injury resulting from loss of resting membrane potential in subendocardial cells. (C) Systolic and diastolic currents of injury resulting from decreased action potential amplitude and duration and reduced resting membrane potential. See text.

waveform recorded from a unipolar chest wall electrode. In the normal heart, electrical activation spreads from endocardium to epicardium; the endocardial cells depolarize first, the epicardial cells depolarize last, and the QRS complex is positive (upright), reflecting an activation sequence toward the (+)ECG electrode. The normal sequence of recovery, however, is from epicardium to endocardium; the epicardial cell action potentials complete their repolarization before the endocardial cells, and the corresponding T wave is upright. It should be noted that both the ST segment and the TQ segment are on the isoelectric baseline, since the two action potentials are at the same voltage level during phases 2 (the plateau) and 4 (resting membrane potential).

In Figure 5–6B the endocardial cells have become ischemic resulting in a decrease in resting membrane potential. Activation still spreads from endocardium to epicardium; recovery, from epicardium to endocardium, and the ST segment remains on the isoelectric baseline. The TQ segment, however, has become elevated above the baseline because of the potential difference during phase 4 created by the injured endocardial cells relative to the nonischemic epicardial cells. This potential difference is called a *diastolic current of injury*, because it occurs during ventricular diastole. Modern ECG amplifiers are designed (condenser coupled) to correct baseline shifts involving the TQ segment, because these changes are usually due to artifacts. As a result, when the ischemic TQ segment elevation is electronically moved back to the baseline, the rest of the ECG waveform is shifted downward, including the ST segment, which drops below the baseline. This ECG change is not considered "true" ST segment depression, because it is not caused by a repolarization abnormality.

In Figure 5–6C, additional alterations in action potential morphology associated with subendocardial ischemia have oc-

curred. Both amplitude and duration of the ischemic action potentials have been reduced, resulting in a potential difference relative to the nonischemic epicardial cells during phase 2. This is called a *systolic current of injury*. The ECG manifestation of this new current of injury is "true" ST segment depression, which becomes added to the already existing ST depression previously described. In addition, because repolarization now spreads from endocardium to epicardium, the T wave becomes inverted. These changes in the ECG, resulting from systolic and diastolic currents of injury, are typical of the changes recorded during a positive exercise test.

Figure 5–7 illustrates what happens when the location of ischemia involves the subepicardial region of the ventricle. In either pure subepicardial ischemia (Fig. 5–7A) or transmural ischemia (Fig. 5–7B), systolic and diastolic currents of injury exist between the ischemic regions and the normal nonischemic myocardium. Because of the location of the ischemia relative to the ECG electrode, opposite shifts in TQ segments and ST-T waves create an ECG pattern of ST segment elevation with increased T wave amplitude.

In summary the displacement of ST segments above or below the isoelectric baseline is the result of two very distinct electrophysiologic events. The most specific change is the diastolic current of injury due to a decrease in phase-4 resting membrane potential in ischemic myocardium. The second mechanism is related to a systolic current of injury that develops between ischemic and normal myocardial cells and results in ST segment and T wave changes. The magnitude and direction of the ST-T wave changes are determined by the location of the ischemic region relative to the position of the (+)ECG electrodes on the body surface. ST segment elevation occurs when the ischemic myocardium and ECG electrodes are in close proximity without intervening normal tissue. ST segment depression is more likely to reflect suben-

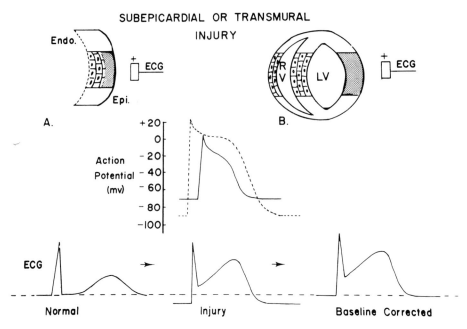

Fig. 5–7. *(A)* Subepicardial and *(B)* transmural injury as viewed from a body surface unipolar (+) ECG electrode. Systolic and diastolic currents of injury are generated between the injured and normal myocardium, causing ST segment elevation and increased T wave amplitude. See text.

docardial ischemia with normal heart muscle superimposed between the ischemic region and the ECG electrodes.

It should be realized that the preceding discussion is an oversimplification of a very complex geometric relationship between ventricular anatomy and the ECG leads on the body surface.[35] Nevertheless, it should suffice to facilitate a more comprehensive understanding of the ECG changes occurring with myocardial ischemia, especially those involving the ST segment and the T wave.

ECG Manifestations of Myocardial Ischemia

From the preceding discussion it is clear that the most important changes in ECG morphology resulting from myocardial ischemia are changes in the relationship between ST and TQ segments of the ECG. Unfortunately, the more specific changes involving the TQ segment cannot be differentiated from those that primarily affect the ST segment and the T wave. Primary ST-T wave abnormalities that mimic ischemia may be due to a number of other conditions including drugs, electrolyte abnormalities, mitral valve prolapse, and the like, all of which contribute to false-positive errors in exercise ECG.

Figure 5–8 illustrates the various ECG changes that have been associated with exercise-induced myocardial ischemia. In Figure 5–8A the normal resting ECG as might be recorded from lead V_5 is shown. Note the smooth transition from ST segment to T wave and the asymmetric T wave characteristic of the normal ECG. During exercise the initial portion of the ST segment normally drops below the baseline, as illustrated in Figure 5–8B, but the smooth transition between ST segment and T wave persists with return of the ST segment to baseline rather quickly. This normal response is called *J junctional* or *J point* depression. The J point defines the onset of the ST segment.

In Figure 5–8, the diagrams *C, D,* and

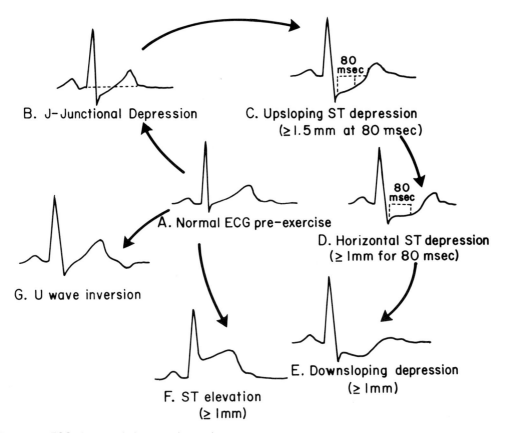

B. J–Junctional Depression

C. Upsloping ST depression
(≥1.5 mm at 80 msec)

80 msec

A. Normal ECG pre-exercise

80 msec

D. Horizontal ST depression
(≥ 1mm for 80 msec)

G. U wave inversion

E. Downsloping depression
(≥ 1mm)

F. ST elevation
(≥ 1mm)

Fig. 5–8.   ECG changes during exercise testing.

E, show the various types of ST segment changes that reflect subendocardial ischemia and characterize the "positive" exercise test. In Figure 5–8*C* the ST segment is still upsloping as in J junctional depression, but the transition between ST and T is sharp, and the ST segment remains significantly depressed (>1.5 mm) below the baseline at 80 msec beyond the J point. In Figure 5–8*D* the more typical horizontal ST segment depression is noted, where the ST segment is at least 1 mm (0.1 mV) depressed and flat for 80 msec or longer. Finally, in Figure 5–8*E* downsloping ST depression is illustrated, where the J point is 1 mm or more depressed, and the ST segment slopes downward. This may also be associated with T wave inversion.

Many patients with CHD develop all three ST segment abnormalities during ex-

ercise testing, although any one is sufficient to define a "positive" test. During exercise upsloping ST depression is first to appear, followed by horizontal and sometimes downsloping ST segment changes; usually the latter are only seen postexercise. In general left precordial leads V_4 to V_6 or unipolar leads using the V_5 chest position are the most sensitive recording sites for detecting ischemic ST segment changes. In approximately 10% of cases, however, the ischemic abnormalities are only seen in vertically oriented ECG leads such as lead II or aV_F.[12] These patients are more likely to have isolated right coronary artery lesions.

The ECG diagram in Figure 5–8*F* shows ST segment elevation, which is an unusual manifestation of exercise-induced myocardial ischemia and reflects transmural injury. This is a more serious ECG abnormality, because a greater mass of myocardium is involved. Chaitman et al.[37] have reviewed the pathogenesis of ST segment elevation during exercise and described three clinically different subsets of patients with this abnormality. One group of patients has the syndrome of variant angina characterized by rest pain, episodic ST segment elevation, and coronary artery spasm. Exercise-induced ST segment elevation may occur in 10% to 30% of these patients and is thought to be caused by alpha-adrenergic stimulation of the coronary vasculature.[38] A second group with exercise ST segment elevation has severe obstructive CAD. ST segment elevation in the right precordial leads or lead aV_L during exercise has been correlated with anterior wall ischemia and disease of the left anterior descending coronary artery.[39,40] Finally, ST segment elevation in leads with pathologic Q waves (patients with previous MIs) is not thought to be an ischemic finding but rather a manifestation of the wall motion abnormality in infarcted myocardium.[41] This is a common observation in testing post-MI patients and, unless associated with other abnormal findings, should not cause concern.

The most unusual and least understood ECG manifestation of ischemia is U wave inversion, illustrated in Figure 5–8G. Although originally described in the early exercise testing literature of the 1940s, this interesting abnormality did not reappear in the medical literature until 1979, when Gerson et al.[42] published their data. They described 36 patients with U wave inversion after exercise testing in a population of 248 patients undergoing coronary angiography. Thirty-five patients (97%) had significant CAD and, in 33 patients (92%) the disease involved either the left-main or left anterior descending coronary artery. Although inverted U waves may occasionally be detected during exercise, they are more likely to be seen immediately after exercise when the heart rate is slowing down. U wave inversion is defined as a negative dip below the isoelectric baseline that occurs after the end of the T wave and usually before the next P wave. It is seen most often in the precordial leads, 1 to 3 minutes after exercise. A return to an upright U wave several minutes later is helpful in verifying that U wave inversion truly occurred. U wave inversion is sometimes observed in resting ECGs but this is not a specific finding for coronary disease.

Examples of actual exercise ECG data illustrating the previously discussed ischemic abnormalities are shown in Figures 5–9 to 5–11.

Conduction Disturbances During Exercise Testing

Although unusual, atrioventricular (AV) and intraventricular heart block may occur during exercise testing. These abnormalities are not necessarily manifestations of myocardial ischemia unless accompanied by anginal symptoms or preceded by ST-T wave changes.

Atrioventricular block is rare during exercise testing. Type I second-degree AV block (Wenckebach) is usually a benign condition associated with increased vagal tone. It has been reported in very athletic individuals but has no clinical significance.[43] Mobitz II AV block, on the other hand, is a more serious manifestation of conduction system disease and usually occurs in the presence of preexisting bundle branch block. Type II AV block is associated with presyncopal and syncopal episodes. When detected during exercise testing or ambulatory monitoring, a permanent artificial pacemaker is indicated.

Exercise-induced bundle branch block is most often rate related and becomes apparent when the heart rate exceeds a critical value. It is almost always anxiety producing for the laboratory staff, because the sudden transition from narrow to wide QRS complexes suggests ventricular tachycardia. Unless the patient is well-known

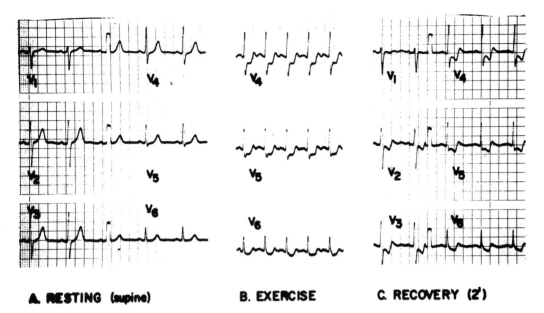

A. RESTING (supine)   **B. EXERCISE**   **C. RECOVERY (2′)**

Fig. 5–9.   Abnormal exercise ECG illustrating ST segment depression. *(A)* Resting (supine), *(B)* exercise *(C)* recovery (2′).

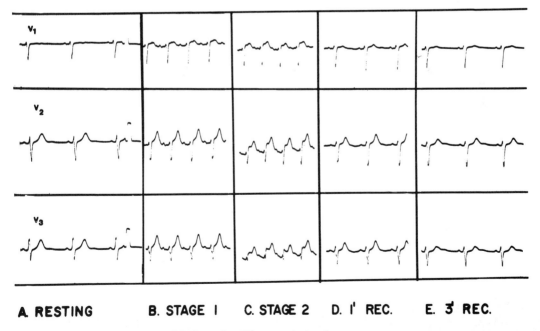

A. RESTING   **B. STAGE 1**   **C. STAGE 2**   **D. 1′ REC.**   **E. 3′ REC.**

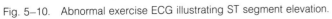

Fig. 5–10.   Abnormal exercise ECG illustrating ST segment elevation.

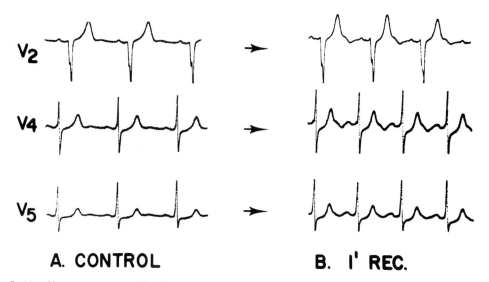

A. CONTROL   **B. 1' REC.**

Fig. 5–11. Abnormal exercise ECG illustrating U wave inversion.

to the staff for this problem, the test should be terminated to determine the nature of the sudden QRS change. Unlike ventricular tachycardia, the P wave to QRS relationship in bundle branch block remains constant, and as the heart rate slows down, the recognition of normal sinus rhythm is possible. The heart rate at which the bundle branch block disappears is always much lower than the rate at which it appeared during exercise (hysteresis). The development of bundle branch block during exercise is usually indicative of underlying conduction system disease but is not to be considered a "positive" test for ischemia unless there are other findings supporting a diagnosis of coronary disease. Although some of these patients may later develop permanent bundle branch block, exercise-induced block in asymptomatic individuals is considered a benign phenomenon.

The recognition of myocardial ischemia in the presence of intraventricular conduction abnormalities may be difficult, especially in left bundle branch block. Ventricular conduction defects cause the sequence of muscle activation to be altered, thus changing the shape and duration of the QRS complex. This change in activation necessitates an obligatory change in

the sequence of recovery, resulting in "secondary" ST-T wave changes. As a general rule, the direction of the ST-T deflection in bundle branch block is opposite to the terminal portion of the QRS complex. Figure 5–12 illustrates right and left bundle branch block as viewed in lead V_5. In left bundle branch block, the ST-T deflection is normally depressed below the baseline in the lateral precordial leads, which prevents recognition of myocardial ischemia with any degree of certainty. In right bundle

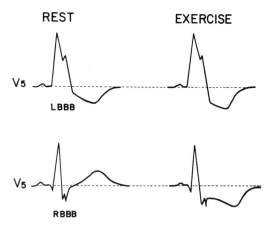

Fig. 5–12. Schematic drawing of rest and exercise lead V_5 in left bundle branch block (LBBB) and right bundle branch block (RBBB).

branch block, however, the ST-T wave configuration is similar to the normal ECG in lead V_5, therefore permitting adequate recognition of myocardial ischemia in most cases; similar ST-T wave changes in the right precordial leads or in other leads with terminal R' waves would not necessarily be indicative of ischemia. Because of the difficulties in recognizing ischemic ST-T wave changes in patients with left bundle branch block, it may be more cost-effective to utilize radionuclide techniques when ischemia is suspected.

Exercise Test Arrhythmias

One of the more challenging aspects of exercise testing is the recognition and management of exercise-induced cardiac arrhythmias. Various supraventricular and ventricular arrhythmias have been observed in clinically healthy subjects as well as in patients with heart disease. Their occurrence should not be considered a specific manifestation of any particular disease process such as myocardial ischemia, although it is well recognized that patients with ischemic heart disease are at greater risk for exercise-induced arrhythmias.

The mechanisms of cardiac arrhythmias vary somewhat from patient to patient but generally are related to either enhanced automaticity, delayed conduction, or both. Exercise may create a favorable environment for cardiac arrhythmias because of increased sympathetic activity, which accelerates phase 4 depolarization of ectopic pacemaker cells. In addition, the increased myocardial oxygen needs brought on by exercise may lead to ischemic arrhythmias in susceptible individuals. Myocardial ischemia induces an increased temporal dispersion of recovery potentials, delayed conduction, and enhanced automaticity, all of which may facilitate arrhythmogenesis.

Exercise may also cause ectopic atrial or ventricular activity to disappear due to the increase in sinus rate, which may result in overdrive suppression of ectopic foci. The suppression of a particular arrhythmia by increased heart rates, however, should not be used as evidence that the arrhythmia is benign. Conversely, an increase in frequency of ectopic beats with exercise is not necessarily an indication that the arrhythmia is due to serious underlying heart disease. Each arrhythmia should be analyzed according to the clinical context within which it occurs.

Table 5–9 lists the common arrhythmias that may occur during exercise testing. It is recommended that exercise testing personnel become familiar with the ECG characteristics of each arrhythmia, so that they may be recognized both on hard-copy rhythm strips as well as on the oscilloscope. A brief atlas of common cardiac arrhythmias is presented in Chapter 3. In addition a number of excellent textbooks and review articles are available on this subject.[44–46]

Supraventricular Arrhythmias

Exercise-induced premature atrial complexes (PACs) are quite common and generally pose no serious threat to the patient. Occasionally, however, they may precipitate one of the supraventricular tachyarrhythmias such as paroxsymal supraventricular tachycardia (PSVT), atrial fibrillation, or atrial flutter. When this oc-

Table 5–9. Exercise-Induced Cardiac Arrhythmias

Supraventricular arrhythmias
  Premature atrial complexes
    Isolated
    Couplets
    With or without aberration
  Paroxysmal supraventricular tachycardia
  Atrial fibrillation
  Atrial flutter

Ventricular arrhythmias
  Premature ventricular complexes
    Isolated
    Couplets
    Unifocal or multifocal
    R-on-T phenomenon
  Ventricular tachycardia
    Nonsustained
    Sustained
  Ventricular fibrillation

curs the test should be terminated. Most often the arrhythmia is transient and usually resolves within several minutes. The restoration of sinus rhythm in patients with sustained PSVT may be facilitated by having the patient perform the Valsalva maneuver or by carefully massaging the right or left carotid sinus (assuming clinical competency in performing this technique). Rarely will it be necessary to use pharmacologic intervention. The drug of choice is intravenous verapamil.

Atrial fibrillation and atrial flutter are unusual exercise-induced cardiac arrhythmias and rarely found in clinically healthy individuals. Most often these arrhythmias are due to cardiac dysfunction and associated increased pressure (stretch) in the right or left atrium. If they do not resolve spontaneously with cessation of exercise, it may be necessary to treat pharmacologically with a digitalis preparation, beta-blockers, or verapamil.

Ventricular Arrhythmias

Exercise-induced premature ventricular complexes (PVCs) are extremely common and have received a great deal of attention in the literature.[47–51] Although more frequent in CAD, these arrhythmias are found in all populations undergoing exercise testing. They tend to be more common with increasing age and at increasing heart rates during exercise. In CAD, however, they may occur at lower heart rates and work loads. Patients with previous MIs, multivessel disease, and left ventricular dysfunction are at greatest risk for PVCs and more serious ventricular arrhythmias.[48,49] In general the more severe the disease the greater the frequency of ventricular arrhythmias. Multifocal PVCs and R-on-T phenomena are considered to be more serious PVCs, although they are frequently found in both healthy and diseased populations. It is usually not necessary to terminate exercise in patients with frequent PVCs unless associated with limiting symptoms, manifestations of ischemia, or left ventricular dysfunction (exertional hypotension). In some patients PVCs appear to be related to a particular heart rate range, below and above which they disappear.

Ventricular tachycardia during exercise testing is always of great concern and necessitates immediate termination of the test. Defined as three or more consecutive PVCs, this arrhythmia may be brief, lasting only several seconds, or it may become sustained. Although most often seen in patients with organic heart disease, this arrhythmia may occasionally occur in clinically normal individuals. In patients with coronary disease, ventricular tachycardia is often associated with left ventricular dysfunction and is especially prone to develop during the postexercise period. It is recommended, therefore, that patients with ischemic ECG abnormalities be monitored for longer periods of time during recovery (8 to 10 minutes). In addition sitting after exercise may be less arrhythmogenic than the supine position in these patients.

Ventricular tachycardia during exercise testing usually reverts spontaneously to normal sinus rhythm without treatment. If the arrhythmia becomes sustained, however, emergency cardiac support may become necessary. For patients who are hemodynamically stable, intravenous lidocaine is the treatment of choice. If, on the other hand, the patient is unstable with hypotension and obtundation, direct-current (DC) cardioversion should be carried out under physician supervision. Fortunately this is an extremely rare complication of exercise testing.

Exercise-induced ventricular fibrillation is the least frequent and most serious of cardiac arrhythmias. When it occurs it is always a humbling experience for the laboratory staff, since it is so uncommon and, therefore, completely unexpected. The clinical setting is usually complicated CAD with ischemic ECG manifestations, left ventricular dysfunction, and chest pain. Figure 5–13 shows an occurrence of postexercise ventricular fibrillation in a 57-year-old man with mild stable angina pectoris 5 years post-MI. One year prior to this episode, he exercised into stage IV of the Bruce protocol with ischemic ST segment depression, U wave inversion, and mild anginal symptoms. Because of normal functional capacity and mild symptoms, he was managed medically. One year later, with stable symptoms, he again exercised into stage IV with similar ST segment and U wave abnormalities. In the fourth minute of recovery and after his symptoms had subsided, ventricular fibrillation occurred very unexpectedly. Within seconds he was successfully defibrillated, and several minutes later his ECG was back to the resting control configuration. This patient subsequently underwent coronary artery bypass surgery but has refused to undergo further exercise testing.

CLINICAL JUDGMENT IN EXERCISE TESTING

There is considerable controversy in the medical literature regarding the diagnostic value of exercise ECG testing in screening for CAD. Of particular concern is the extent to which the exercise test improves the ability to recognize coronary disease as compared to the routine clinical assessment. Chapter 3 emphasized the logical sequence of steps in establishing a cardio-vascular diagnosis, beginning with the history and physical examination and adding additional tests as necessary to answer *clinically important* questions. The detection of CAD in high-risk asymptomatic individuals is of major importance to our society, since the complications of this disease head the list of causes of death and disability. Clearly, there is a hierarchy of diagnostic tests for detecting significant coronary atherosclerosis, ranging from the low-cost, low-risk clinical assessment to the high-cost, technically complex coronary angiogram. Exactly where the exercise test fits into the hierarchy is the subject of this section.

Exercise Test Accuracy

The diagnostic accuracy of the exercise ECG test can only be discussed within a predefined, clinically relevant framework. If an abnormal or positive ECG response to exercise is to be considered evidence for significant coronary atherosclerosis, the definition of "abnormal" and "significant" must first be considered.

The ECG manifestations of myocardial ischemia have been described in the preceding section. The usual criteria for an abnormal ECG response to exercise are summarized in Table 5–10 and generally assume that the resting ECG is within normal limits. Most studies in the literature that have correlated exercise ECG data with coronary angiographic anatomy have

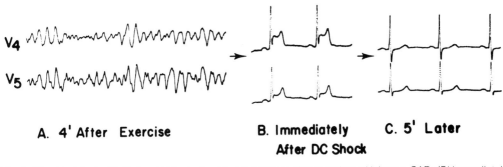

A. 4' After Exercise   **B. Immediately After DC Shock**   **C. 5' Later**

Fig. 5–13.   Ventricular fibrillation *(A)* 4 minutes after exercise testing in patient with known CAD. *(B)* Immediately after defibrillation there is ST segment elevation in leads V_4 and V_5, *(C)* which resolved within 5 minutes.

Table 5–10.   ECG Criteria For An
"Abnormal" Exercise Test[a]

ST segment depression
  Upsloping: ≥1.5 mm (0.15 mV) depression at 80
    msec from J point
  Horizontal: ≥1.0 mm (0.1 mV) depression for 80
    msec
  Downsloping: ≥1.0 mm (0.1 mV) depression at J
    point
ST segment elevation: ≥1.0 mm (0.1 mV) elevation
    above control resting ST segment
U wave inversion during or after exercise

[a]Assumes resting electrocardiogram (ECG) is within
normal limits.

only considered ST segment depression as
evidence for a positive exercise test. This
is clearly an oversimplification of the diagnostic utility of the exercise ECG, although a useful starting point for discussion.

The definition of a "significant" coronary lesion on angiography is also somewhat arbitrary, although it is based on experimental data relating changes in blood
flow and pressure gradients across stenotic
lesions.[52] There is a general consensus that
coronary blood flow is impaired, at rest,
when there is a 90% reduction in cross-
sectional area of a major coronary blood
vessel. This corresponds to a 75% reduction in luminal diameter. During exercise,
when there is an increased myocardial oxygen demand, a 75% reduction in cross-
sectional area (50% diameter reduction)
may be sufficient to impair oxygen delivery
to the myocardium. There are a number
of other factors such as anemia, coronary
collaterals, location of lesions, and superimposed coronary artery spasm that may
complicate the relationship between lesion
size and adequacy of myocardial blood supply. These confounding factors plus the
well-recognized limitations of angiographic assessment of lesion size make any
absolute definition of what is a "significant"
lesion almost impossible. Nevertheless, it is
clinically important to evaluate the exercise
ECG test in terms of its ability to differentiate patients with significant coronary

disease from those with insignificant lesions or normal arteries.

Table 5–11 is a standard table for determining the accuracy of the exercise test.
Data from 102 patients studied at the LDS
Hospital in Salt Lake City are shown. The
angiographic definition of coronary disease (CAD+) was 75% or greater reduction in the luminal diameter of a major
coronary vessel. The definition of an abnormal exercise test (T+) was greater than
or equal to 0.1 mV horizontal or downsloping ST segment depression. Using
these definitions there were 45 patients
with CAD+, of which 36 (80%) had an
abnormal exercise test (T+), and 9 (20%)
had a normal test (T−). Similarly, there
were 57 individuals who did not have angiographically significant coronary disease
(CAD−), of which 49 (86%) had a negative
test (T−), and 8 (14%) had an abnormal
test (T+).

The *sensitivity* of a diagnostic test reflects
the percentage of patients with documented disease who have abnormal test
findings (Table 5–12). In the preceding example 80% of the coronary disease group
had abnormal ST-segment depression, giving a sensitivity, or *true-positive* rate of 80%.
The 20% of patients with normal exercise
test findings define the *false-negative* rate.
Note that the true-positives and false-negatives add up to 100% of the coronary disease patients.

The *specificity* of a diagnostic test is a
measure of the test's ability to rule out disease in nondiseased individuals. In this example 86% of individuals without significant angiographic lesions had a normal
ECG response to exercise. The specificity
or *true-negative* rate was 86% with 14% *false-
positives*. The true-negatives and false-positives add up to 100% of the nondiseased
population.

The data presented in Table 5–11 are
comparable to many similar studies published in the literature. Froelicher[53] summarized six such studies involving over
1,400 patients and found an average spec-

Table 5–11. Treadmill–Angiographic Correlation in 102 Patients

Treadmill Test	CAD+ (%)	CAD- (%)	Totals
Abnormal (T+)	36 (80%)	8 (14%)	44
Normal (T-)	9 (20%)	49 (86%)	58
Totals	45 (100%)	57 (100%)	102

CAD+, significant coronary lesions on angiogram; CAD-, no significant coronary lesions on angiogram; T+, positive treadmill test; T-, negative treadmill test.

ificity of 90% and sensitivity of 70%. The sensitivity was lowest for patients with one-vessel disease (45%) and highest for three-vessel disease (86%).

There are a number of limitations to be found in exercise test–angiographic correlation studies. Most, if not all, of the patients participating in these studies are symptomatic (or else they would not have undergone angiographic procedures). The applicability of these data to the general population and especially to asymptomatic patients with coronary disease is open to question.[54] Another serious problem is related to the fact that the exercise ECG detects myocardial ischemia, whereas the coronary angiogram identifies anatomic obstructions. A more ideal evaluation of the exercise test would be to correlate the ECG findings with some other independent measure of myocardial ischemia. Unfortunately, other tests of myocardial ischemia still use the coronary angiogram as the gold-standard definition of disease. Finally, the exercise ECG test is limited to those patients whose resting ECGs are normal. In patients with resting ECG abnormalities such as bundle branch blocks and old MIs, other tests for ischemia that do

not rely on the ECG may be more appropriate.

Having defined the accuracy of the exercise test in terms of sensitivity and specificity based on angiographic assessment, it is clear that there are two kinds of errors associated with the test. The false-negative error refers to the percentage of normal tests in patients with significant coronary disease; the false-positive error reflects the percentage of abnormal tests in the non-diseased population. Like sensitivity and specificity, both of these errors depend on the criteria chosen for ischemic ECG abnormalities as well as the definition of "significant" CAD on angiography. Table 5–13 lists the causes of false-negative and false-positive errors.

Table 5–12. Sensitivity, Specificity, and Predictive Value

Treadmill Test	CAD+	CAD-
Abnormal (T+)	TP	FP
Normal (T-)	FN	TN

Sensitivity = TP/(TP + FN)

Specificity = TN/(TN + FP)

Predictive Value (+ test) = TP/(TP + FP)

TP, true-positives; FP, false-positives; FN, false-negatives; TN, true-negatives.

Table 5–13. Errors in Exercise ECG

False-negative errors
  CAD without myocardial ischemia
    Single-vessel disease with adequate collaterals
    Post-MI patients without ischemia
    Postcoronary artery bypass surgery patients
    Overestimation of angiographic lesion size
  Myocardial ischemia without ECG abnormalities
    Inadequate ECG lead system
    Preexisting ST-T wave changes on resting ECG
    Insufficient ischemia to affect the ECG

False-positive errors
  Myocardial ischemia without significant CAD
    Underestimation of lesion size
    Other conditions leading to ischemia
      Valvular heart disease with LVH
      Hypertensive heart disease
      Cardiomyopathy
      Severe anemia
  ECG changes that mimic ischemia
    Digitalis therapy
    Hypokalemia
    Hyperventilation-induced ECG changes
    Mitral valve prolapse syndrome
    Pectus excavatum chest deformity
    Neurocirculatory (vasoregulatory) asthenia

CAD, coronary artery disease; ECG, electrocardiogram; LVH, left ventricular hypertrophy.

The false-negative errors are found in 20% to 40% of the coronary disease population and depend somewhat on the clinical and angiographic characteristics of the patients being studied. Because the angiogram is used as the gold-standard for defining disease, most of the false-negatives are found in patients who *do not have* myocardial ischemia, although they may have "significant" lesions. Adequate collaterals in patients with single-vessel disease account for a large proportion of false-negatives. Most of these patients do not, in fact, have angina pectoris and are at low risk for future clinical events such as myocardial infarction or sudden death. This also applies to a large percentage of post-MI and postcoronary artery bypass surgery patients who no longer have myocardial ischemia. Finally, overestimation of angiographic lesion size may define "significant" disease in patients who do not have ischemic symptoms or ECG abnormalities.

There are, however, a small number of patients who have both significant coronary disease and myocardial ischemia but normal exercise ECG findings. These patients represent a potentially more serious false-negative error, since they are truly misdiagnosed by the exercise test. In some patients the standard ECG lead placement may be inadequate to detect the ischemic abnormality. Fox and his colleagues,[55] using a 16-lead precordial mapping system, showed improved recognition of ischemic ECG abnormalities in patients with single-vessel disease when compared with using the 12-lead ECG. In these patients the false-negative error was reduced from 58% using the 12-lead ECG to 26% with the precordial map. In some patients with significant coronary disease, there may not be sufficient ischemia to affect the ECG waveform, although the ischemia may be recognized with other more sensitive techniques (thallium perfusion defects or segmental wall motion abnormalities). This may occur in patients with preexisting ECG abnormalities or those taking beta-blocking drugs.

The false-positive errors occur in 10% to 15% of the nondiseased population undergoing exercise testing. Again, the percentage of errors is related to the characteristics of the population being studied. One group of false-positives are patients with other forms of heart disease who get ischemic ECG changes because of increased myocardial oxygen demands that are greater than the available supply. Valvular heart disease, severe hypertension with left ventricular hypertrophy, and cardiomyopathies may all be associated with exercise-induced ischemia. Severe anemia may also be associated with ischemic ECG abnormalities due to the inadequate oxygen-carrying capacity of the coronary blood. It is unlikely, however, that this is clinically important, because these patients rarely undergo maximal exercise testing.

Other patients with false-positive exercise tests include those with whom the ECG only mimics ischemia. Drugs and electrolyte abnormalities head the list of false-positive errors. Digitalis preparations are the major offending drugs. There are characteristic resting ECG changes in digitalized patients consisting of sagging ST segment depression with flat to slightly inverted T waves and shortened QT intervals. During exercise the ST segment becomes more depressed and often meets criteria for a positive test. Unlike true ischemic ECG abnormalities, patients on digitalis may have more positive ECG abnormalities early in exercise that become less abnormal with increasing heart rates and work loads.[56] If at all possible it is recommended that patients be taken off digitalis for at least 3 weeks prior to diagnostic testing. Otherwise, exercise radionuclide studies may be more appropriate in these patients.

The major electrolyte abnormality associated with false-positive exercise tests is hypokalemia, frequently the result of thiazide diuretic therapy. The resting ECG in these patients often shows slight ST segment depression, low amplitude T waves, and prominent U waves. Again, these patients are often easy to recognize, and they should not undergo diagnostic testing until their potassium deficits have been corrected.

Mitral valve prolapse is a common and often benign abnormality of the mitral valve apparatus with characteristic auscultatory and echocardiographic findings. Auscultation at the cardiac apex in these patients often reveals a midsystolic click with or without a late systolic murmur. The murmur is due to mitral regurgitation associated with the prolapsed mitral valve leaflet. For reasons that are unclear, these patients often have resting and exercise ST-T wave abnormalities that mimic ischemia. There is also an increased tendency for cardiac arrhythmias to occur. This condition is more common in women and may account for a portion of the increased false-positives in women.

Another category of patients with false-positive ECG changes are those with labile, positional, and/or hyperventilation-induced ST-T wave changes. This also seems to be more common in women and in individuals who have a vertically oriented frontal plane QRS axis (+90 degrees). Ellestad[57] believes that some of these patients may have ECG changes because of alterations in sympathetic tone and has labeled this phenomenon "Reynolds syndrome." Another condition that may be related to sympathetic nervous system imbalance has been called neurocirculatory (or vasoregulatory) asthenia. Also known as the hyperkinetic heart syndrome, these patients often complain of dyspnea, palpitations, nervousness, and vague nonanginal chest pains. Friesinger et al.[58] have described exercise ECG abnormalities in these patients that mimic ischemia. Beta-blocking drugs may block the ST-T changes associated with those conditions, further supporting a sympathetic nervous system etiology. These patients do not generally experience anginal symptoms during testing, and their ECG abnormalities are minimal.

APPLICATION OF BAYES' THEOREM TO EXERCISE TESTING

The sensitivity and specificity of the exercise test define the accuracy of the test in differentiating patients with known CAD from nondiseased individuals. As discussed in the preceding section, the exercise test is far from perfect, having both false-positive and false-negative errors. Because of this clinical reality, it is useful to express the descriptors of exercise test accuracy in term of probabilities, as this will enhance an understanding of the value of diagnostic exercise testing in various populations.

The sensitivity (percentage of true-positives) can be thought of as the probability that a patient with known coronary disease will have an abnormal test. This can be expressed as a *conditional probability*, $P(T+|CAD+)$. Similarly, the specificity of the test defines the probability that a normal individual will have a negative test; that is, $P(T-|CAD-)$. The false-negative probability can be expressed as $P(T-|CAD+)$; the false-positive, as $P(T+|CAD-)$. In all of these probabilities, the condition that is known is the clinical state of the person being tested (i.e., either CAD+ or CAD-), and the unknown is whether the test will be positive or negative. Although these terms are useful in characterizing the diagnostic accuracy of the exercise test, they do not answer the questions being asked in a diagnostic laboratory.

When a patient undergoes diagnostic exercise testing, the known condition is the outcome of the test, that is, "positive" or "negative" for ischemia. The unknown is whether or not the patient has coronary disease. The conditional probability, $P(CAD+|T+)$, is called the *predictive value of a positive test* and is the probability that coronary disease is present if the test is abnormal. Similarly, the *predictive value of a negative test* can be expressed as P(CAD−|T−) and is the probability that coronary disease is not present when the test is normal.

Bayes' theorem of conditional probability states that the predictive value of a test depends on the descriptors of test accuracy (sensitivity and specificity) as well as the prevalence of disease in the population being tested. Using the terminology described previously, this important relationship can be expressed as follows:

From this example it can be seen that the number of false-positives and false-negatives in a population depends greatly on the characteristics of the population. In a population where there is very little disease, most of the positive tests will be false-positives. In a population of high disease prevalence, most of the negative tests will be false-negatives. In both of these extremes, the test adds little new diagnostic information.

How does all this apply to the individual

$$P(CAD+|T+) = \frac{P(CAD+)\,P(T+|CAD+)}{P(CAD+)\,P(T+|CAD+)\,+\,P(CAD-)\,P(T+|CAD-)}$$

The terms P(CAD+) and P(CAD−) are called *pretest* or *prior* probabilities and reflect the probability of coronary disease (CAD+) or no coronary disease (CAD−) before testing. From a population perspective, these terms define the prevalence of disease in that particular population. Together, they add up to 100% of the population. For example, if 10% of the population has underlying coronary disease, P(CAD+) is 10% and P(CAD−) is 90%.

A similar Bayes' theorem formula can be expressed for the predictive value of a negative test result:

person who is undergoing diagnostic exercise testing? The prevalence of coronary disease in the population is not of immediate concern. What is of interest, however, is the patient's pretest probability of coronary disease. A clinical assessment prior to testing is necessary for determining the prior risk, P(CAD+). In a classic publication, Diamond and Forrester[59] discuss how age, sex, risk factors, and symptoms can be used to determine the pretest probability of coronary disease. If the patient is asymptomatic, P(CAD+) can be estimated from the *Coronary Risk Handbook*,[60] published by

$$P(CAD-|T-) = \frac{P(CAD-)\,P(T-|CAD-)}{P(CAD-)\,P(T-|CAD-)\,+\,P(CAD+)\,P(T-|CAD+)}$$

These two equations for predictive value can best be understood from a population example illustrated in Table 5–14. In population A only 10% have coronary disease; the predictive value of a positive test is 39% (61% of the positive tests are false-positives). The predictive value of a negative test is 97% (only 3% of the negative tests are false-negatives). The same test applied to population B, where coronary disease prevalence is 90%, yields strikingly different predictive values. The predictive value of a positive test becomes 98% (only 2% false-positives); the predictive value of a negative test is 32% (68% false-negatives).

the AHA and distributed by its state affiliates. This set of probability tables is based on statistics from the Framingham heart disease study[2] and is used to estimate an individual's risk of developing CHD based on age, sex, and risk factors. Diamond and Forrester[59] show how these probabilities of coronary disease incidence can be equated to the actual prevalence of disease in the population. For example, an asymptomatic patient with a 10% probability of developing clinical manifestations of coronary disease in 6 years also has approximately the same risk of having angiographically significant disease at the time of study.

Table 5–14.   The Predictive Value of a Positive and Negative Exercise Test in Two Hypothetical Populations

Test Accuracy:	1. Sensitivity = 80% = P(T+	CAD+)
	2. False (−) = 20% = P(T−	CAD+)
	3. Specificity = 86% = P(T−	CAD−)
	4. False (+) = 14% = P(T+	CAD−)

Population A: Coronary disease prevalence of 10%
P(CAD+) = 10%); P(CAD− = 90%

$$P(CAD+|T+) = \frac{10 \times 80}{(10 \times 80) + (90 \times 14)} = \frac{800}{2,060} = 39\%$$

$$P(CAD-|T-) = \frac{90 \times 86}{(90 \times 86) + (10 \times 20)} = \frac{7,740}{7,940} = 97\%$$

Population B: Coronary disease prevalence of 90%
P(CAD+) = 90%; P(CAD−) = 10%

$$P(CAD+|T+) = \frac{90 \times 80}{(90 \times 80) + (10 \times 14)} = \frac{7,200}{7,340} = 98\%$$

$$P(CAD-|T-) = \frac{10 \times 86}{(10 \times 86) + (90 \times 20)} = \frac{860}{2,660} = 32\%$$

In patients who are having symptoms of chest discomfort, Diamond and Forrester[59] present data for pretest likelihoods of coronary disease based on age, sex, and classification of symptoms into three categories: Nonanginal chest pain, atypical angina, or typical angina. The clinical descriptions of these symptoms are discussed in Chapter 3.

Figure 5–14 illustrates a graphic representation of Bayes' theorem, relating pretest probabilities, ranging from 0% to 100%, to the predictive value of the exercise test result. The actual shape of the two curves is dependent on the sensitivity and specificity of the test. For this illustration, a sensitivity of 80% and specificity of 86% were chosen to correspond to the data presented in Table 5–11. The two examples illustrated in Table 5–14 are also indicated on the predictive value curves.

It should be apparent that Bayes' theo-

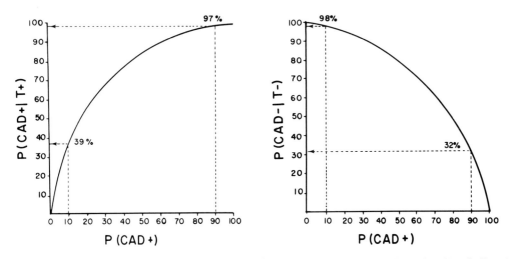

Fig. 5–14.   Bayesian analysis of diagnostic exercise ECG testing. The predictive values of positive (left) and negative (right) tests are related to the pretest probabilities of coronary artery disease, P(CAD+). See text.

rem is applicable to just about every diagnostic test in medicine. The message of Bayes' theorem is that the interpretation or significance of a given test result requires a knowledge of *both* the accuracy of the test for diagnosing the disease in question *and* the patient's pretest likelihood of having that disease before the test is performed. For patients with very low pretest risk (<10%), an abnormal test is most often a false-positive; for patients with very high pretest risk (>75%), a negative test is usually a false-negative. The diagnostic test offers the most information content in patients with an intermediate risk for disease. In screening for occult CAD, the exercise test is most useful in patients with significant coronary risk factors (pretest risk >10%) and in patients with atypical chest pain symptoms.

The preceding examples using Bayes' theorem represent rather simplistic illustrations of the application of information theory to diagnostic testing. In these examples the exercise test response was dichotomized into "positive" or "negative" categories based on a single criterion of 0.1 mV ST segment depression. A mathematically more sophisticated version of Bayes' theorem has been described by Diamond et al.,[61] which permits calculating the predictive values for different degrees of ST segment depression. This approach results in a significant increase in the diagnostic content of the exercise ECG when the specific magnitude of the ST segment depression is used instead of categoric criteria such as 0.1 mV depression. The predictive value of a "positive" test becomes progressively greater with increasing degrees of ST segment depression.

Rifkin and Hood[62] have also analyzed exercise test data published in the literature and constructed Bayesian graphs relating pretest probabilities to predictive values for half-millimeter partitions of ST segment depression. They too concluded that the predictive value depends on the degree of ST segment depression. They also thought

that the terms *positive* and *negative* are inappropriate descriptors of exercise test results; instead, they suggested that the test be interpreted as a continuum of risk based on the degree of ST segment abnormality.

These concepts have important implications for relatively low-risk, asymptomatic subjects who are being screened for CAD. A positive test in this population should be interpreted only as *another risk factor* for coronary disease that increases that patient's probability of having disease. If a patient with a 10% pretest risk has a certain degree of ST segment depression such that the predictive value becomes 40%, this represents a fourfold increase in risk. The predictive value can now become the *new* pretest risk for a subsequent diagnostic test such as a radionuclide study.

Patterson et al.[63] have published nomograms for diagnosing the presence or absence of CAD based on sequential Bayesian analyses applied to a series of tests. Using this approach, a cost-effective strategy can be designed for each patient undergoing diagnostic testing, beginning with the low-cost risk factor assessment and symptom classification, moving next to the exercise ECG test and then, if necessary, the more expensive exercise thallium test. Each test result becomes the new pretest probability for the subsequent test until a degree of certainty has been achieved that allows for the appropriate treatment decision to be made.

DIAGNOSTIC EXERCISE TESTING

The decision to perform a diagnostic test in medicine is one that should be made only after careful consideration of the cost/benefit ratio to the patient. This is especially important in cardiovascular medicine, where recent technologic advances have given us a plethora of new and expensive procedures. As these procedures become increasingly more available, there is a natural tendency to want the most up-to-date quantitative assessment for our patients.

Exercise ECG testing, although less expensive than many cardiovascular procedures, has become rather routine in screening for coronary disease. There has been some concern that the test may be over-utilized, especially in low-risk populations. The following sections will focus on the diagnostic applications of exercise testing and indicate those clinical situations where exercise testing is likely to contribute to patient management.

Screening of Asymptomatic Individuals

This is the most controversial area of diagnostic testing because of the false-positive problem. Bayes' theorem implies that the lower the pretest risk, the more likely an abnormal test result is a false-positive. Yet, clinical CHD often strikes catastrophically with acute MI or sudden death as the first manifestations. The challenge in screening the asymptomatic population is to identify a high-risk subset who are most likely to benefit from exercise testing.

There is an unfortunate tendency to use age as the only cutoff for when to recommend exercise testing in asymptomatic subjects. The ACSM, for example, recommends that all apparently healthy individuals over age 44 undergo maximal exercise testing before starting an exercise training program.[6] The *Coronary Risk Handbook*,[60] however, states that 45-year-old men in the Framingham Study without major coronary risk factors only had 2% to 3% probability of developing CHD in 6 years. Bayes' theorem indicates that in this population, over 85% of positive tests are likely to be false-positives. Even if the age cutoff were increased to age 50, the false-positive problem would be substantial and preclude any cost-effective application of the exercise ECG test.

A more practical approach is to establish a pretest probability threshold below which exercise testing would generally not be indicated and above which it would be. Using conventional ECG analysis techniques, a pretest probability of coronary disease greater than 10% is a useful indication for diagnostic exercise testing, since a positive test has a predictive value approaching 50% or greater depending on the degree of ST segment depression. Figure 5–15 illustrates the serum cholesterol and systolic blood pressure values associated with a 10% coronary disease risk for men and women using *Coronary Risk Handbook* data.[60] Figure 5–15A and B represent nonsmokers; C and D represent smokers. These data are applicable only to nondiabetics and those with normal resting ECGs. For each age group the values of systolic blood pressure and serum cholesterol that fall on the age-specific lines indicate a pretest probability of approximately 10%. Values falling to the right of or above the age-specific lines reflect pretest probabilities greater than 10%; values to the left and below indicate pretest probabilities less than 10%. For each age group males and cigarette smokers are at increased risk compared to females and nonsmokers at comparable blood pressure and cholesterol levels.

It must be emphasized that the plots in Figure 5–15 represent, at best, only general guidelines for diagnostic exercise testing in asymptomatic subjects. For each age group other factors such as diastolic hypertension, diabetes mellitus, resting ECG abnormalities, and family history of premature CAD should influence the decision. It is also likely that using more sophisticated computerized criteria will improve the sensitivity and specificity of the exercise test, thereby increasing the predictive value of a positive test in subjects with less than 10% pretest risk. Nevertheless, it should be clear that guidelines for testing must be carefully considered in order to avoid indiscriminate testing of individuals who are not likely to benefit from the test. These guidelines need to be flexible and will most certainly evolve as the state of the art improves.

In addition to defining guidelines for

NONSMOKERS

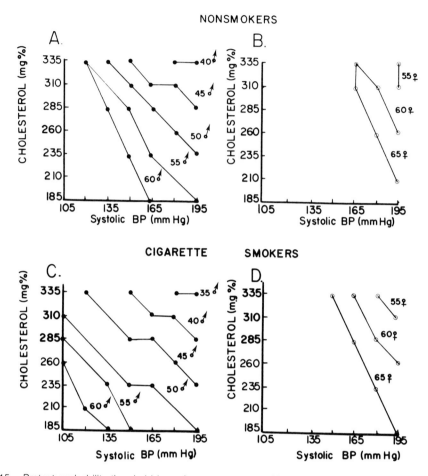

Fig. 5–15. Pretest probability threshold based on age, sex, smoking habits, cholesterol, and systolic blood pressure. Values above and to the right of the age-specific lines indicate P(CAD+) greater than 10%. A. Nonsmokers, men; B. Nonsmokers, women; C. Cigarette smokers, men; D. Cigarette smokers, women.

testing asymptomatic subjects, a strategy for managing the positive responder needs to be considered.[64,65] In the absence of symptoms, an abnormal ECG response to exercise increases that individual's risk for coronary disease, although the majority of positive tests in asymptomatic subjects are false-positives.

There are basically three degrees of abnormal responses that occur when testing for CAD: (1) the high-risk positive test; (2) the intermediate-risk response; and (3) the low-risk response. One basis for this classification was published by McNeer et al.[66] in a study of over 1,400 patients undergoing exercise testing, coronary angiography,

and long-term follow-up. The ability to exercise into stage IV of the Bruce protocol (>10 METs) or achieve a maximal heart rate greater than 160 beats per minute (bpm) was associated with an excellent prognosis and low probability for three-vessel or left main coronary disease. In contrast, patients with ECG abnormalities in stage I or II or at heart rates less than 120 bpm had a poor prognosis with a high probability of triple vessel or left main coronary disease. The intermediate-risk group fell in between these two extremes.

Based on these data, it seems reasonable to recommend coronary angiography for those patients with high-risk abnormalities, since they are more likely to be candidates for coronary artery bypass surgery or coronary angioplasty. Similarly, patients with low-risk abnormalities can be managed conservatively with serial exercise testing and treatment of coronary risk factors. The data indicate that these patients are very unlikely to experience coronary events during short-term follow-up (12 months). The intermediate-risk responder should probably undergo further noninvasive testing such as thallium 201 scintigraphy and, if positive, be followed by coronary angiography. Patients with triple-vessel or left-main disease are good candidates for surgery.

Differential Diagnosis of Chest Pain

In the symptomatic population the exercise test is of proven value. Diamond and Forrester[59] have provided data on pretest probabilities for men and women whose symptoms can be categorized as nonanginal chest pain, atypical angina, and typical angina (Table 5–15). In men over age 40 and women over age 60, symptoms of *typical angina* are associated with pretest probabilities of 90% or greater. Exercise testing would not be expected to add significant diagnostic information in these patients, athough testing might be useful in assessing cardiovascular functional capacity and disease severity.

When symptoms are less than typical for angina pectoris, or when typical angina occurs in younger patients, the exercise test can contribute important diagnostic information. Patients able to achieve high work loads and heart rates greater than 85% of their age-predicted maximum without significant chest discomfort or ECG abnormalities are very unlikely to have obstructive coronary lesions as the basis for their symptoms. On the other hand patients who develop anginal symptoms during exercise along with diagnostic ECG changes have a very high probability of underlying CAD. Further treatment decisions can be made by classifying the abnormal responses into low-risk, intermediate-risk, and high-risk abnormalities as defined by McNeer et al.[66] Symptomatic patients with low-risk abnormalities have a good short-term prognosis and can usually be managed conservatively with antianginal medications and risk-factor modification. The intermediate-risk and high-risk responders who have exercise-induced angina and ECG abnormalities should proceed directly to coronary angiography and be considered for angioplasty or surgery.

The subset of symptomatic patients who have exercise-induced chest pain *without* ECG abnormalities is uncommon. Weiner et al.[67] determined that the predictive value of exercise-induced angina for coronary disease was 90% in their series of 302 patients. This is comparable to the predictive value of typical angina by history as reported by Diamond and Forrester[59] for men over age 40 and women over age 60. In Weiner's study,[67] exercise-induced angina was also as predictive as ST segment

Table 5–15.   Pretest Probability (%) of Coronary Disease According to Age, Sex, and Symptoms

Age	Nonanginal Chest Pain		Atypical Angina		Typical Angina	
	Men	Women	Men	Women	Men	Women
30–39	5	1	22	4	70	26
40–49	14	3	46	13	87	55
50–59	22	8	59	32	92	79
60–69	28	19	67	54	94	91

Modified from Diamond, G.A., and Forrester, J.S.: Analysis of probability as an aid in the clinical diagnosis of coronary artery disease. N. Engl. J. Med., *300*:1350, 1979.

depression and, therefore, can be used as another criterion for a positive test. Using a similar management strategy as described for asymptomatic subjects and symptomatic patients with ECG abnormalities, high-risk patients whose symptoms are limiting at low work loads (≤4 METs) and/or low heart rates (<120 bpm) should undergo coronary angiographic studies. Low-risk patients with good exercise tolerance and normal heart rate responses to exercise can be followed with periodic exercise testing and antianginal medication. The intermediate-risk subgroup should undergo further noninvasive testing and, if abnormal, followed by coronary angiography.

Evaluation of Syncope and Palpitations

Although ambulatory ECG monitoring is usually the preferred diagnostic test for evaluating patients with symptoms of syncope, presyncope, or palpitations, exercise testing is useful if the symptoms are clearly exercise related. Many patients complaining of intermittent palpitations do not have significant cardiac findings on history or physical examination; the symptoms can often be related to episodes of sinus tachycardia or benign premature beats. These patients usually do not need sophisticated diagnostic studies.

In patients with known heart disease, especially those with ischemic manifestations, provocative testing to induce arrhythmic events is often necessary for optimal management. Many of these patients are at increased risk for sudden death and require complex antiarrhythmic therapies. Arrhythmias associated with ST segment abnormalities or decreased physical working capacity are bad prognostic signs and indicate the need for aggressive management strategies including cardiac catheterization and surgical procedures.

There are no particular exercise testing methods that are specifically designed for evaluating arrhythmias or transient conduction defects. The exercise protocol should be chosen according to the patient's ability to exercise and clinical status. The decision to terminate an exercise test because of arrhythmias provoked by exercise is determined by the characteristics of the arrhythmia and the clinical state of the patient. Serious ventricular arrhythmias such as paroxysmal ventricular tachycardia, frequent multifocal PVCs, couplets or R-on-T phenomenon, as well as rapid atrial tachyarrhythmias require terminating the test prematurely. Isolated PVCs that develop during exercise in the absence of other ECG or clinical abnormalities do not necessitate terminating the test.

The interpretation of the exercise test prematurely terminated by an arrhythmia is often difficult. If the patient achieved at least 85% to 90% of the predicted maximal heart rate without ST-T changes or chest pain, it is unlikely that the arrhythmia was caused by myocardial ischemia. Termination of the test at lower work loads makes the test inadequate to rule out ischemia, unless there are ischemic ECG abnormalities. If the patient has no other manifestations of heart disease and the arrhythmia is not reproducible on repeat testing, it is unlikely that the arrhythmia is clinically important.

Occasionally, serious exercise-induced ventricular arrhythmias have been observed in clinically healthy individuals who have either smoked cigarettes or consumed caffeine-containing drinks prior to testing. Repeat testing after avoiding these noxious stimulants is often normal, and further cardiac workup usually fails to uncover underlying heart disease.

ADVANCES IN DIAGNOSTIC EXERCISE TESTING

In the preceding sections the diagnostic utility of the exercise test was discussed primarily from the viewpoint of ST-T wave changes visually observed in selected ECG leads. This was the state of the art in exercise testing up to the 1970s and is still the primary method of exercise ECG analysis. In recent years, however, there have been a number of interesting advances in diagnostic testing that have significantly improved the predictive accuracy of the test for detecting CAD. In selected patient populations these advanced methods have resulted in more accurate detection of myocardial ischemia as well as more quantitative assessment of ischemic size and location. Although most exercise testing laboratories continue to rely on visual ST-T wave analysis, it is likely that many of these new concepts will eventually become incorporated into routine exercise testing. Table 5–16 lists several important advances that have improved the diagnostic accuracy of the exercise test.

Computer Processing of the Exercise ECG

This is, perhaps, the most established of the "new" advances in exercise testing, having been introduced over 20 years ago. Computer applications to the analysis of resting ECGs have become increasingly utilized in medical centers where a large number of ECGs are processed daily. It was only natural to extend these techniques to the exercise testing laboratory where signal/noise ratio problems often interfere with accurate visual interpretation of the exercise ECG. In addition, advances in microcircuit technology have resulted in the development of relatively inexpensive but powerful microcomputers, which are affordable by most clinical testing laboratories. Many of the commercially available exercise testing systems already have digi-

Table 5–16. Advances in Diagnostic Exercise Testing

1. Computer analysis of the exercise ECG
2. Multivariate analysis of exercise test data
3. Quantitative ST segment analysis
4. Precordial and body surface ECG mapping
5. Cardiokymography

tal processing features, although the full potential of computerized analyses of exercise ECG data has yet to be explored.

Bhargava et al.[68] have reviewed the literature on computer processing of exercise ECG data and discussed different approaches taken by the commercially available systems. Most systems use signal-averaging techniques to reduce random noise and compute averaged complexes for quantitative ST segment analysis. Various computer-derived criteria of ST segment amplitude, slope, and area have been proposed, although optimal criteria for detecting myocardial ischemia have yet to be determined. Several studies, summarized by Simoons et al.,[69] have compared visual with computer-assisted exercise ECG interpretation and showed improved sensitivity and specificity for coronary disease with the computer systems. Only small numbers of patients and highly selected populations were evaluated in these studies. It is unlikely that computer processing of ECG data derived from the usual exercise ECG leads will significantly improve the predictive accuracy of the diagnostic exercise test, unless other clinical and hemodynamic variables are taken into consideration in the classification process.

Multivariate Analysis of Exercise Test Data

The ECG response to exercise is only one indicator of myocardial ischemia that can be obtained from the exercise test. A number of studies have been reported that demonstrate a significant improvement in the diagnostic accuracy of exercise testing by incorporating more quantitative information from the exercise ECG along with hemodynamic and other clinical variables. Using multivariate linear discriminant analyses, the relative weights of exercise test variables can be calculated, and a treadmill score computed that indicates the severity of coronary disease. The higher the overall score the more likely a particular test will be indicative of severe CAD.

Cohn et al.[70] derived treadmill scores in 405 patients undergoing both exercise testing and coronary angiographic studies. Variables included in the score were ST segment parameters (maximum depth, slope, time of onset of ischemic change, duration of changes in recovery), severity of ventricular arrhythmias, blood pressure and heart rate responses to exercise, presence or absence of chest pain during exercise, and age and sex of the patient. Of all these variables, the depth and configuration of ST segment depression and the patient's age were the most influential in predicting the presence and severity of CAD. In addition, there was a 10% to 15% improvement in predictive accuracy using the treadmill score compared to simple ST segment criteria.

A major advantage of using exercise test "scores" for diagnosing CAD is that each exercise test result falls into a spectrum of possible responses rather than being simply dichotomized into "positive" or "negative" based on a single criterion of ST segment depression. In addition, a more accurate assessment of disease severity can usually be made from the magnitude of the total score for a given patient.

Using similar multivariate techniques in a study of 608 patients, Kansal et al.[71] derived treadmill scores from a slightly different set of exercise test variables. They also reported improved diagnostic accuracy compared to ST-segment criteria alone. The additional variables considered included maximal heart rate achieved, maximal double product, and total treadmill time. For male patients the most significant variables were scored as follows: (1) maximal exercise heart rate less than 80% of predicted maximum (9 points); (2) ST segment change greater than 1 mm from baseline control (6 points); (3) age greater than 55 years (5 points); and (4) treadmill time less than 8 minutes using the Bruce protocol (3 points). Using these variables optimal diagnostic accuracy was achieved when CAD was defined by a score of 7 or greater. In women the most significant exercise test variables for predicting coronary disease were maximal heart rate less than 90% of predicted (4 points), and treadmill time less than 6 minutes (3 points). Age and ST segment changes were less important but contributed slightly to the diagnostic accuracy of the test. This study emphasized the importance of including non-ST-T variables in the diagnostic assessment for CAD.

Quantitative ST Segment Analyses

Hollenberg et al.[72] described a computerized technique for quantitating continuous changes in the ST segment response to exercise in leads aV_F and V_5. A score for each patient was computed that took into consideration the ST segment deviation from baseline (measured at the J point), ST segment slope, duration of exercise, and the percentage of maximal predicted heart rate achieved. In their study population the sensitivity (the percentage of true-positives) increased by 10% to 15% compared to visual ST segment analyses with no loss in specificity. The score was also very accurate in distinguishing a group of patients with three-vessel or left main coronary disease from those with less severe disease. The disadvantage of this technique was the necessity for continuous computer processing of the ECG signals.

More recently, Hollenberg et al.[73] compared the accuracy of the computerized treadmill score with standard ECG criteria in 377 asymptomatic men with low prevalence of coronary disease. Using standard visual criteria 12% of subjects had a positive test, whereas less than 1% had a "positive" treadmill score. Coronary angiography in the 10 subjects with the highest scores revealed only 1 subject with significant single-vessel disease. The authors concluded that the computerized score improved the specificity of the exercise test in asymptomatic subjects by eliminating most of the false-positives.

A completely different approach to quantitating the ST segment response to exercise was taken by Elamin et al.[74] From each of 13 leads of ECG data, these investigators plotted ST segment depression against increasing heart rates during exercise. The plots were evaluated to determine the maximum slope of the regression line relating ST segment depression to heart rate. This "maximum ST/HR slope" was used as an index of myocardial ischemia and compared to coronary angiographic findings in 206 patients with anginal symptoms. In this population, the ranges of maximum ST/HR slopes were completely different (no overlap) in patients without significant coronary disease, and in patients with single-, double-, and triple-vessel disease. A major disadvantage of this technique was the time required to compute the maximum ST/HR slope (average of 3 hours per test), because the measurements were all made by visual analysis of the raw ECG data. Nevertheless, the strikingly accurate prediction of coronary disease and the number of obstructed arteries demands that this approach be explored in other patient populations using computer techniques to simplify the measurements.

Precordial and Body Surface ECG Mapping

Because exercise-induced myocardial ischemia is a localized phenomenon that depends on the anatomic distribution of obstructive coronary lesions, more extensive ECG lead sets have been investigated in an attempt to improve the predictive accuracy of the exercise ECG.

Fox et al.[55] have developed a simple but accurate 16-lead precordial grid illustrated in Figure 5–16. ECG signals from each lead during exercise were analyzed visually for ST segment depression, and regions of increasing ST segment depression were plotted on diagrams of the precordial grid. A typical plot of a patient with isolated right

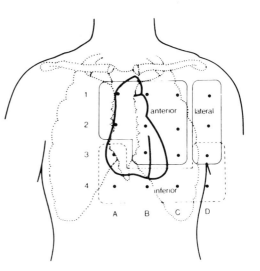

Fig. 5–16.   Sixteen-lead precordial grid used by Fox et al.[55] From Fox, K.M., Selwyn, A., Oakley, D., and Shillingford, J.P.: Relation between the precordial projection of S-T segment changes after exercise and coronary angiographic findings. Am. J. Cardiol., 44:1068, 1979.

CAD is shown in Figure 5–17, illustrating ST segment depression localized to the inferior region of the precordium. Precordial maps were compared with standard exercise ECG leads in 100 symptomatic patients undergoing coronary angiography studies.[55] Using 0.1-mV ST segment depression as criteria for a positive test, the precordial grid technique increased the sensitivity from 80% (standard ECG leads) to 96% with no change in specificity (90% for both lead systems). Of interest, the reduction in false-negatives was entirely due to improved detection of localized ischemia in patients with single-vessel disease. In these patients, ST segment depression was confined to leads other than the standard 12-lead ECG. Furthermore, the location of the ischemic abnormalities on the grid accurately identified the diseased coronary artery. Right coronary lesions involved inferior regions of the grid; left anterior descending (LAD) lesions, the superior-located ECG leads; left circumflex, the lateral regions. If these findings can be reproduced in other populations of patients, this

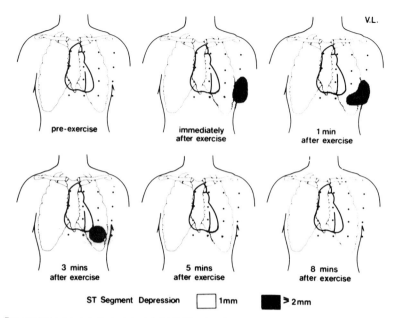

Fig. 5–17. Precordial grid plots in isolated right CAD, showing localized ST segment depression in the inferior regions of the precordium. From Fox, K.M., Selwyn, A., Oakley, D., and Shillingford, J.P.: Relation between the precordial projection of S-T segment changes after exercise and coronary angiographic findings. Am. J. Cardiol., *44*:1068, 1979.

lead system will represent a major advance in diagnostic exercise ECG testing.

More extensive body surface ECG mapping techniques have been evaluated during exercise, athough, to date, the published studies have been primarily concerned with methodologic issues.[75,76] It is likely, however, that the more quantitative ECG information provided by these systems will advance the state of the art in exercise testing.

Cardiokymography

Because of the diagnostic limitations of the standard exercise ECG test, other noninvasive techniques for detecting exercise-induced manifestations of myocardial ischemia have been under investigation. Regional left ventricular wall motion abnormalities are well recognized early indicators of ischemia that often precede the specific ECG changes. The cardiokymograph (CKG) was designed as an inexpensive device to detect regional wall motion using changes in an induced electromag-

netic field as a measure of underlying tissue movement. The CKG device is a circular, capacitive disk held in a plastic ring, which is strapped to the chest approximately over the V_3 ECG electrode position. Cardiac motion beneath the disk distorts the CKG's electromagnetic field, which in turn, causes a change in the frequency of an external oscillator. A voltage change proportional to cardiac wall motion is generated and recorded as an analog signal on a strip chart recorder.

Figure 5–18 illustrates the three distinct types of CKG waveforms as described by Silverberg et al.[77] The type I tracing shows the normal systolic inward motion throughout ejection. Types II and III waveforms demonstrate two abnormal responses characterized by ischemia-induced paradoxic outward motion during systole. The CKG is recorded in the supine position before and within 2 to 3 minutes after exercise. An abnormal response is defined when a type I waveform at rest becomes a type II or III waveform after exercise *or* a type II waveform at rest becomes a type

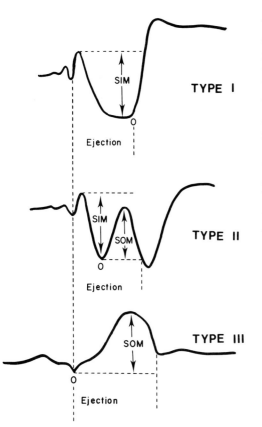

TYPE I

TYPE II

TYPE III

Fig. 5–18. Cardiokymographic tracings showing normal systolic inward motion (SIM, type I), abnormal midsystolic outward motion (type III). From Silverberg, R.A., et al.: Noninvasive diagnosis of coronary artery disease: The cardiokymographic stress test. Circulation, 62:632, 1980. By permission of the American Heart Association, Inc.

III after exercise and then returns to the control configuration.

Validation studies comparing the noninvasive CKG recordings with direct measurements from the epicardial surface of open-chest dog hearts have been published by Vas et al.,[78] showing excellent correlation between the two methods. In addition the CKG tracing closely resembled the direct recordings from the surface of the heart before, during, and after myocardial ischemia was induced by coronary artery constriction.

Several clinical studies have now been published by independent groups of investigators comparing the CKG findings with exercise ECG data and thallium 201 scintigraphy in patients undergoing coronary angiographic studies.[77,79,80] Summary results from three studies are tabulated in Table 5–17. In all three studies the sensitivity and specificity of the CKG test were similar to or better than the exercise ECG; in one study, the CKG results were comparable to the thallium 201 stress tests. Furthermore, tests with concordant CKG and exercise ECG findings (i.e., both positive or both negative) were much more accurate in predicting the presence or absence of coronary disease than either test alone or thallium 201 scintigraphy.

The major limitation of the CKG stress test is that in 10% to 20% of tests there is either interobserver variability in interpreting the data or inability to obtain reproducible tracings for interpretation.[79] Nevertheless, the low cost of this procedure coupled with its high accuracy makes it an attractive adjunct to exercise ECG testing. Combining the two tests would be expected to yield significant improvements in the detection of CAD. Furthermore, it is likely that the percentage of technically inadequate CKG tests will decrease with improvements in instrumentation and continued experience with this new procedure.

Radionuclide Stress Testing

Radionuclide methods of stress testing for CAD were initially developed because of the diagnostic errors associated with exercise ECG testing. There are, in addition, a variety of resting ECG abnormalities, listed in Table 5–18, that preclude accurate recognition of myocardial ischemia during exercise testing. Two radionuclide imaging techniques, thallium 201 perfusion imaging and radionuclide ventriculography, have become increasingly popular exercise methods for evaluating patients with known or suspected coronary disease.[81] The major disadvantages of radionuclide techniques are that they are expensive, require sophisticated equipment, and de-

Table 5–17.   Comparison of Several Noninvasive Tests for Detecting Coronary Artery Disease

Study	No. Patients	Exercise ECG		CKG		Thallium	
		Sens.	Spec.	Sens.	Spec.	Sens.	Spec.
Silverberg[77]	122	59%	69%	74%	94%	—	—
Weiner[79]	188	66%	86%	73%	95%	—	—
Burke[80]	99	68%	62%	76%	90%	79%	88%

CKG, cardiokymography; ECG, electrocardiogram; sens., sensitivity; spec., specificity.

mand a great deal of technical and interpretive expertise. Nevertheless, in select patient populations these tests provide valuable noninvasive clinical information needed for patient management.

Thallium 201, a potassium analog, is a perfusion-limited radioactive tracer that is distributed within the myocardium in proportion to myocardial blood flow and cellular viability. In normally perfused heart muscle, there is rapid accumulation of thallium in an evenly distributed pattern throughout the myocardium when imaged with a scintillation camera. Ischemic myocardium is initially underperfused and appears as a defect or "cold-spot" surrounded by normally perfused heart muscle. In exercise-induced myocardial ischemia, the defect is usually transient; after several hours there is delayed uptake of thallium into the previously ischemic zones and efflux of thallium from the nonischemic zones. Repeat imaging during this "redistribution" phase will show a uniform distribution of the radiotracer within the myocardium. In this way ischemic myocardium can be differentiated from old MI, which is identified by a persistent defect on the redistribution scans.

Table 5–18.   Problem Cases in Exercise ECG

1. Right or left ventricular hypertrophy
2. Bundle branch block and other intraventricular conduction defects
3. Previous myocardial infarctions
4. Hyperventilation-induced ST-T wave changes
5. Drug effects (digitalis, quinidine, beta-blockers)
6. Electrolyte abnormalities (hypokalemia)
7. Pre-excitation syndromes (Wolff-Parkinson-White)
8. Artificial ventricular pacemakers
9. Nonspecific ST-T wave changes

The thallium stress test is performed in conjunction with a standard symptom-limited exercise ECG test. During the final minute of exercise, 2 mCi of thallium 201 is injected intravenously; approximately 1 minute later exercise is terminated, and imaging begun immediately thereafter. The images are obtained in the anterior, left anterior oblique, and left lateral positions. Three to four hours after the postexercise images are obtained, imaging is repeated to evaluate the redistribution patterns. Interpretation usually involves both visual analyses of the immediate and delayed images as well as computer-processed quantification of regional thallium 201 activity and kinetics. Figure 5–19 illustrates an example of immediate and redistribution thallium scans.

Okada et al.[82] reviewed the nuclear cardiology literature up to 1980 and summarized studies involving over 1,800 patients undergoing both thallium 201 and exercise ECG tests. Coronary angiography was used to define the presence or absence of disease in these studies. Visually interpreted thallium scans had an average sensitivity of 82% and a specificity of 91%, compared to 60% and 81%, respectively, for exercise ECG testing. Much of the improvement in predictive accuracy occurred in patients with abnormal resting ECGs or in patients unable to achieve 85% of predicted maximal heart rates.

More recently, computer-enhanced imaging techniques along with quantitative analysis of thallium washout and redistribution have resulted in sensitivities of over 90% for detecting patients with CAD.[83]

Exercise radionuclide ventriculography

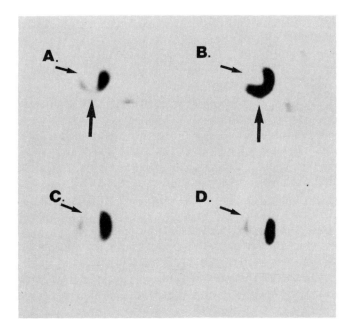

Fig. 5–19.   Immediate post-exercise and redistribution thallium scans in a patient with coronary artery disease. *(A)* Mid-ventricular short-axis tomographic view immediately after exercise. Note marked reduction in count activity in the anterior wall and septum (small arrow) and inferior wall (large arrow). *(B)* Corresponding short-axis view after 3-hour delay. Note the persistent defect in the anterior wall and septum (small arrow), representing infarction, and the marked redistribution in the inferior wall (large arrow), demonstrating reversible ischemia. *(C)* Mid-ventricular horizontal long-axis tomographic view immediately after exercise. Note the marked reduction in count activity in the anterior wall and septum (small arrow). *(D)* Corresponding horizontal long-axis view after 3-hour delay. Note the persistent defect in the anterior wall and septum (small arrow), representing infarction. (Courtesy of Gary Cuputo, M.D.)

is an imaging technique comparable to contrast ventriculography obtained during cardiac catheterization. This technique is used to evaluate cardiovascular performance at rest and during exercise and provides information regarding the functional consequences of myocardial ischemia. Two methods have been developed which use technetium 99m bound to red blood cells as the radiotracer. The multiple-gated equilibrium (MUGA) imaging technique uses the ECG signal to control the temporal sequences of imaging throughout the cardiac cycle. Data are acquired over several hundred cycles until a sufficient count density is achieved to create a well-defined sequence of images spanning the entire cardiac cycle. Angiographic images are obtained at rest and during supine bicycle ergometer exercise. The first-pass radionuclide technique requires a rapid bolus injection of radiotracer, and only the initial pass through the central circulation is analyzed. This method is suitable for upright bicycle ergometry and generally permits more maximal exercise levels to be achieved while imaging.

Both methods of radionuclide ventriculography generate information regarding left ventricular volumes at end systole and end diastole, global ventricular function (ejection fractions), and segmental or regional wall motion. Ejection fractions may be computed using either geometric analysis of end-systolic and end-diastolic silhouettes to calculate volumes or, more commonly, from background-corrected time–activity curves relating changes in radioactive counts from end diastole to end systole. Normal subjects increase their ejection fractions by at least 5% during exercise without developing regional wall motion abnormalities.[82] Failure of ejection fraction to increase by at least 5% during exercise is considered evidence for CAD.[82] Regional wall motion is usually quantitated by scoring the left ventricular segments using a 5-point scale: normal motion (3 points), mild hypokinesia (2 points), moderate to severe hypokinesia (1 point), akinesia (0 points), dyskinesia (−1 point). A decrease of one or more points in a particular region during exercise, or a segmental score of less than 1.5 at rest is considered evidence for CAD.[82]

Okada et al.[82] have summarized the reported experience up to 1980 using radionuclide angiography for detecting CAD in over 400 patients. Exercise-induced regional wall motion abnormalities had an overall sensitivity of 73% and a specificity of 100%. Failure to increase left ventricular ejection fraction during exercise had a sensitivity of 87% and specificity of 93% for CAD. The predictive accuracy of these two descriptors of myocardial ischemia were significantly better than the exercise ECG in the reported studies.

There are definite advantages in radionuclide exercise testing over the standard exercise ECG. The thallium 201 scans are not only more accurate in detecting CAD but also permit more exact localization of significant coronary lesions. This may be particularly important in individuals with previous MIs and in those with multivessel disease, where the clinical significance of an angiographic lesion may be in question. Exercise radionuclide ventriculography, in addition to being a more sensitive method for detecting coronary disease, permits more quantitative functional assessments to be made, which may have important therapeutic implications in certain patients. However, because of the increased costs and technical requirements, it is unlikely that radionuclide procedures will ever replace more standard exercise ECG studies for the large majority of patients undergoing diagnostic exercise testing. Furthermore, advances in exercise ECGs and im-provements in the CKG technique have significantly increased the sensitivity and specificity of the exercise test. As a result, indications for radionuclide studies are likely to decrease, except in situations where specific anatomic information is needed.

IDENTIFICATION OF HIGH-RISK AND LOW-RISK PATIENTS

Risk stratification is an important prerequisite for both effective prevention and optimal management of CAD. The ECG and hemodynamic responses to exercise testing are of proven value in identifying high-risk and low-risk patients. The following discussion will focus on three clinical areas of interest where exercise testing provides valuable prognostic information: (1) risk assessment in asymptomatic individuals; (2) assessment of CAD severity; and (3) risk stratification after acute MI. In each of these areas various treatment decisions are likely to be influenced by the results of the exercise test.

Risk Assessment in Asymptomatic Populations

The diagnostic role of exercise testing in evaluating asymptomatic subjects has already been discussed. From Bayes' theorem it was shown that the predictive value of ischemic ST segment abnormalities for CAD was dependent on the pretest or prior probability of disease. In low-risk individuals the predictive value of isolated ST segment depression is quite limited, since the majority of positive tests are false-positives. From a prognostic point of view, however, the implications of a positive exercise test are somewhat different. The issue is not so much the presence or absence of coronary disease as defined angiographically, but whether or not an individual with a positive test is at greater risk for future coronary events (MI, angina pectoris, or sudden death).

There have been a number of reports investigating the prognostic value of exercise test findings in clinically healthy individuals. Allen et al.[84] followed 888 asymptomatic men and women for 5 years after maximal treadmill testing and found significant age and sex differences for the predictive power of the exercise test. Exercise test abnormalities in men under age 40 were not indicative of increased risk for CAD. Over age 40, however, ischemic ST segment abnormalities, exercise duration less than 6 minutes (Ellestad protocol), and no change or increase in R wave amplitude immediately after exercise were associated with new coronary events during the follow-up period. In women only exercise duration less than 4 minutes correlated with increased coronary disease incidence. In this study no attempt was made to control for other risk factors.

Using case-control epidemiologic methods, Giagnoni et al.[85] studied 135 asymptomatic normotensive subjects with supine exercise-induced ST segment depression and 379 controls matched for age, sex, coronary risk factors, and occupation who had negative exercise tests. In the 6-year follow-up, the relative risk for new coronary events attributed only to ST segment depression was 5.5; that is, there was a 5.5 times greater incidence of disease events in those with abnormal tests compared with carefully matched controls without ST segment depression. The data suggest that exercise-induced ST segment depression is an independent risk factor for predicting coronary disease events in asymptomatic subjects.

Finally, in the large Seattle Heart Watch project reported by Bruce et al.,[86] several other exercise test predictors including chest pain during exercise, inability to complete stage II (Bruce protocol), and maximal heart rate less than 90% of predicted maximum were important prognostic variables along with ST segment depression. In a 10-year follow-up of asymptomatic healthy men, the presence of any major

coronary risk factors combined with at least two exercise test variables was associated with a 6-year coronary disease incidence of 24%. In the absence of coronary risk factors, however, the predictive value of exercise test abnormalities was limited. The investigators concluded that exercise testing for risk assessment was *not* cost-effective in the absence of conventional coronary risk factors. They recommend, instead, a stepwise approach to risk assessment in the clinically healthy population beginning with low-cost risk factor assessment and symptom classification and including exercise testing only in men with positive risk factors. Recommendations for asymptomatic women were not given because of insufficient data.

Evaluating the Severity of Coronary Artery Disease

The diagnosis of CAD is only the first step in the process of developing an optimal management plan. Many of the techniques used for diagnostic studies including the history, physical examination, noninvasive procedures, and cardiac catheterization also provide information regarding disease severity. The ECG, hemodynamic, and clinical responses to exercise testing can be used to distinguish high-risk from low-risk patients with coronary disease.[87–89] Table 5–19 lists the exercise test abnormalities that have been associated with severe CAD, usually defined angiographically as triple-vessel or left main disease. A test is considered to be strongly positive for severe disease when one or more of these findings are detected. In addition, a strongly positive test in a patient being worked up for known or suspected coronary disease is usually an indication for angiographic studies to further define the extent of disease.

The predictors of disease severity listed in Table 5–19 include both ECG parameters, which describe the ischemic process, and hemodynamic parameters, which bet-

Table 5-19.   Exercise Test Predictors of Severe CAD

ECG parameters
  ST segment depression
    Marked ST segment depression (≥3 mm)
    Early onset (≤4 METs)
    Downsloping configuration
    Prolonged ST segment depression (>7 min after
      exercise)
    Global changes (inferior and anterior leads)
    Max ST/HR slope (>6.0 µV/bpm)
  ST segment elevation
  U wave inversion
Low maximal workload (≤4 METs)
Abnormal blood pressure response
  Inadequate blood pressure rise with exercise
  Exertional hypotension
Chronotropic incompetence
Anginal symptoms during exercise

ECG, electrocardiographic; MET, metabolic equivalent; ST/HR, ST segment depression to heart rate.

ter define the functional consequences of the heart disease. Global ST segment abnormalities are characterized by the simultaneous occurrence of ST segment depression in both anterior- and inferior-oriented ECG leads. Blumenthal et al.[87] found that almost 60% of their patients with global ischemia on exercise had left main coronary disease. Marked ST segment depression occurring early in exercise and persisting long after exercise was also predictive of severe CAD.

Okin et al.[90] used a simplified version of the maximal ST/HR slope, described in the previous section, limited to leads V_5, V_6, and aV_F, and found that a peak slope greater than 6.0 µV/bpm identified three-vessel coronary disease (predictive value, 93%) more accurately than standard ST segment criteria (predictive value, 50%). These data suggest that more sophisticated analyses of exercise ECG data can improve the prognostic accuracy in identifying severe coronary disease.

Exercise-induced ST segment elevation in the absence of previous MI not only indicates severe transmural ischemia but also predicts the location of the ischemic process within the myocardium.[91] ST segment elevation confined to inferior-oriented leads is strongly suggestive of right CAD; anterior ST segment elevation predicts left main or left anterior descending disease; lateral ST segment elevation is somewhat predictive of left circumflex disease. It must be remembered, however, that coronary artery spasm in the absence of severe CAD may also be responsible for exercise-induced ST segment elevation.[41]

Exercise test parameters of left ventricular dysfunction include low maximal workload (≤ 4 METs), inadequate blood pressure rise with exercise and exertional hypotension. Although not specific for CAD, these parameters are often associated with severe coronary lesions and are predictors of increased morbidity and mortality.

Exertional hypotension, defined as a fall in systolic blood pressure during exercise of 10 mm Hg or more, may be indicative of severe CAD, especially if accompanied by chest pain. Morris et al.[92] feel that this is a reliable predictor of multivessel disease only if the following five conditions are met: (1) the fall in blood pressure persists on repeated measurements over 15- to 20-second intervals; (2) there is absence of cardiomyopathy, valvular heart disease, orthostatic hypotension, hypovolemia, or congestive heart failure; (3) cardiac arrhythmias are not present during the blood pressure recordings; (4) exercise is at least 1 minute in duration; and (5) the patient is not on drugs that would impair the cardiac output response to exercise. The increased use of beta-blocking drugs after uncomplicated MI may occasionally be responsible for exercise-induced hypotension in the absence of severe coronary disease.

Failure of the systolic blood pressure to rise above 130 to 140 mm Hg during maximal exercise testing may also be prognostically significant. Bruce et al.[93] found this to be an important predictor of sudden death in the Seattle Heart Watch study of ambulatory men with CHD.

An impaired heart rate response to exercise has been defined differently by different investigators but is generally considered to be indicative of severe coronary disease. Ellestad and Wan[94] coined the term *chronotropic incompetence* as a heart rate below the 95% confidence limits for any given work load based on age and sex. In their long-term follow-up studies, an inadequate heart rate response was associated with severe left ventricular dysfunction, triple-vessel coronary disease, and increased morbidity or mortality. In the study by McNeer et al.,[66] maximal heart rates below 120 bpm were also associated with increased risk for future coronary events.

Finally, anginal symptoms occurring at low work loads have been correlated with severe CAD and increased morbidity.[95] Weiner et al.[67] found that angina during exercise testing was as sensitive a predictor of cardiac mortality and multivessel disease as ST segment depression alone. This is an important observation, since many patients may be limited by anginal symptoms during exercise testing before diagnostic ECG changes have occurred. These patients should not be pushed beyond symptoms of moderate severity.

Exercise Testing After MI

Exercise testing soon after acute MI is a relatively recent addition to the list of clinical indications for exercise testing. Initial studies in the United States, published in the late 1970s, documented the safety and clinical utility of this technique in the post-MI patient population.[96–98] As physicians gained more experience with low-level exercise studies, the predischarge or early postdischarge exercise test became a routine procedure for the relatively uncomplicated post-MI patients.

Th objectives of post-MI exercise testing and the benefits to the patients are listed in Table 5–20. Not all post-MI patients are candidates for early exercise testing, especially when risk assessment is being considered. Patients with significant inhospital complications such as cardiogenic shock, congestive heart failure, intractable arrhythmias, heart block, and postinfarction angina are already at increased risk (Table 5–21). Exercise testing would not be expected to contribute to subsequent management in these patients.

Epstein et al.[4] have developed an effective strategy for evaluating the post-MI patient that places exercise testing in a proper perspective relative to other invasive and noninvasive procedures. Their strategy is based on the probable outcome of 100 hypothetical post-MI survivors categorized by clinical and noninvasive methodologies, as illustrated in Figure 5–20. The initial classification uses clinical criteria (rales, S3 gallop, radiographic findings) to identify approximately 30 patients (30% of all post-MI patients) with clinical heart failure and 70 patients without manifestations of failure. The next stratification identifies approximately 20 patients from both clinical subsets with radionuclide left ventricular ejection fractions of less than 30%. The last assessment utilizes exercise testing in the remaining 80 less complicated patients to identify 25 patients with exercise test ab-

Table 5–20. Post-MI Exercise Testing

Objectives	Patient Benefits

Risk Assessment
  Identification of ischemic
    abnormalities
  Evaluation of cardiac
    rhythm
  Assessment of functional
    cardiovascular capacity
Exercise prescription
	Contributes to patient management
	Helps determine prognosis
	Determines rate of physical rehabilitation
	Provides psychological benefits to patient and family

Table 5–21.　Contraindications to Early Post-MI Exercise Testing

1. Clinical left ventricular failure (S3 gallop, pulmonary rales, sinus tachycardia, etc.)
2. Uncontrolled ventricular arrhythmias
3. Continued ischemic symptoms at rest within 5 days of test
4. Uncontrolled hypertension (blood pressure >180/100)
5. Active pleurisy or pericarditis
6. Any complicating illness that precludes exercise testing
7. Any physical or mental handicap that would preclude cooperation during testing

normalities and 55 patients with normal responses to exercise. These 55 patients (assumed to represent 55% of all post-MI patients) have a very low 1-year mortality.

From these considerations, Epstein et al.[4] have recommended the strategy diagrammed in Figure 5–21. Patients with recurrent symptoms of angina pectoris should proceed directly to cardiac catheterization to define the extent of coronary disease and determine the need for bypass

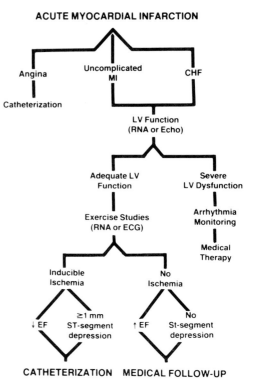

Fig. 5–21.　Recommended strategy of Epstein et al.[4] for post-MI evaluation. CHF, congestive heart failure; EF, ejection fraction; LV, left ventricle; RNA, radionuclide angiography. Reprinted, by permission of the New England Journal of Medicine (307:1487, 1982).

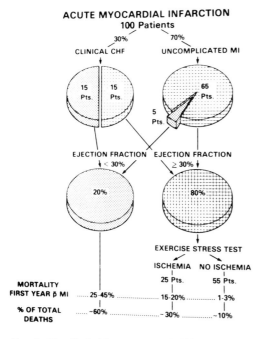

Fig. 5–20.　Probable outcome of 100 consecutive acute MI survivors categorized by clinical and non-invasive methodologies. Reprinted, by permission of the New England Journal of Medicine (307:1487, 1982).

surgery or angioplasty. The small subset of patients with severe left ventricular dysfunction should receive medical management, unless surgically correctable defects such as ventricular septal rupture, mitral regurgitation, or ventricular aneurysms are identified. Exercise studies are recommended for the majority of patients who are relatively uncomplicated in order to identify a high-risk subset with exercise-induced abnormalities. These high-risk patients are candidates for further invasive studies to better define optimal treatment. The remaining patients are considered to be low-risk and do not need further diagnostic studies unless their clinical status changes.

Post-MI exercise testing is usually carried out just prior to hospital discharge or within several weeks following discharge.

Because of the proximity to the onset of acute MI, the predischarge exercise test should be a low-level, submaximal evaluation. For patients not on beta-blocking drugs, exercise testing is usually terminated when the heart rate reaches 120 or 130 bpm, depending on age, unless symptoms or other abnormalities occur first. Patients on beta-blocking drugs are generally limited to work loads of 5 METs or below. The modified Naughton treadmill protocol described in Table 5–6 is recommended for predischarge evaluations, although the 2-mph speed may be too fast for some patients. Low-level bicycle protocols are also applicable for this purpose.

If exercise testing is performed at approximately 3 weeks post-MI, a symptom-limited protocol may be utilized in patients who are considered to be uncomplicated. Limiting symptoms include chest pain, dyspnea, leg fatigue, or dizziness. Tests may also be terminated for exertional hypotension, significant arrhythmias, conduction abnormalities, and marked ST segment depression. Debusk and Haskell[99] have compared heart rate-limited and symptom-limited protocols in patients 3 weeks post-MI for both safety and diagnostic utility and found no significant differences between the two protocols.

In the evaluation of post-MI patients, symptom-limited protocols have several advantages over submaximal tests with arbitrary end points. They more accurately reflect the patient's functional cardiovascular capacity and provide better guidelines for return to work and recreational activities. At approximately 3 weeks post-MI, a symptom-limited test may be more cost-effective by eliminating the need for a second exercise test 4 to 8 weeks later in those patients who have a normal exercise response. Finally, as recently shown by Ewart et al.,[100] symptom-limited testing may have a significant positive impact on the patient's confidence for performing physical activities at home. The explanation of the exercise test findings to the patient and spouse can often be of therapeutic value by alleviating anxieties associated with physical exertion.

The use of beta-blocking drugs in post-MI patients may present problems in interpreting the ECG and blood pressure responses to exercise testing. The effects of beta-blockers on the cardiovascular system include decreased contractility, heart rate and blood pressure responses to exercise, all of which may minimize or mask symptoms and ST segment changes of myocardial ischemia. While these effects may have obvious therapeutic benefits for post-MI patients, the prognostic value of exercise testing may be decreased. It is recommended, therefore, that patients be taken off beta-blocking drugs 2 days prior to exercise testing, unless there are patient-specific contraindications to doing so. In the population of post-MI patients for whom beta-blockers are used as prophylaxis against recurrent coronary events, sudden withdrawal for 2 days prior to exercise testing would not be expected to have adverse effects. The other alternative is not to begin prophylactic beta-blocker therapy until after the results of exercise testing are known. Patients with normal exercise test findings may not even need long-term beta-blocker therapy, since their risk for recurrent coronary events is extremely low.

The exercise test variables that have important prognostic and therapeutic values include new ST segment depression, exertional hypotension, poor exercise tolerance, and anginal symptoms. Weiner[3] has recently reviewed the post-MI exercise testing literature, analyzing results from five studies involving almost 900 patients. Exercise-induced ST segment depression was the most predictive single parameter, identifying 20% to 60% of those patients who subsequently developed recurrent MI, unstable angina, or sudden death. Angina pectoris, exertional hypotension, and low functional capacity were also predictive of recurrent disease events. Cardiac arrhythmias during exercise, however, did not contribute to the coronary disease risk in these studies, although it is likely that patients with arrhythmic complications were excluded from participating because of poor ventricular function.

The predictive power of the post-MI exercise test can be further improved by using more sophisticated analytic techniques such as multivariate or discriminant function analysis. Davidson and Debusk,[101] using these techniques, found that ST segment depression (≥ 0.2 mV), angina pectoris, and a maximal work load of less than 4 METs were most predictive of future coronary events. Of interest, ST segment depression of less than 0.2 mV was not prognostically important unless associated with angina or low maximal workload. Madsen and Gilpin[102] evaluated several multivariate methodologies to identify the best exercise test variable for predicting morbidity and mortality post-MI. Using a symptom-limited bicycle ergometer protocol (50-watt increments every 6 minutes) they found that exercise duration was the most important single variable for predicting death within the first year post-MI. Other important variables included sex, age, PVCs, and double product. Their data suggest that multivariate analyses can correctly identify 65% of patients who will die or develop new MIs within 1 year post-MI.

The results of exercise testing have important implications for the subsequent management of post-MI patients. Abnormal ECG findings indicative of myocardial ischemia should be followed-up with coronary angiography to identify surgically correctable lesions or lesions suitable for angioplasty. Patients who have severe functional limitations should undergo further workup to better characterize their hemodynamic and anatomic abnormalities. The widespread use of beta-blockers after MI may be responsible for some of these functional abnormalities.

Approximately 50% of post-MI survivors will have neither hemodynamic nor ECG abnormalities during exercise testing.[4] These asymptomatic patients can be classified as low-risk and encouraged to return to productive life-styles as soon as possible. It is likely that many of these uncomplicated patients can return to occupational activities at 3 to 4 weeks post-MI and avoid the prolonged convalescence previously recommended after acute MI.

EVALUATION OF CARDIOVASCULAR FUNCTIONAL CAPACITY

The functional assessment of the cardiovascular system is a necessary prerequisite for making a number of important therapeutic decisions in the practice of cardiovascular medicine. Functional exercise testing is also of value in the workup of dyspnea, easy fatigability, weakness, and other symptoms related to decreased working capacity. The particular responses to exercise testing are often helpful in differentiating cardiovascular impairment from respiratory, skeletal muscle, and other causes of disability. Finally, the rehabilitation of patients with cardiovascular and other disabling diseases requires exercise testing to determine safe and effective exercise prescriptions. The following discussion considers physiologic concepts and practical methods for measuring functional capacity in the exercise laboratory.

The term "cardiovascular functional capacity" is, in a sense, a misnomer, since the exercise test response is more a measure of the patient's total physical working capacity than it is an isolated test of cardiovascular function. The ability to perform physical work on a treadmill or bicycle requires the coordinated interactions of the respiratory system, central nervous system, hematologic system, skeletal muscles, and cardiovascular system. A breakdown within one or more of these organ systems often results in a decreased physical working capacity.

In the exercise laboratory the gold-standard measure of physical working capacity is the *maximal oxygen uptake* or $\dot{V}O_2$

max. Also called the *maximal aerobic capacity*, this is the maximal uptake of oxygen per minute measured during an incremental work exercise test. The $\dot{V}O_2$ max, in turn, is determined by the maximal capacity of the cardiovascular system to transport oxygenated blood to the exercising muscles (central factors) and the maximal ability of the skeletal muscles to extract and utilize the oxygen for work (peripheral factors). The Fick equation, under conditions of maximal exercise, expresses the relationship between oxygen uptake, oxygen transport, and oxygen utilization:

$$\dot{V}O_2 \text{ max} = (max\ HR \times max\ SV)$$
$$\times (max\ CaO_2 - min\ C\overline{v}O_2)$$

where *max HR* is maximal heart rate (bpm), *max SV* is maximal stroke volume (ml/beat), max CaO_2 is maximal arterial oxygen content (ml O_2/ml blood), min $C\overline{v}O_2$ is the minimal mixed venous oxygen content. $\dot{V}O_2$ max is expressed as ml O_2/min. When normalized for body weight and expressed as ml O_2/kg/min, $\dot{V}O_2$ max becomes a parameter that reflects aerobic fitness.

From the Fick equation it is apparent that, in addition to cardiac function (heart rate and stroke volume), $\dot{V}O_2$ max is determined by pulmonary factors (ventilation, diffusing capacity); arterial blood factors (hemoglobin concentration and saturation); and skeletal muscle factors (fiber type, mitochondria, aerobic enzymes). In the absence of respiratory, hematologic, or neuromuscular disorders, however, $\dot{V}O_2$ max can be used as an index of cardiac function.[103]

The oxygen uptake during progressive exercise is almost linearly related to the workload until $\dot{V}O_2$ max is achieved. This relationship is illustrated in Figure 5–22, taken from a review by Mitchell and Blomqvist.[104] During exercise oxygen uptake increases until a workload is reached beyond which oxygen uptake cannot rise. This limit represents the maximal ability of the exercising subject to transport and uti-

lize oxygen. $\dot{V}O_2$ max is somewhat determined by the type of exercise being performed and the total mass of skeletal muscle used during exercise. Treadmill exercise, for example, may be associated with a 10% to 15% greater $\dot{V}O_2$ max than bicycle ergometer exercise in the same subject. Also shown in Figure 5–22 is the exponential-like rise in blood lactate during progressive exercise. Low levels of exercise use aerobic mechanisms predominately; with increasing levels of work, however, there is a progressively greater contribution of anaerobic metabolism, which is superimposed on the linear increase in aerobic metabolism. Beyond $\dot{V}O_2$ max, the increased work performed relies entirely on anaerobic mechanisms.

The responses of cardiac output, heart rate, stroke volume, and arteriovenous oxygen content difference to progressive exercise and $\dot{V}O_2$ are illustrated in Figure 5–23, taken from Mitchell and Blomqvist.[104] In a physically fit subject, there is a four- to fivefold increase in cardiac output from rest to maximal exercise. Approximately two thirds of this increase is accounted for by increases in heart rates (approximately threefold increase), and one third is due to an increase in stroke volume ($\sim$ 1.5-fold increase), which mostly occurs early during exercise. With increasing exercise the arteriovenous oxygen content difference widens three to four times, largely due to increased extraction of oxygen by the exercising skeletal muscles.

From these relationships the various factors influencing physical working capacity can be readily appreciated. Table 5–22 lists factors that both increase and decrease aerobic capacity. As shown in Figure 5–24, these factors exert their influence at different sites in the Fick equation. The factors responsible for a given individual's ability or inability to perform physical work can usually be determined by a careful clinical evaluation followed by exercise testing. For accurate interpretation of the exercise test response, it is important to appreciate

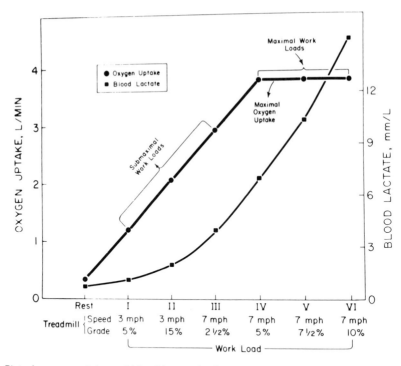

Fig. 5–22.   Plot of oxygen uptake and blood lactate (ordinates) against exercise work loads (abscissa). Reprinted, by permission of the New England Journal of Medicine (284:1018, 1974).

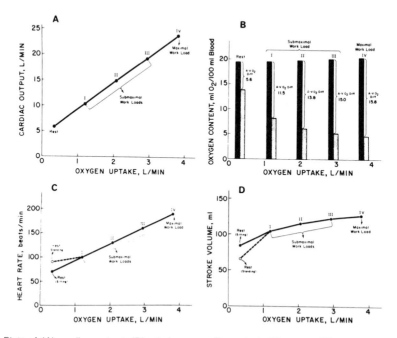

Fig. 5–23.   Plots of (A) cardiac output, (B) arteriovenous O_2 content difference, (C) heart rate, and (D) stroke volume, versus oxygen uptake from rest to maximal exercise. Reprinted, by permission of the New England Journal of Medicine (284:1018, 1974).

Table 5–22.   Factors Affecting Aerobic Capacity ($\dot{V}O_2$ max)

Factors That Decrease	*Factors That Increase*
1. Aging	1. Aerobic conditioning
2. Deconditioning	2. Increased muscle mass
3. Acute illness	3. Genetic factors
4. Bronchopulmonary disease	4. Psychological factors
5. Cardiovascular diseases	5. Increased PO_2 of inspired air
6. Anemia	
7. Carbon monoxide exposure	
8. High altitude	
9. Skeletal muscle disease	
10. Drugs	

the complex interactions of the various organ systems responsible for the performance of physical work.

Measurement of Maximal Oxygen Uptake

The essential requirement for assessing a person's functional capacity is the determination of maximal oxygen uptake. There are three types of exercise testing procedures for this purpose: (1) direct measurements of ventilation and respiratory gases during maximal exercise testing; (2) estimation of $\dot{V}O_2$ max from maximal exercise performance; and (3) prediction of $\dot{V}O_2$ max from submaximal exercise. Techniques for predicting $\dot{V}O_2$ max from submaximal tests are discussed in Chapter 4.

The direct measurement of oxygen up-

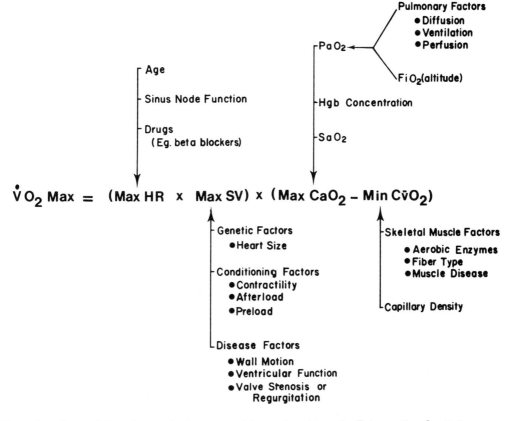

Fig. 5–24.   Factors influencing maximal oxygen uptake as viewed from the Fick equation. See text.

take during exercise requires a great deal of time and effort from the laboratory staff, considerable motivation and some discomfort from the exercising subject, and expensive, sophisticated equipment. For these reasons, direct measurement techniques are largely confined to research laboratories where the necessary expertise is readily available and where more accurate measurements are required for scientific investigations. In the future, however, it is likely that fully automated systems for respiratory gas analyses will be more utilized in clinical laboratories.

The direct measurement techniques for quantitating airflow and calculating minute ventilation, oxygen uptake, and carbon dioxide output require on-line computer processing of the signal outputs from gas analyzers, pneumotachometers or turbine air flow meters. Various methods for analyzing these signals and displaying the computed results have been published.[105–108] In general these methods are complex, expensive, and demand careful calibrations and equipment maintenance. Commercially available, automated systems have significantly improved the ease with which respiratory data are obtained and analyzed, although these systems also require considerable professional expertise.

For many clinical applications the indirect methods of estimating or predicting $\dot{V}O_2$ max are reasonable alternatives to the more complex and expensive direct measurement techniques. Submaximal tests for predicting $\dot{V}O_2$ max are suitable for fitness assessments and exercise prescriptions in the healthy population, although there are many limitations to these tests (Chapter 4). The tests, however, can usually be supervised by less experienced and lower salaried personnel than required for maximal testing. Estimations of $\dot{V}O_2$ max from maximal treadmill or bicycle tests are more accurate, but they require more careful supervision, take longer to complete, and demand much greater effort from the individual being evaluated.

The oxygen cost during treadmill work can be calculated using the equations presented in Table 5–23, depending on whether the subject is walking (1.9 to 3.7 mph) or running (>5 mph).[6] The total oxygen cost (ml O_2/kg/min) for a given treadmill speed (mph) and elevation (percent grade expressed as a fraction) is the sum of the horizontal and vertical components. It follows that an estimated $\dot{V}O_2$ max can be calculated from the maximal speed and elevation achieved during treadmill exercise, providing the subject does not hold on to the side rails. These formulas can also be used for estimating the oxygen costs associated with outdoor activities, but the vertical component for running needs to be multiplied by 2. Estimates of $\dot{V}O_2$ for walking or running speeds from 3.7 to 5.0 mph are less accurate because of individual variations in walking and running patterns during fast walking or slow running.

Montoye et al.[109] compared the equations in Table 5–23 with directly measured exercise $\dot{V}O_2$ in 656 male subjects (all age groups) participating in the Tecumseh Community Health Study. The equations were most accurate in estimating $\dot{V}O_2$ in adult males during grade walking, but slightly underestimated $\dot{V}O_2$ during horizontal walking. The formulas also underestimated $\dot{V}O_2$ in subjects under age 18. It must be emphasized, however, that the estimates of $\dot{V}O_2$ using these formulas are for steady-state exercise and may not be as accurate at high treadmill work loads and maximal exercise because the anaerobic component associated with these work loads is not taken into consideration.[6]

The standard treadmill protocols described in Table 5–6 have estimated $\dot{V}O_2$ values for each stage of exercise. These values are only applicable if the subject is in a steady state and not holding on to the handrails during exercise. There is a substantial reduction in the $\dot{V}O_2$ and heart rate response to exercise when handrails are used for support.[110] This enables the exercising subject to significantly extend the

Table 5–23.   Estimations of Oxygen Costs (ml O_2/kg/min) for Treadmill Walking 1.9 to 3.7 mph) or Running (>5 mph)

Walking
- horizontal component: $\dot{V}O_2$ = (speed × 2.68) + 3.5
- vertical component: $\dot{V}O_2$ = (speed × 48.28) × % grade expressed as a fraction

Running
- horizontal component: $\dot{V}O_2$ = (speed × 5.36) + 3.5
- vertical component: $\dot{V}O_2$ = (speed × 24.14) × % grade

total duration of exercise and falsely elevate the estimated $\dot{V}O_2$ max. In some individuals who are unable to maintain balance on the treadmill, resting one or two fingers on the rails may still permit a reasonable estimate of $\dot{V}O_2$ max. The use of handrails for most people can be minimized by the exercise test technician. A careful explanation of the proper techniques for walking on the treadmill followed by a demonstration will usually enable most patients to walk without using the handrails.

The range of normal $\dot{V}O_2$ values for the various treadmill protocols was established primarily on healthy adults. There is some question regarding the applicability of these estimates of $\dot{V}O_2$ in patients with cardiovascular disease, especially those with recent MIs. Sullivan and McKirnan[111] have compared oxygen uptake values measured directly during a modified Bruce protocol in post-MI patients and healthy subjects. Oxygen uptake values were approximately 10% lower in the post-MI patients than in the normal subjects at comparable work loads. In addition post-MI patients had higher respiratory exchange ratios indicating increased CO_2 production and suggesting a greater reliance on anaerobic metabolism during exercise. Haskell et al.,[112] on the other hand, have shown that $\dot{V}O_2$ max can be reliably predicted from the treadmill work load in early post-MI patients, if the exercise intensity is slowly progressive (1 MET increase per stage) and if the patients avoided holding on to the handrails. More rapid increases in exercise intensity, however, resulted in the measured $\dot{V}O_2$ max being approximately 10% below predicted.

These studies suggest that the assessment of functional capacity in post-MI patients using published data derived from healthy adults needs to be done with caution. Slowly progressive protocols such as the modified Naughton (Table 5–6) are likely to be associated with a minimum of error. If more rapidly progressive protocols are used in post-MI patients, it is recommended that the estimated $\dot{V}O_2$ max be reduced by 10%.

Estimates of maximal oxygen uptake can be determined from bicycle ergometric testing (Table 5–24).[113] The following formula can also be used for calculating the oxygen cost for upright bicycle work:[6]

$$\dot{V}O_2 \text{ (ml/min)} = \text{(kgm/min} \times 2 \text{ ml/kgm)} + 3.5 \text{ ml/kg/min} \times \text{kg (BW)}$$

The calculation is reasonably accurate for work rates between 300 and 1,200 kgm/min. For estimating an individual's maximal aerobic capacity, the maximal work load in kgm/min should be used in the above formula, and the calculated $\dot{V}O_2$ max should be divided by the body weight (BW) in kg.

Classification of Physical Fitness

In apparently healthy subjects, $\dot{V}O_2$ max depends on a number of factors including age, sex, body size, genetic endowment, and habitual level of physical activity.[104] Table 5–25, taken from an AHA publication,[113] provides an aerobic fitness classification system based on $\dot{V}O_2$ max for men and women of various ages. Individuals

Table 5–24.   Oxygen Requirements for Bicycle Ergometric Work Loads

Body Weight		Oxygen Cost								
(lbs)	(kg)	(ml O₂/kg/min)								
88	40	22.5	30.0	37.5	45.0	52.5	60.0	67.5	82.5	97.5
110	50	18.0	24.0	30.0	36.0	42.0	48.0	54.0	66.0	78.0
132	60	15.0	20.0	25.0	30.0	35.0	40.0	45.0	55.0	65.0
154	70	13.0	17.0	21.5	25.5	30.0	34.5	38.5	47.0	55.5
176	80	11.0	15.0	19.0	22.5	26.0	30.0	34.0	41.0	49.0
198	90	10.0	13.3	16.7	20.0	23.3	26.7	30.0	36.7	43.3
220	100	9.0	12.0	15.0	18.0	21.0	24.0	27.0	33.0	39.0
242	110	8.0	11.0	13.5	16.5	19.0	22.0	24.5	30.0	35.5
264	120	7.5	10.0	12.5	15.0	17.5	20.0	22.5	27.5	32.5
Work load										
kgm/min		300	450	600	750	900	1050	1200	1500	1800
Watts		50	75	100	125	150	175	200	250	300

The oxygen cost is expressed in $ml\ O_2/kg/min$.

who are clinically healthy but fall into the "low" or "fair" fitness categories are most likely deconditioned as a result of chronic inactivity. These people are ideal candidates for exercise training programs such as those described in Chapter 14. The extent to which $\dot{V}O_2$ max can be improved by physical training is dependent on the initial fitness level, the quality and duration of the exercise training program, and the genetic endowment of the individuals being trained.

Values of $\dot{V}O_2$ max in the average or good range are found in individuals who may or may not exercise regularly. Some people are physically fit because of occupational activities; others are genetically predisposed to have average or above average exercise tolerance. Values of $\dot{V}O_2$ max over 55 ml/kg/min are primarily observed in highly trained individuals.[104] Most world-class endurance athletes have $\dot{V}O_2$ max values above 75 ml/kg/min.[114] These extremely high values are likely to be due to the combination of intense training regimens coupled with an exceptional genetic endowment.

Functional Capacity of Patients With Cardiac Disease

The assessment of maximal aerobic capacity in patients with heart disease re-

Table 5–25.   Cardiorespiratory Fitness Classification[113]

Age (years)	Women Maximal Oxygen Uptake (ml/kg/min)				
	Low	Fair	Average	Good	High
20–29	<24	24–30	31–37	38–48	49+
30–39	<20	20–27	28–33	34–44	45+
40–49	<17	17–23	24–30	31–41	42+
50–59	<15	15–20	21–27	28–37	38+
60–69	<13	13–17	18–23	24–34	35+

Age (years)	Men Maximal Oxygen Uptake (ml/kg/min)				
	Low	Fair	Average	Good	High
20–29	<25	25–33	34–42	43–52	53+
30–39	<23	23–30	31–38	39–48	49+
40–49	<20	20–26	27–35	36–44	45+
50–59	<18	18–24	25–33	34–42	43+
60–69	<16	16–22	23–30	31–40	41+

Exercise Testing and Training of Apparently Healthy Individuals: A Handbook for Physicians. The Committee on Exercise, Dallas, American Heart Association, 1972. By permission of the American Heart Association, Inc.

quires an understanding of the limiting factors to exercise in both normal and diseased individuals. The cardiac patient's disability is often the result of both central and peripheral factors. Central factors are related to the underlying disease process and may or may not be reversible, depending on the specific nature of the cardiac abnormalities. Peripheral factors, on the other hand, are frequently the result of physical inactivity or deconditioning. An important rationale for cardiac rehabilitation is the ability to reverse the deconditioning effects through exercise training. Even though the basic cardiac abnormality may not be improved, the peripheral adaptations to an exercise program will enhance the patient's overall functional capacity.

Symptom-limited exercise testing of cardiac patients often provides the necessary functional information for determining the extent and nature of the disability. The parameters of particular interest include measured or estimated $\dot{V}O_2$ max, blood pressure, and cardiac output (heart rate, stroke volume) responses to exercise. In most clinical laboratories where oxygen uptake is not directly measured, $\dot{V}O_2$ max can be estimated from the maximal work load achieved during slowly progressive exercise.[112] Direct measurements of cardiac outputs during exercise require radionuclide angiography or very complex gas analyses techniques usually only found in research laboratories.

Patterson et al.[115] have studied $\dot{V}O_2$ max in patients with a variety of chronic cardiac diseases and found that the onset of limiting symptoms in these patients occurred when $\dot{V}O_2$ max was below 22 ml/kg/min. Patients who were severely limited usually had $\dot{V}O_2$ max below 16 ml/kg/min. When there was a discrepancy between the measured functional capacity and the patients' subjective reporting of symptoms, the exercise test better reflected the actual degree of cardiac impairment. This is an important observation, since treatment decisions

in cardiovascular medicine are frequently determined by the patient's functional class (New York Heart Association functional class I, II, III, and IV). This clinical classification system is based on the patient's subjective reporting of limiting symptoms, which may not be as accurate an assessment of $\dot{V}O_2$ max as that determined by exercise testing.

A more objective functional grading system for classifying patients with chronic heart disease has been proposed by Weber et al.[116] Using directly measured $\dot{V}O_2$ max during treadmill testing, four functional classes were defined (Table 5–26). As the severity of heart failure increased from class A to class D, there was a progressive decline in maximal cardiac output and maximal stroke volume. Class B and C patients were able to increase both stroke volumes and heart rates during exercise. Class D patients were entirely dependent on increases in heart rates to raise cardiac output.

In order to appreciate the functional limitations of cardiac patients as evaluated in the exercise laboratory, normal standards in healthy men and women of various ages need to be defined. Because of the technical difficulties in quantitating the hemodynamic and ventilatory responses to maximal exercise testing, there have not been many studies that have measured cardiac outputs and $\dot{V}O_2$ during exercise in clinically normal subjects. Approximately normal standards have been published by Hossack et al.[117] using small numbers of subjects. These normal limits of maximal cardiac output, stroke volume, and $\dot{V}O_2$ in sedentary, healthy men have been used as

Table 5–26. Functional Classification of Patients with Chronic Congestive Heart Failure[116]

Class	$\dot{V}O_2$ Max (ml/kg/min)
A	>20
B	16–20
C	10–15
D	<10

a reference data base from which to evaluate the functional capacity of cardiac patients.

Hossack[117] and his colleagues first established a linear relationship between the directly measured exercise cardiac outputs and $\dot{V}O_2$ in 10 normal subjects. The regression equation for this relationship was expressed as:

$$\dot{Q} \text{ (L/min)} = 5.31 + 4.6 \text{ (}\dot{V}O_2 \text{ in L/min)}$$

There was an excellent correlation coefficient ($r = .94$) for this relationship, and the standard error of the estimate was 1.24 L/min. This equation was used to estimate the maximal cardiac output response to exercise from $\dot{V}O_2$ max. The maximal stroke volume in these patients was determined by dividing the maximal cardiac output by maximal heart rate. Figure 5–25 illustrates the "normal" age-adjusted range for $\dot{V}O_2$ max, maximal cardiac output, maximal stroke volume, and maximal heart rate established by Hossack.[117] In comparison, the

values of these parameters in a group of medically managed patients with CAD are shown in Figure 5–26. Many coronary patients fell below this normal range in all four parameters. Catheterization studies showed that patients with depressed left ventricular ejection fractions (below 50%) at rest were most likely to have decreased $\dot{V}O_2$ max and maximal cardiac outputs.

CONCLUSIONS

Exercise testing is an important clinical tool for detecting myocardial ischemia, evaluating cardiovascular function and physical working capacity, assessing prognosis and risk for future cardiac disease events, and determining optimal treatment strategies for patients with cardiovascular diseases. The successful use of this tool, however, requires a broad knowledge of cardiovascular structure and function, electrocardiography, clinical characteristics of cardiac diseases, basic and advanced

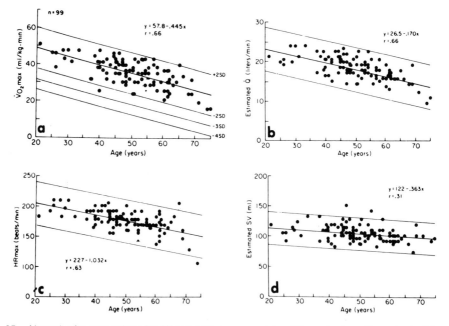

Fig. 5–25.   Normal reference values for (A) maximal oxygen uptake, (B) maximal cardiac output, (C) maximal heart rate, and (D) maximal stroke volume versus age, as reported by Hossack et al.[117] From Hossack, K.F., et al.: Maximal cardiac output during upright exercise: Approximate normal standards and variations with coronary heart disease. Am. J. Cardiol., 46:204, 1980.

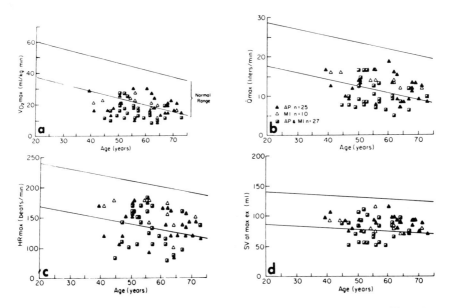

Fig. 5–26.   Medically managed patients with CAD. Values for *(A)* maximal oxygen uptake, *(B)* maximal cardiac output, *(C)* maximal heart rate, and *(D)* maximal stroke volume versus age. The normal range is between the two parallel lines. From Hossack, K.F., et al.: Maximal cardiac output during upright exercise: Approximate normal standards and variations with coronary heart disease. Am. J. Cardiol., *46*:204, 1980.

cardiac life-support techniques, and the principles of clinical judgment. Individuals working in exercise testing laboratories, moreover, need to keep up with rapidly advancing changes in exercise testing methodology and applications. Finally, the cost/benefit ratio must always be considered when determining the need for clinical exercise testing in order to avoid the inappropriate and, at times, potentially harmful use of this procedure. The test is only as good as the mental processes and technical expertise of the professional staff using it.

REFERENCES

1. Levy, R.I., and Moskowitz, J.: Cardiovascular research: Decades of progress, a decade of promise. Science, *217*:121, 1982.
2. Kannel, W.B., and Gordon, T. (eds.): The Framingham Study: An epidemiological investigation of cardiovascular disease. Vol. 12. Bethesda, Md., National Heart, Lung, and Blood Institute, 1968.
3. Weiner, D.A.: Prognostic value of exercise testing early after myocardial infarction. J. Cardiac Rehab., *3*:114, 1983.
4. Epstein, S.E., Palmeri, S.T., and Patterson, R.E.: Evaluation of patients after acute myocardial infarction. Indications for cardiac catheterization and surgical intervention. N. Engl. J. Med., *307*:1487, 1982.
5. Ellestad, M.B., Blomqvist, C.G., and Naughton, J.: Standards for adult exercise testing laboratories. Circulation, *59*:421A, 1979.
6. Guidelines for Graded Exercise Testing and Exercise Prescription. American College of Sports Medicine. 3rd Ed. Philadelphia, Lea & Febiger, 1986.
7. Fardy, P.S., Webb, D., and Hellerstein, H.K.: Benefits of arm exercise in cardiac rehabilitation. Phys. Sports Med., *5*:33, 1977.
8. Franklin, B.A.: Exercise testing, training and arm ergometry. Sports Med., *2*:100, 1985.
9. Mellerowicz, H., and Smodalaka, V.N.: Ergometry: Basics of Medical Exercise Testing. Baltimore, Urban & Schwarzenberg, 1981.
10. Chaitman, B.R., and Hanson, J.S.: Comparative sensitivity and specificity of exercise electrocardiographic lead systems. Am. J. Cardiol., *47*:1335, 1981.
11. Mason, R.E., and Likar, I.: A new system of multiple lead exercise electrocardiography. Am. Heart J., *71*:196, 1966.
12. Blackburn, H., and Katigbak, R.: What electrocardiographic leads to take after exercise? Am. Heart J., *67*:184, 1964.
13. Phibbs, B.P., and Buckels, L.J.: Comparative yield of ECG leads to multistage stress testing. Am. Heart J., *90*:275, 1975.

14. Mason, R.E., Likar, I., Biern, R.Q., and Ross, R.S.: Multiple lead exercise electrocardiography. Experience in 107 normal subjects and 67 patients with angina pectoris and comparison with coronary arteriogrpahy in 84 patients. Circulation, 36:517, 1967.

15. Froelicher, V.F., et al.: A comparison of two bipolar exercise electrocardiographic leads to lead V_5. Chest, 70:611, 1976.

16. Chaitman, B.R., et al.: Improved efficiency of treadmill exercise testing using a multiple lead ECG system and basic hemodynamic exercise response. Circulation, 57:71, 1978.

17. Tam, H.W., and Webster, J.G.: Minimizing electrode motion artifact by skin abrasion. IEEE Trans. Biomed. Eng., 24:134, 1977.

18. Buchfuhrer, M.J., et al.: Optimizing the exercise protocol for cardiopulmonary assessment. J. Appl. Physiol., 55:1558, 1983.

19. Bruce, R.A., Kusumi, F., and Hosmer, D.: Maximal oxygen intake and nomographic assessment of functional aerobic impairment in cardiovascular disease. Am. Heart J., 85:346, 1973.

20. Balke, B., and Ware, R.W.: An experimental study of "physical fitness" of Air Force personnel. U.S. Armed Forces Med. J., 10:675, 1959.

21. Wolthuis, R.A., et al.: New practical treadmill protocol for clinical use. Am. J. Cardiol., 39:697, 1977.

22. Ellestad, M.H., Allen, W.A., Wan, M.L.K., and Kemp, G.L.: Maximal treadmill stress testing for cardiovascular evaluation. Circulation, 39:517, 1969.

23. Naughton, J., Sevellus, G., and Balke, B.: Physiological responses of normal and pathologic subjects to a modified work capacity test. J. Sports Med., 31:201, 1963.

24. Starling, M.R., Crawford, M.H., Kennedy, G.T., and O'Rourke, R.A.: Exercise testing early after myocardial infarction: Predictive value for subsequent unstable angina and death. Am. J. Cardiol., 46:909, 1980.

25. Detry, J.M., et al.: Diagnostic value of history and maximal exercise electrocardiography in men and women suspected of coronary heart disease. Circulation, 56:756, 1977.

26. Levine, H.J.: Difficult problems in the diagnosis of chest pain. Am. Heart J., 100:108, 1980.

27. Constant, J.: The classical diagnosis of nonanginal chest pain: The differentiation of angina from nonanginal chest pain by history. Clin. Cardiol., 6:11, 1983.

28. Glasser, S.P., and Ramsey, M.R.: An automated system for blood pressure determination during exercise. Circulation, 63:348, 1981.

29. Hossack, K.F., et al.: Evaluation of automated blood pressure measurements during exercise testing. Am. Heart J., 104:1032, 1982.

30. Koppes, G., McKiernan, T., Bassan, M., and Froelicher, V.F.: Treadmill exercise testing. Part 1. Curr. Probl. Cardiol., 7(8):1, 1977.

31. Stuart, R.J., and Ellestad, M.H.: National survey of exercise testing. Chest, 77:94, 1980.

32. Vincent, G.M., Abildskov, J.A., and Burgess, M.J.: Mechanisms of ST-segment displacement: Evaluation by direct current recordings. Circulation, 56:559, 1977.

33. Holland, R.P., and Brooks, H.: Precordial and epicardial surface potentials during myocardial ischemia in the pig. Circ. Res., 37:471, 1975.

34. Elharrar, V., and Zipes, D.P.: Cardiac electrophysiologic alterations during myocardial ischemia. Am. J. Physiol., 233:H329, 1977.

35. Holland, R., and Arnsdorf, M.F.: Solid angle theory and the electrocardiogram: Physiologic and quantitative interpretation. Prog. Cardiovasc. Dis., 19:431, 1977.

36. Cohen, D., and Kaufman, I.: Magnetic determination of the relationship between the S-T segment shift and the injury current produced by coronary artery occlusion. Circ. Res., 36:414, 1975.

37. Chaitman, B.R., Waters, D.D., Theroux, P., and Hanson, J.S.: S-T segment elevation and coronary spasm in response to exercise. Am. J. Cardiol., 47:1350, 1981.

38. Specchia, G., et al.: Significance of exercise-induced ST-segment elevation in patients without myocardial infarction. Circulation, 63:46, 1981.

39. Dunn, R.F., et al.: Exercise-induced ST-segment elevation in leads V_1 or aV_L. A predictor of anterior myocardial ischemia and left anterior descending coronary artery disease. Circulation, 63:1357, 1981.

40. Longhurst, J.C., and Kraus, W.L.: Exercise-induced ST elevation in patients without myocardial infarction. Circulation, 60:616, 1979.

41. Chahine, R.A., Raizner, A.E., and Ishimori, T.: The clinical significance of exercise induced ST segment elevation. Circulation, 54:209, 1976.

42. Gerson, M.C., Phillips, J.F., Morris, S.N., and McHenry, P.L.: Exercise-induced U-wave inversion as a marker of stenosis of the left anterior descending coronary artery. Circulation, 60:1014, 1979.

43. Meytes, L., et al.: Wenckebach A-V block: A frequent feature following heavy physical training. Am. Heart J., 90:426, 1975.

44. Chou, T.: Electrocardiography in Clinical Practice. Orlando, Fla., Grune & Stratton, 1979.

45. Schamroth, L.: Ventricular extrasystoles, ventricular tachycardia, and ventricular fibrillation: Clinical-electrocardiographic considerations. Prog. Cardiovasc. Dis., 23:13, 1980.

46. Marriott, H.J., and Myerburg, R.J.: Recognition of arrhythmias and conduction abnormalities. In The Heart. 5th Ed. Edited by J.W. Hurst. New York, McGraw-Hill, 1982.

47. Blackburn, H., et al.: Premature ventricular complexes induced by exercise: Their frequency and response to physical conditioning. Am. J. Cardiol., 31:441, 1973.

48. Goldschlager, N., Cake, D., and Cohn, K.: Exercise-induced ventricular arrhythmias in patients with coronary artery disease. Am. J. Cardiol., 31:434, 1973.

49. McHenry, P.L., Morris, S.N., Kavalier, M., and Jordan, J.W.: Comparative study of exercise-induced ventricular arrhythmias in normal sub-

jects and patients with documented coronary artery disease. Am. J. Cardiol., *37*:609, 1976.

50. Faris, J.V., McHenry, P.L., Jordan, J.W., and Morris, S.N.: Prevalence and reproducibility of exercise-induced ventricular arrhythmias during exercise testing in normal men. Am. J. Cardiol., *37*:617, 1976.

51. Sami, M., Kraemer, H., and DeBusk, R.J.: Reproducibility of exercise-induced ventricular arrhythmias after myocardial infarction. Am. J. Cardiol., *43*:724, 1979.

52. Hurst, J.W., et al.: Atherosclerotic coronary heart disease, angina pectoris, myocardial infarction, and other manifestations of myocardial ischemia. *In* The Heart. 5th Ed. Edited by J.W. Hurst. New York, McGraw-Hill, 1982.

53. Froelicher, V.F.: Exercise Testing & Training. New York, LeJacq Publishing, 1983.

54. Philbrick, J.T., et al.: The limited spectrum of patients studied in exercise test research: Analyzing the tip of the iceberg. JAMA, *248*:2467, 1982.

55. Fox, K.M., Selwyn, A., Oakley, D., and Shillingford, J.P.: Relation between the precordial projection of S-T segment changes after exercise and coronary angiographic findings. Am. J. Cardiol., *44*:1068, 1979.

56. Tonkon, M.J., et al.: Effects of digitalis on the exercise electrocardiogram in normal adult subjects. Chest, *72*:714, 1977.

57. Ellestad, M.H.: Stress Testing: Principles and Practice. 2nd Ed. Philadelphia, F.A. Davis, 1980.

58. Friesinger, G., et al.: Exercise ECG and vasoregulatory abnormalities. Am. J. Cardiol., *30*:733, 1972.

59. Diamond, G.A., and Forrester, J.S.: Analysis of probability as an aid in the clinical diagnosis of coronary artery disease. N. Engl. J. Med., *300*:1350, 1979.

60. Coronary Risk Handbook. American Heart Association, Dallas, Texas, 1973.

61. Diamond, G.A., et al.: Application of information therapy to clinical diagnostic testing: The electrocardiographic stress test. Circulation, *63*:915, 1981.

62. Rifkin, R.D., and Hood, W.B.: Bayesian analysis of electrocardiographic exercise stress testing. N. Engl. J. Med., *297*:681, 1979.

63. Patterson, R.E., Eng, C., and Horowitz, S.F.: Practical diagnosis of coronary artery disease: A Bayes' theorem nomogram to correlate clinical data with noninvasive exercise tests. Am. J. Cardiol., *53*:252, 1984.

64. Turner, J., and Goldschlager, N.: No symptoms, positive stress test: What next? J. Cardiovasc. Med., 521, May, 1983.

65. Laslett, L.J., Amsterdam, E.A., and Mason, D.T.: Evaluating the positive exercise stress test in the asymptomatic individual. Chest, *81*:364, 1982.

66. McNeer, J.F., et al.: The role of the exercise test in the evaluation of patients for ischemic heart disease. N. Engl. J. Med., *57*:64, 1978.

67. Weiner, D.A., et al.: The predictive value of anginal chest pain as an indicator of coronary disease during exercise testing. Am. Heart. J., *96*:458, 1978.

68. Bhargava, V., Watanabe, K., and Froelicher, V.F.: Progress in computer analysis of the exercise electrocardiogram. Am. J. Cardiol., *47*:1143, 1981.

69. Simoons, M.L., et al.: Quantitation of exercise electrocardiography. Circulation, *63*:471, 1981.

70. Cohn, K., et al.: Use of treadmill score to quantify ischemic response and predict extent of coronary disease. Circulation, *59*:286, 1979.

71. Kansal, S., Roitman, D., Bradley, E.L., and Sheffield, L.T.: Enhanced evaluation of treadmill tests by means of scoring based on multivariate analysis and its clinical application: A study of 608 patients. Am. J. Cardiol., *52*:1155, 1983.

72. Hollenberg, M., Budge, W.R., Wisneske, J.A., and Gertz, E.W.: Treadmill score quantifies electrocardiographic response to exercise and improves test accuracy and reproducibility. Circulation, *61*:276, 1980.

73. Hollenberg, M., et al.: Comparison of a quantitative treadmill exercise score with standard electrocardiographic criteria in screening asymptomatic men for coronary artery disease. N. Engl. J. Med., *313*:600, 1985.

74. Elamin, M.S., et al.: Accurate detection of coronary heart disease by new exercise test. Br. Heart J., *48*:311, 1982.

75. Yanowitz, F.G., et al.: Application of body surface mapping to exercise testing: S-T80 isoarea maps in patients with coronary artery disease. Am. J. Cardiol., *50*:1109, 1982.

76. Miller, W.T., Spach, M.S., and Warren, R.B.: Total body surface potential mapping during exercise: QRS-T wave changes in normal young adults. Circulation, *62*:632, 1980.

77. Silverberg, R.A., et al.: Noninvasive diagnosis of coronary artery disease: The cardiokymographic stress test. Circulation, *61*:579, 1980.

78. Vas, R., et al.: Noninvasive analysis of regional wall motion: Cardiokymography. Am. J. Physiol., *233*:H700, 1977.

79. Weiner, D.A., et al.: Cardiokymography during exercise testing: A new device for detection of coronary artery disease and left ventricular wall motion abnormalities. Am. J. Cardiol., *51*:1307, 1983.

80. Burke, J.F., et al.: The cardiokymography exercise test compared to the thallium-201 perfusion exercise test in the diagnosis of coronary artery disease. Am. Heart J., *107*:718, 1984.

81. Strauss, H.W., McKusick, K.A., and Bingham, J.B.: Cardiac nuclear imaging: Principles, instrumentation, and pitfalls. Am. J. Cardiol., *46*:1109, 1980.

82. Okada, R.D., Boucher, C.A., Strauss, H.W., and Pohost, G.M.: Exercise radionuclide imaging approaches to coronary artery disease. Am. J. Cardiol., *46*:1188, 1980.

83. Pitt, B., et al.: Impact of radionuclide techniques in evaluation of patients with ischemic heart disease. J. Am. Coll. Cardiol., *1*:63, 1983.

84. Allen, W.H., Aronow, W.S., Goodman, P., and Stinson, P.: Five-year follow-up of maximal

treadmill stress test in asymptomatic men and women. Circulation, *62*:522, 1980.

85. Giagnoni, E., et al.: Prognostic value of exercise ECG testing in asymptomatic normotensive subjects. N. Engl. J. Med., *309*:1085, 1983.

86. Bruce, R.A., Hossack, K.F., DeRouen, T.A., and Hofer, V.: Enhanced risk assessment for primary coronary heart disease events by maximal exercise testing: 10 years' experience of Seattle Heart Watch. J. Am. Coll. Cardiol., *2*:565, 1983.

87. Blumenthal, D.S., Weiss, J.L., Mellits, E.D., and Gerstenblith, G.: The predictive value of a strongly positive stress test in patients with minimal symptoms. Am. J. Med., *70*:1005, 1981.

88. Weiner, D.A., McCabe, C.H., and Ryan, T.J.: Prognostic assessment of patients with coronary artery disease by exercise testing. Am. Heart. J., *105*:749, 1983.

89. Thompson, P.D., and Kelemen, M.G.: Hypotension accompanying the onset of exertional angina. Circulation, *52*:28, 1975.

90. Okin, P.M., et al.: Improved accuracy of the exercise electrocardiogram: Identification of three-vessel coronary disease in stable angina pectoris by analysis of peak rate-related changes in ST segments. Am. J. Cardiol., *55*:271, 1985.

91. Dunn, R.F., Bailey, I.K., Uren, R., and Kelly, D.T.: Exercise-induced ST-segment elevation. Correlation of thallium-201 myocardial perfusion scanning and coronary arteriography. Circulation, *61*:989, 1980.

92. Morris, S.N., Phillips, J.F., Jordan, J.W., and McHenry, P.L.: Incidence and significance of decreases in systolic blood pressure during graded treadmill exercise testing. Am. J. Cardiol., *41*:221, 1978.

93. Bruce, R.A., et al.: Noninvasive prediction of sudden cardiac death in men with coronary heart disease. Predictive value of maximal stress testing. Am. J. Cardiol., *39*:833, 1980.

94. Ellestad, M.H., and Wan, M.K.C.: Predictive implications of stress testing. Circulation, *51*:363, 1975.

95. Cole, J.P., and Ellestad, M.H.: Significance of chest pain during treadmill testing: Correlation with coronary events. Am. J. Cardiol., *41*:227, 1978.

96. Markiewicz, W., Houston, N., and Debusk, R.F.: Exercise testing soon after myocardial infarction. Circulation, *56*:26, 1977.

97. Theroux, P., et al.: Prognostic value of exercise testing soon after myocardial infarction. N. Engl. J. Med., *301*:341, 1979.

98. Starling, M., Crawford, M.H., Kennedy, G., and O'Rourke, R.A.: Exercise testing early after myocardial infarction: Predictive value for subsequent unstable angina. Am. J. Cardiol., *46*:909, 1980.

99. Debusk, R.F., and Haskell, W.: Symptom-limited vs. heart-rate-limited exercise testing soon after myocardial infarction. Circulation, *61*:738, 1980.

100. Ewart, C.K., Taylor, C.B., Reese, L.B., and Debusk, R.F.: Effects of early postmyocardial infarction exercise testing on self-perception and

subsequent physical activity. Am. J. Cardiol., *51*:1076, 1983.

101. Davidson, D.M., and Debusk, R.F.: Prognostic value of a single exercise test 3 weeks after uncomplicated myocardial infarction. Circulation, *61*:236, 1980.

102. Madsen, E.B., and Gilpin, E.: Prognostic value of exercise test variables after myocardial infarction. J. Cardiac. Rehab., *3*:481, 1983.

103. Weber, K.T., Janicki, J.S., and Likoff, M.J.: Exercise testing in the evaluation of cardiopulmonary disease. Clin. Chest Med., *5*:173, 1984.

104. Mitchell, J.H., and Blomqvist, G.: Maximal oxygen uptake. N. Engl. J. Med., *284*:1018, 1971.

105. Beaver, W.L., Wasserman, K., and Whipp, B.J.: On-line computer analysis and breath-by-breath graphical display of exercise function tests. J. Appl. Physiol., *34*:123, 1973.

106. Wilmore, J.H., Davis, J.A., and Norton, A.C.: An automated system for assessing metabolic and respiratory function during exercise. J. Appl. Physiol., *40*:619, 1976.

107. Kannagi, T., et al.: An evaluation of the Beckman Metabolic Cart for measuring ventilation and aerobic requirements during exercise. J. Cardiac Rehab., *3*:38, 1983.

108. Sue, D.Y., Hansen, H.E., Blais, M., and Wasserman, K.: Measurement and analysis of gas exchange during exercise using a programmable calculator. J. Appl. Physiol., *49*:456, 1980.

109. Montoye, H.J., Ayen, T., Nagle, F., and Howley, E.: The oxygen requirement for horizontal and grade walking on a motor driven treadmill. Med. Sci. Sports Exerc., *17*:640, 1985.

110. Ragg, K.E., Murray, T.F., Karbonit, L.M., and Jump, D.A.: Errors in predicting functional capacity from a treadmill exercise test. Am. Heart J., *100*:581, 1980.

111. Sullivan, M., and McKirnan, M.D.: Errors in predicting functional capacity for postmyocardial infarction patients using a modified Bruce protocol. Am. Heart J., *107*:486, 1984.

112. Haskell, W.L., Savin W., Oldridge, N., and Debusk, R.F.: Factors influencing estimated oxygen uptake during exercise testing soon after myocardial infarction. Am. J Cardiol., *50*:299, 1982.

113. Exercise Testing and Training of Apparently Healthy Individuals: A Handbook for Physicians. The Committee on Exercise. Dallas, American Heart Association, 1972.

114. Astrand, P.O., and Rodahl, K.: Textbook of Work Physiology. 2nd Ed. New York, McGraw-Hill, 1977.

115. Patterson, J.A., Naughton, J., Pietras, R.J., and Gunnar, R.M.: Treadmill exercise in assessment of the functional capacity of patients with cardiac disease. Am. J. Cardiol., *30*:757, 1972.

116. Weber, K.T., Kinasewitz, G.T., Janicki, J.S., and Fishman, A.P.: Oxygen utilization and ventilation during exercise in patients with chronic cardiac failure. Circulation, *65*:1213, 1982.

117. Hossack, K.F., et al.: Maximal cardiac output during upright exercise: Approximate normal standards and variations with coronary heart disease. Am. J. Cardiol., *46*:204, 1980.

6

FORMULATING THE EXERCISE PRESCRIPTION

The exercise prescription is generally the responsibility of an exercise specialist.[1] In cardiac rehabilitation the program director, medical director, or physician supervising the exercise test is responsible for formulating the prescription, although the exercise specialist may also be actively involved.[1]

The exercise prescription is a "dosage" of exercise that is given in quantifiable units of work and consists of intensity, frequency, duration, and mode of activity. The exercise prescription is established from the results of the patient evaluation and the medical history. Guidelines for prescribing exercise have been developed from numerous studies,[1-5] and are discussed in greater detail later in the chapter.

PURPOSE

The purpose of the exercise prescription is to provide a specific amount or dose of exercise that is safe and beneficial for the individual. In particular the exercise prescription is devised to improve cardiovascular function and a sense of well-being and, hopefully, to lessen the risk for coronary heart disease (CHD). The prescription takes into account the individual's physical condition and adjusts intensity, frequency, and duration accordingly. The mode of exercise is important to ensure that activities are enjoyable as well as beneficial. Making activities more pleasurable helps to ensure long-term program adherence,[6] which is essential if the program is to have real benefits.

PHYSIOLOGIC BASIS

The intensity of exercise is established as a percentage of functional aerobic capacity, which is best reflected by maximal oxygen uptake, $\dot{V}O_2$ max.[7,8] However, because direct measurement of oxygen uptake is not performed in most clinical testing facilities, accurate determination of the heart rate response to exercise is generally substituted for $\dot{V}O_2$ measurements.[9,10] The intensity of training required for physiologic improvement is between 57% and 78% of maximal aerobic capacity ($\dot{V}O_2$ max), which is equivalent to an exercise heart rate of 70% to 85% of maximal heart rate.[11-13] A heart rate range permits the selection of the most appropriate intensity according to physical condition, age, and other factors.[14-16] Individuals with poorer physical fitness at entrance can expect greater improvement with less effort compared to more highly trained persons, who require a greater intensity for comparable gains.[17-19] The relationship of oxygen uptake and heart rate as a percentage of maximum is consistent for normal persons, cardiac patients, athletes, men, and women,[20-22] as well as for exercising upper or lower extremities (Fig. 6-1).[21,23,24]

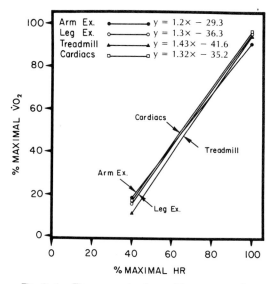

Fig. 6–1. The regression lines of two groups of normal persons and one of CAD subjects show similar relationship between submaximal oxygen intake expressed as percentage of maximum and heart rates as percentage of maximal heart rate. In the formula Y = percentage of maximal oxygen intake, and X = percentage of maximal heart rate. (Data from Hellerstein, et al.[9] and Fardy, et al.[21])

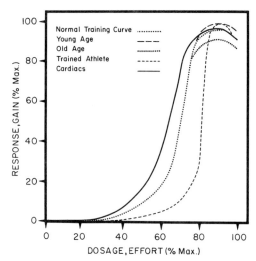

Fig. 6–2. Improvement anticipated from effort expended. A conceptual diagram illustrating training curves in various populations. Note that the trained athlete is required to exercise at a greater intensity to make gains similar to those of normal persons or cardiacs. Also, note that age of onset of training affects the maximal physiologic gain. From Fardy, P.S.: Train for aerobic power. In Toward an Understanding of Human Performance. Edited by E.J. Burke. Ithaca, New York, Mouvement Publication, 1977.

In order that exercise elicit a therapeutic effect, it is necessary to evoke the overload principle.[25,26] This means that the dosage of effort must exceed that of normal daily activity, but fall short of producing prolonged or excessive fatigue, breathlessness, or mental confusion.[27] The degree of improvement is related to the dosage, although the relationship is not linear (Fig. 6–2)[28] and is affected by age,[7,29] level of fitness,[1,30,31] and genetic predisposition.[7] The rate of improvement in men and women is the same.[32–34]

The dose–response curve shifts to the right with increased fitness. A greater training stimulus is required for more highly trained individuals.[1] The rate of improvement is gradual at first, increasing more rapidly up to an intensity of approximately 90% of maximal effort. The curve then flattens[8,28] and can assume a downward trend representing fatigue if the exercise is too intense and recovery time is insufficient. Training gains are subject to considerable individual variation.[8,16,34] Some individuals improve rapidly whereas others require a longer training period.

HEART RATE DETERMINATION

Adherence to the exercise heart rate prescription is necessary for both maximal benefits and safety. Therefore, heart rate measurements should be made regularly during an exercise session. Heart rates can be obtained manually, with telemetry, with an electrocardiogram (ECG) recorder, or with an accurate cardiotachometer. In a cardiac rehabilitation program, short ECG rhythm strips provide accurate heart rates and can also ensure a safe level of effort by detecting ventricular arrhythmias, conduction defects, and ST segment changes. Occurrences of ischemic ST segment displacement, or marked rhythm alterations frequently are asymptomatic. They may also occur at low levels of physical exertion,[35,36] which illustrates the fallacy that a safe level of effort can be perceived subjectively in cardiac patients. Monitoring equipment is discussed more completely in Chapters 7 and 11. Procedures for determining heart rate by palpation are discussed later in this chapter.

INTENSITY OF TRAINING

The single most important factor in the exercise prescription is intensity,[16,31,34] which is expressed as a percentage of aerobic capacity or maximal heart rate. The exercise heart rate reflects a percentage of $\dot{V}O_2$ max,[37] as well as giving an indication of myocardial oxygen demand.[38]

Early investigations to determine the threshold of exercise intensity indicated that an absolute heart rate of 130 to 150 beats per minute (bpm) was required for improvement.[11,39,40] Other studies, however, have found that improvements are possible with lower rates.[41,42] The fallacy of using a fixed target heart rate for everyone is the failure to consider differences in age and physical condition. Because maximal heart rate decreases with age (Table 6–1),[37,43] the actual heart rate during exercise may vary considerably and still result in significant improvements in cardiovascular fitness. A heart rate of 130, for example, is approximately 65% of the age-predicted maximal heart rate for a 20-year-old person and about 81% of age-predicted maximal heart rate for a 60 year old. In the former example the training stimulus is probably too little, whereas in the latter

it might be too strenuous. The initial level of fitness also influences the effectiveness of the training stimulus. Favorable adaptive changes are observed with a lower training stimulus in less fit individuals.[1,30,31]

It should be apparent from this discussion that less than maximal activity (aerobic) brings about favorable cardiovascular change and is most recommended for endurance training and cardiac rehabilitation.[2,3] Maximal or near maximal activity (anaerobic) is not necessary for beneficial results and may subject the person to unnecessary risk. Even a modest level of activity—for example, regular walking at a brisk pace—can be of sufficient intensity to have beneficial results.[2,3,44] If the intensity of training is excessive, there may be undue cardiovascular and musculoskeletal stress[45,46] including heart block,[46] muscle injury or soreness, and decreased program adherence.[37,45] Many documented coronary events have been observed during such circumstances.[47] A modest level of exercise is especially suggested at the outset of a new program for persons who were formerly athletes. These individuals tend to over exert themselves,[48] as they reflect on past accomplishments and think that their physical condition has little changed. As a rule of thumb, one should not become excessively out of breath while exercising; that is, one should be able to pass the "talk test."[48] This can be ensured reasonably well by close adherence to the training heart rate. This level of exertion usually pro-

Table 6–1.   Relationship of Age and Maximal Heart Rate[a]

Age	Average Max HR	85% Max	70% Max
20	200	170	140
25	195	166	137
30	190	162	133
35	185	158	129
40	180	153	126
45	175	149	123
50	170	145	119
55	165	140	115
60	160	136	112
65	155	132	109

[a]With maximal heart rate equal to 220 minus age in years.

duces perspiration, an increase in breathing, and a not unpleasant sense of fatigue.[48]

Alternative approaches to prescribing the appropriate intensity of exercise include the Karvonen method of using heart rate, the metabolic equivalent (MET) method, or the perceived exertion scale. With the Karvonen system, resting heart rate is subtracted from maximal rate, and a percentage of the difference is added to the resting rate to yield the training rate.[11,49] This approach takes into account the variability in resting heart rate. For example, if two individuals have identical maximal heart rates, the one with a lower resting heart rate might conceivably have a lower absolute exercise heart rate, although the percentage of difference could be the same. If the Karvonen system is used, 60% of the difference between resting and maximal heart rates has been found necessary for improvement. As an example of this method:

Maximal heart rate	170
Resting heart rate	70
Heart rate prescription is equal to 170 minus 70 × 0.60 (% required for improvement) plus 70 (resting heart rate).	
Heart rate prescription	130

The Karvonen method is sometimes advantageous in patients who are taking beta-blockers that significantly lower maximal heart rate, or for those persons whose resting heart rates are abnormally high, resulting in an exercise prescription barely above the resting level. For example, a 65-year-old man with a resting heart rate of 90 might have the following prescription:

Maximal heart rate		155
Target heart rate	70% maximal heart rate	
or		108

If this person is taking a beta-blocker medication, the following could be anticipated:

Maximal heart rate		100
Target heart rate	70% maximal heart rate	
or		70
Resting heart rate		65

In either example the exercise prescrip-

tion is not much above the resting rate and might preclude any physical exertion beyond standing. Since elevated resting heart rates are common in patients with coronary disease, particularly those who have had bypass surgery, the Karvonen system should be considered. The methods used for determining target heart rates apply for normal persons and postinfarct and post bypass surgery patients.[2-4]

Prescribing exercise using METs is another method to indicate exercise intensity. A MET is equivalent to the amount of oxygen required at rest in a sitting position and equals approximately 3.5 ml O_2/kg/min.[50] Multiples of this value reflect respective levels of energy expenditure (Tables 6–2 and 6–3). Prescribing exercise by METs is popular because of the numeric simplicity. The concept is easy to understand, and the numbers are easily related to other measures of work (Table 6–4).

There are several limitations with prescribing exercise by METs.[3] Its apparent simplicity as a representation of exercise intensity has often resulted in its use without a thorough understanding of meaning. As a result, there is a tendency to overestimate the accuracy of METs. At best, the METs method represents an estimate of energy expenditure that is easily understood and convenient to adopt. Its limitations are failure to consider variations in energy expenditures among individuals according to size, physical condition, level of skill, environmental factors, and so on; activities that require high levels of skill are subject to a wide range of MET values; the element of competition can significantly alter METs. The use of METs to prescribe exercise can be improved by modifying the prescription according to the level of physical condition of the individual (Table 6–5).

A final limitation in using METs to prescribe exercise is determining the oxygen uptake equivalency of a MET. Usually, a MET is equivalent to 3.5 ml O_2/kg/min. In upright exercise, however, standing rest oxygen uptake is closer to 4.0 ml O_2/kg/

Table 6–2.   Leisure Activities: Sports, Exercise Classes, Games, Dancing—Approximate Range in Energy Cost (METs)[a]

Archery (target or field)	3–4	Horseshoe pitching	2–3
Backpacking	5–11	Hunting (bow or gun)	3–7
Badminton	4–9	Small game (walking,	
Basketball		carrying light load)	3–7
Nongame	3–9	Hunting (bow or gun)	
Game play	7–12	Big game (dragging	
Bed exercise		carcass, walking)	3–14
(arm movement, supine		Jogging (running)	7–15
or sitting)	1–2	Mountain climbing	5–10
Bicycling		Paddleball	
(pleasure or to work)	3–8	(or racquetball)	8–12
Bowling	2–4	Sailing	2–5
Canoeing, rowing, and		Scuba diving	5–10
kayaking	3–8	Shuffleboard	2–3
Conditioning exercises		Skating, ice and roller	5–8
(calisthenics)	3–8	Skiing, snow	
Dancing		Downhill	5–8
(social and square)	3–7	Cross-country	6–12
Fencing	6–10	Sledding	
Fishing		(and tobogganing)	4–8
From bank, boat, or ice	2–4	Snowshoeing	7–14
Stream (wading)	5–6	Squash	8–12
Football, touch	6–10	Soccer	5–12
Golf		Softball	3–6
Using power cart	2–3	Stair-climbing	4–8
Walking (carrying bag		Swimming	4–8
or pulling cart)	4–7	Table tennis	3–5
Handball	8–12	Tennis	4–9
Hiking, cross-country	3–7	Volleyball	3–6
Horseback riding	3–8		

[a]Adapted from Fox, S.M., Naughton, J.P., and Gorman, P.A.: Physical activity and cardiovascular health. III. The exercise prescription: Frequency and type of activity. Mod. Concepts Cardiovasc. Dis., *41*:25, 1972.

min.[51] The 3.5 ml O_2/kg/min value eliminates the oxygen uptake attributed to the change from sitting to standing that is not part of the activity. Furthermore, it should be understood that the value of 3.5 ml O_2/kg/min is only an average and that resting $\dot{V}O_2$ should be measured to increase accuracy. A comparison between MET values using estimated resting $\dot{V}O_2$ and actual resting $\dot{V}O_2$ is shown in Table 6–6. At upper levels of exercise, there is a difference of two METs according to which baseline value is adopted.

Ratings of perceived exertion (RPE) constitute another technique used for prescribing intensity of exercise. The concept of perceived exertion was originally devised by Borg.[52,53] The RPE scale (Table 6–7) was subsequently developed to quantify perceived exertion and to test its reliability and validity for use in prescription of exercise and evaluating the stress of physical activity. The Borg scale ranges from 6 to 20 and assigns subjective estimates of effort to numeric scores. The numeric scale was purposely devised to represent approximately 10% of the heart rate range in healthy young and middle-aged men.[52,53] RPE has also become very popular as a method for determining the level of effort in both functional and diagnostic exercise stress testing.

Research shows that RPE correlates well with several physiologic functions (e.g., heart rate, oxygen uptake, ventilation, respiratory rate, body temperature, lactate levels) and is useful and accurate for prescribing exercise both in healthy individuals and in cardiacs.[54–57] Other work, however, has described the potential for serious limitations if exercise is prescribed for cardiac patients solely on the basis of per-

Table 6–3. Leisure Activities: Nonsports Approximate Range in Energy Cost (METs)[a]

	METs
Carpentry	2–7
Electric vibrator	2
Gardening	
Hoeing	4–8
Digging, shoveling, and pushing	4–8
Wheelbarrow	4–10
Weeding	3–5
Raking	3–6
Home improvement (painting, plumbing)	3–8
Heavy housework (scrubbing floors, making beds)	3–6
Light housework (sweeping, polishing, ironing)	2–4
Mowing lawn	
On cart	2
Power mower	4–5
Hand mower	4–6
Splitting and sawing wood or cutting trees	
Hand	5–10
Power	2–4
Snow shoveling	
Wet snow	8–15
Powder snow	6–9
Walking	
Horizontal or slight grade	3–5
Steep grade	6–8
Upstairs	6–8
Downstairs	4–5

[a]Adapted from Fox, S.M., Naughton, J.P., and Gorman, P.A.: Physical activity and cardiovascular health. III. The exercise prescription: Frequency and type of activity. Mod. Concepts Cardiovasc. Dis., 41:25, 1972.

Table 6–4. Comparison of Work Output During Bicycle Ergometry and Treadmill Work[a]

Bicycle Ergometer External Work Output			Energy Expenditure of an Average Individual (70-kg body weight)			Treadmill Work Loads[e]	
METs	(kpm/min[b])	(Watts[c])	O_2 Uptake (L/min)	O_2 Uptake (ml/kg × min)	Calories[d] (per min)	Speed (mph)	Grade (%)
2.4	150	25	0.6	8.5	3.0	2.0	0.0
3.7	300	50	0.9	13.0	4.5	3.0	0.0
5.0	450	75	1.2	17.0	6.0	3.0	5.0
6.0	600	100	1.5	21.0	7.5	3.0	7.5
7.0	750	125	1.8	26.0	9.0	3.0	10.0
8.5	900	150	2.1	30.0	10.5	3.0	15.0
						4.0	10.0
10.0	1050	175	2.4	36.0	12.0	4.0	14.0
11.0	1200	200	2.7	39.0	14.0	7.0 (running)	0.0
						3.5	16.0
12.0	1350	225	3.0	43.0	15.0	4.0	18.0
						3.5	20.0
13.5	1500	250	3.3	47.0	17.0	8.0 (running)	0.0
						4.2	16.0
14.5	1650	275	3.8	51.0	18.0	3.5	26.0
						4.0	22.0
16.0	1800	300	3.9	56.0	20.0	10.0 (running)	0.0
						5.0	18.0

[a]Adapted from Exercise Testing and Training of Apparently Healthy Individuals: A Handbook for Physicians. New York, American Heart Association, 1972.
[b]Kilopond-meter: Energy necessary to lift a 1-kg mass 1 m against the normal gravitational force.
[c]Watt: A unit of power equal to 6.12 kpm/min.
[d]Calorie: A unit of energy based on heat production. One calorie equals 200 ml of O_2 consumed.
[e]Steady state required.

Table 6–5. Prescribing Exercise According to Individual Functional Capacity

Functional Capacity (METs)[a]	Percentage plus Functional Capacity	Average Conditioning Intensity (METs)
3	60[b] + 3 = 63	1.90
5	60 + 5 = 65	3.25
10	60 + 10 = 70	7.00
15	60 + 15 = 75	11.25
20	60 + 20 = 80	16.00

[a]As determined from exercise stress test.
[b]60% is the minimal rx intensity.

Table 6–6. A Comparison of Estimated METs (using 3.5 ml/kg × min) and Actual METs (utilizing resting $\dot{V}O_2$) During Exercise Testing[a]

Exercise Stage	MPH	% Grade	$\dot{V}O_2$ (ml/kg × min)	Actual METs	Estimated METs
Standing rest			4.2	1.0	1.2
1	2.0	0	10.4	2.5	3.0
2	2.0	3.5	12.6	3.0	3.6
3	2.0	7.0	15.8	3.7	4.5
4	2.0	10.5	19.2	4.5	5.5
5	2.0	14.0	22.2	5.2	6.3
6	2.0	17.5	25.6	6.0	7.3
7	3.0	12.5	28.7	6.8	8.2
8	3.0	15.0	32.4	7.6	9.3
9	3.0	17.5	36.5	8.6	10.4
10	3.0	20.0	40.7	9.6	11.6

[a]Adapted from Fardy, P.S., and Hellerstein, H.K.: Comparison of continuous and intermittent multistage exercise tests. Med. Sci. Sports, *10*:7, 1978.

ceived exertion.[35,36] Cardiac patients should only use perceived exertion to assess exercise intensity in conjunction with a prescribed target heart rate that has been determined from a functional exercise stress test. Low-level heart rate prescrip-

Table 6–7. Borg Scale of Perceived Exertion[52,53]

6	
7	Very, very light
8	
9	Very light
10	
11	Fairly light
12	
13	Somewhat hard
14	
15	Hard
16	
17	Very hard
18	
19	Very, very hard
20	

(Data from G.A. Borg)

tions that are arbitrarily selected and are labeled "safe" and beneficial can also have serious and potentially dangerous limitations. For example, a heart rate of 120 has been suggested as an intensity of effort that can safely be undertaken. For those patients taking beta-blockers, however, a heart rate of 120 may represent an extremely high level of effort and perhaps be unattainable. The patient who is told to exercise until the appearance of symptoms and that "your body will signal when to stop" might also be placed in a compromised position.[35,36]

DURATION OF EXERCISE

Most studies indicate that the duration of exercise must be at least 20 to 30 minutes to be beneficial for the cardiovascular system.[1-4] Nevertheless, it has also been shown that programs of only 5 to 10 minutes have produced favorable results,[37,41,42] particularly for less fit individuals. A minimum of 20 minutes of exercise at the prescribed target heart rate is used in most cardiac rehabilitation and beginning adult fitness programs.

The length of the program is another important factor of program design. Most programs in cardiac rehabilitation are 8 to 12 weeks in duration, which is considered a minimal amount of time for significant changes to occur. Some training adaptation may appear in 4 to 6 weeks,[41,58] especially in persons who exercise at high intensity or those who are unfit initially. In some instances training improvements have been observed after 2 weeks.[8,42] However, in some measures, particularly body composition, it may take many months before changes are noted.[16,59] The rate as well as the magnitude of changes can vary considerably among individuals.[59]

FREQUENCY OF EXERCISE

Even though the frequency of exercise appears less important than intensity or duration,[16,19,39] a minimal number of sessions per week is needed for favorable cardiovascular change or for maintenance. In most studies training 3 to 5 days a week is required to improve cardiovascular function,[39,45] and 2 to 3 days a week is necessary for maintenance,[1,3] although improvements have been demonstrated from as few as 2 days a week.[3,60] Fewer than 2 days of training a week is insufficient for beneficial changes.[2,3,61] It has also been observed that training 5 or more days a week might be no better or even worse than fewer days of training,[8,62] because the incidence of injury is increased when compared to 3 days a week of regular activity. Guidelines for intensity, frequency, and duration of exercise for highly trained and sedentary individuals and cardiac patients are summarized in Table 6–8.

MODE OF EXERCISE

A variety of exercise modalities can be effective as long as intensity, duration, and frequency of exercise meet approved standards and the individual adheres to accepted training principles.[2,3,16] In selecting the most appropriate mode of exercise, the objective of the program needs to be considered. For example the mode is different if the objective is cardiovascular fitness rather than cardiac rehabilitation. For fitness, activities should be planned that improve the cardiovascular system and are enjoyable. If cardiac rehabilitation is the primary objective, then activities that are quantifiable and easily supervised are of equal or greater importance. Because exercise soon after infarct or surgery (phases I and II) is generally conducted in a confined and closely controlled environment, activities are selected that can be performed in limited amount of space. Providing an environment that is enjoyable as well as one that produces beneficial results is extremely important to maintain long-term interest and compliance. Minimizing competition is also important in cardiac rehabilitation,[25] although eliminating competition entirely may neither be possible nor realistic. The exercise specialist needs to be innovative in order to select and develop activities that are designed to best meet all of these needs on an individual basis.

Cardiovascular function and physical work capacity are enhanced best through continuous, rhythmic, and isotonic movements of large muscle groups that are designed to overload the oxygen transport system. Activities such as walking, jogging, swimming, bicycling, rowing, and cross country skiing are all appropriate.[2,3,50] There is no "best" type of exercise, although each of those mentioned has advantages and disadvantages. Swimming and bicycling are good because they are less likely to cause musculoskeletal injury to the lower extremities than are jogging or aero-

Table 6–8. Exercise Requirements for Achieving Cardiovascular Changes in Highly Trained Persons, Sedentary Individuals, and Cardiacs[a]

	Intensity	Frequency	Duration
Highly trained	85%–90% max HR	5–7 days	1–2 hours
Sedentary and cardiac	60%–85% max HR	3–5 days	15–45 min

[a]From Fardy, P.S.: Training for aerobic power. In Toward an Understanding of Human Performance. Edited by E.J. Burke. Ithaca, New York, Mouvement Publications, 1977.

bic dance.[63] An exercise prescription for swimming, however, should be devised from a test mode that is similar to that activity, if not swimming itself. If the prescription is based on treadmill testing, the results could create a metabolic overload that might compromise patient safety.[3,64] Unfortunately, swim test devices are uncommon and seldom used in either cardiac rehabilitation or adult fitness. In addition serious exercise training by swimming requires a degree of competency that few possess, and both swimming and bicycling require special equipment and facilities and are weather dependent if done outdoors.

Walking and jogging can be done almost anywhere and have minimal equipment and facility needs. Avoiding hard surfaces and wearing appropriate shoes help to alleviate musculoskeletal injury from walking, jogging, running, and jumping activities.[13]

Benefits to the cardiovascular system from sudden stop-and-go activities such as handball and racquetball, as well as static isometric and heavy-resistance strength-building exercises, are questionable.[3,25] These exercises can subject the myocardium to undue demands and provoke dangerous Valsalva maneuvers,[28] rhythm alterations,[65] and pressor responses.[66] The strain of heavy lifting can also prevent adequate blood flow through the lungs and contribute to catastrophic results.[28] Some isometric activity is tolerable and may even be beneficial for the patient with normal ventricular function.[67] Otherwise, isometrics and heavy-resistance exercise are generally only recommended for the athlete or

individual whose primary objective is to increase strength and muscle size.

Isokinetic exercise is a popular training technique that emphasizes constant muscle resistance throughout the range of motion at varying speeds of limb movement.[68–70] It appears that strength and cardiovascular function may be improved from isokinetics,[8,71,72] although there is still need for more research. The different types of exercise training programs are defined and summarized in Tables 6–9 and 6–10.

ADDITIONAL CONSIDERATIONS

Continuous versus Intermittent Exercise

The merits of continuous and intermittent or interval exercise have been widely

Table 6–9. Types of Training Programs

Aerobic
Low level to less than maximal intensity exercise

The supply of oxygen to exercising muscles meets the demand

Anaerobic
High-intensity exercise
The demand for oxygen at the muscle cells is greater than the supply

Isotonic
Muscle contraction accompanied by a change in the length of the muscle fibers

Isometric
Muscle contraction that results in increased tension but no change in length of the muscle fibers

Isokinetic
Muscle contraction with constant resistance throughout the range of motion

Continuous
Prolonged exercise that is isotonic and aerobic

Interval (intermittent)
Short bouts of high-intensity anaerobic exercise with periods of rest between
Classic interval training consists of a predetermined and set time and distance of work, number of repetitions, and a predetermined and set time for rest

Table 6–10. Types of Exercise Training Programs

Aerobic		Anaerobic
Continuous		Intermittent
Isotonic	Isometric	Isokinetic
	Training stimulus may be elicited through:	
	Controlled exercises and/or recreational activities	

reported.[16,73,74] Each of these training techniques has inherent advantages, and the ideal program contains elements of both. Nevertheless, there are generally more benefits from interval or intermittent training for most types of conditioning programs. More physical work is possible in the same amount of time, and the same level of work can be undertaken with reduced physiologic demand and with lower levels of metabolic byproducts.[16,74] As a general rule, however, high-intensity interval or intermittent training is not recommended for cardiac patients.[4] Instead, continuous or low-level interval work is emphasized, particularly at the outset to prepare the myocardium, skeletal muscles, ligaments, and tendons for more intense physical exertion.[37,75] Interval and intermittent training are particularly popular because they can easily be applied in carefully regulated doses, can incorporate a variety of exercises to enhance endurance in upper and lower extremity muscle groups, and provide interesting and diverse activities.

Training Specificity

Another important consideration of the exercise prescription is the specificity of training. Since adaptation is muscle specific,[3,8,76] it is necessary to exercise all major muscle groups for a complete conditioning program.[3,77] Furthermore, training response to identical work loads differs markedly according to the muscle groups and even fibers within muscle groups that are recruited.[3,51,78] Those individuals whose leisure interests or occupation require arm work should incorporate arm exercises as a part of their training program.

A program that is limited to leg exercise (e.g., walking–jogging and stationary bicycling) is insufficient to meet the demands imposed by upper extremity effort.

Individualization

In the past, exercise programs often had been conducted as group sessions where everyone performed the same activity in the same dosage. Today, most programs recognize the need for individualization. In particular it is necessary to account for decreases in maximal heart rate with increased age (Table 6–1) and to adjust the training stimulus according to individual ability and actual maximal heart rate.[1–4]

Individualized exercise does not preclude group activity but, rather, reinforces the concept of having each person in the group proceed at the most appropriate pace for that individual. This is important because long-term adherence is generally better with group exercise compared to exercising alone.[79–81]

Counting the Pulse

Palpating the heart at rest is sometimes difficult because of clothing, fatty tissue, and chest cage size. It is usually easier to obtain an accurate heart rate at other sites (Fig. 6–3), most notably the carotid or radial arteries. Following exercise, a pulse at any of these sites can usually be felt easily. Taking the pulse over the carotid artery has created some controversy for fear of exerting too much pressure and evoking a carotid sinus reflex action.[82] Since patients with coronary artery disease (CAD) are more sensitive to carotid sinus reflex,[83,84] they should be especially cautious when palpating at this site.

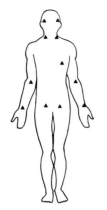

Fig. 6–3. Sites for determining pulsations.

The best method of manually counting heart rate is to determine the number of pulsations in a given time and convert to minute heart rate. This technique requires a stopwatch and a table for rapid conversion (Tables 6–11 and 6–12).[7] The method is as follows:

1. The stopwatch is started on the earliest detectable beat, which is counted as zero.
2. The watch is stopped at the specified number of seconds. Thirty is commonly used, although ten is better.
3. Convert the time to minute rate. Since heart rate decelerates rapidly upon cessation of exercise,[18] the rate during effort is estimated more accurately if the pulse is counted immediately after stopping.

If a stopwatch is unavailable, a large clock or timer with a sweep second hand or even a wristwatch with a second hand will suffice. The technique in this situation is as follows:[85]

1. Locate the pulse as quickly as possible.
2. Count the number of beats for 10 seconds, beginning with zero.
3. Multiply by 6 for the minute rate (Table 6–13).

If the pulse is counted for more than 15 seconds, the heart rate will decelerate in most persons, athough changes are not as great in poorly conditioned individuals.[86] If it takes 20 to 30 seconds to locate and count the pulse, the exercise heart rate will be substantially underestimated. The disadvantage of counting the pulse for less than 10 seconds, unless with a stopwatch, is that the potential for error is magnified, especially at high heart rates. For example, an error of one-half second when taken for 5 seconds means a difference of 20 beats at a heart rate of 200.

The disadvantages of manual heart rate determinations are:

1. It can take too much time to locate the pulse.
2. The accuracy of counting beats is questionable.
3. Accurate timing can present a problem.
4. Recovery pulse rates may not reflect exercise rates.
5. Arrhythmias make counting difficult.

Table 6–11. Conversion of Pulse Beats for 10 Seconds into Minute Heart Rate

10-Second Rate	Minute Rate	10-Second Rate	Minute Rate
10	60	23	138
11	66	24	144
12	72	25	150
13	78	26	156
14	84	27	162
15	90	28	168
16	96	29	174
17	102	30	180
18	108	31	186
19	114	32	192
20	120	33	198
21	126	34	204
22	132	35	210

Table 6–12.   Conversion Table for Time of 30 Pulse Beats to Pulse Rate Per Minute[a]

Time (sec)	Heart Rate (bpm)	Time (sec)	Heart Rate (bpm)	Time (sec)	Heart Rate (bpm)
18.0	100	14.6	123	11.2	161
17.8	101	14.4	125	11.0	164
17.6	102	14.2	127	10.8	167
17.4	103	14.0	129	10.6	170
17.2	105	13.8	130	10.4	173
17.0	106	13.6	132	10.2	176
16.8	107	13.4	134	10.0	180
16.6	108	13.2	136	9.8	184
16.4	110	13.0	138	9.6	188
16.2	111	12.8	141	9.4	191
16.0	113	12.6	143	9.2	196
15.8	114	12.4	145	9.0	200
15.6	115	12.2	148	8.8	205
15.4	117	12.0	150	8.6	209
15.2	118	11.8	153	8.4	214
15.0	120	11.6	155	8.2	220
14.8	122	11.4	158	8.0	225

Using a stopwatch, determine the time required for 30 pulse beats. Move down the respective column to the time obtained and convert to the respective heart rate.

[a]Adapted from Saltin, B., et al.: Physical training in sedentary middle-aged and older men. II. Oxygen uptake, heart rate, and blood lactate concentration at submaximal and maximal exercise. Scand. J. Clin. Lab. Invest., *24*:323, 1969.

Updating the Prescription

Cardiac patients with uncompromised or only moderately compromised left ventricular function can begin to show benefits from exercise in 4 to 6 weeks. As patients and normal persons adapt to exercise, peripheral and central changes occur, which are reflected in reduced heart rates at submaximal levels of effort.[7,8] Consequently, more work can be performed at the same target heart rate. Therefore, work loads must be increased for further training changes.[4]

The staff has the responsibility to update the exercise prescription when appropriate. This can be done in two ways, that is, by increasing work loads so that the relative heart rate remains constant, and by increasing the target heart rate so that relative to maximum one is exercising at a greater intensity. For example, after a few weeks of exercise, a work load on the bicycle ergometer might be increased from 300 to 450 kpm/min to keep the person at

Table 6–13.   Conversion Table for Time of 10 Pulse Beats to Pulse Rate Per Minute[a]

Time (sec)	Heart Rate (bpm)	Time (sec)	Heart Rate (bpm)	Time (sec)	Heart Rate (bpm)
6.0	100	4.8	125	3.6	167
5.9	102	4.7	128	3.5	171
5.8	103	4.6	130	3.4	176
5.7	105	4.5	133	3.3	182
5.6	107	4.4	136	3.2	188
5.5	109	4.3	140	3.1	194
5.4	111	4.2	143	3.0	200
5.3	113	4.1	146	2.9	207
5.2	115	4.0	150	2.8	214
5.1	118	3.9	154	2.7	222
5.0	120	3.8	158	2.6	230
4.9	122	3.7	162	2.5	240

[a]Based on technique of Saltin et al.[17]

the training heart rate. After a few more weeks, the staff might decide to increase the target heart rate from 70% to 75% maximal heart rate, which would result in the need to increase work loads again. Over a 12-week cardiac rehabilitation program, the target heart rate is usually increased to 80% or even 85% of maximal heart rate. However, before relative heart rate is increased, the cardiac rehabilitation staff, including the physician, should assess the patient's progress and then decide the course of action to optimize safety and benefit.

Modifying the Exercise Prescription

The guidelines that have been presented thus far meet the needs of most cardiac patients and normal persons. In some instances, however, modifications are necessary. The compromised cardiac patient is an example of such an individual. These patients generally have limited physical work capacity and very low tolerance for exercise compared to those with normal ventricular function. As a result, these patients usually start at a low intensity and progress slowly. In these examples the amount of exercise is primarily adjusted through alterations in duration or frequency. These patients might exercise a little longer each session or exercise more frequently for their prescription. Exercise sessions might also be interspersed with periods of rest, which could be decreased in duration as adaptation takes place. Each patient must be assessed individually, and the prescription needs to be flexible enough to meet the person's specific needs.

Pharmacologic Agents

Certain medications will affect the exercise prescription. These must be carefully considered in order to maximize the effects of training and of the prescribed medications. In addition it is imperative to determine at each training session that medications were taken in the appropriate dosage and at the time designated. Medi-

cations are discussed in detail in Chapter 3.

Exercise Prescription Form

An exercise prescription form should be designed for cardiac rehabilitation that contains all of the necessary information to conduct the exercise training session safely and effectively. The form should include data and results of the most recent exercise test, medications, comments and recommendations, and the exercise prescription. The prescription form should be signed by the program director or medical director and needs to be accessible to the staff and become part of the patient's exercise training file. Information should be updated at subsequent evaluations.

Prescribing Exercise at the Work Site

Exercise programs conducted at the work site can be beneficial for employees.[87,88] Programs vary in size from small exercise rooms with little equipment, which are designed for a restricted number of persons, usually upper level executives, to large well-equipped facilities designed for large numbers of employees. The guidelines for prescribing exercise are the same as those already discussed, although modes of exercise often vary considerably.

Although programs at the work site have become more common in recent years, most businesses do not have the financial base for expensive programs. Success under these circumstances relies on a creative staff that can develop low-cost programs.

A good example of creative planning is a program that was in a high-rise office building located in an urban setting where space was not available for an exercise room and out-of-house facilities were inconvenient. Yet, the employer was interested in having employees exercise. The result was an organized stair-climbing program that was preceded and followed by a thorough evaluation. The program demonstrated that stair climbing, which was performed at the convenience of the employee, had excellent compliance, improved cardiovascular function, reduced body fat, and enhanced work efficiency.[30] This project demonstrated that a beneficial program could be conducted under restrictive circumstances at low cost and easily scheduled into the regular work routine.

CONCLUSIONS

The exercise prescription is based on the results of the exercise test, taking into consideration age, medical history, and level of physical condition. With this information the exercise specialist or other allied health professional can develop an appropriate intensity, frequency, duration, and mode of exercise to meet each individual's needs. Hopefully, the exercise regimen will become part of a lifelong plan to foster better health and fitness. Sedentary normal persons and cardiac patients need to train a minimum of three times a week, for 20 to 30 minutes per session, at 70 to 85% of the maximal heart rate, determined from a maximal exercise test. The exercise prescription needs to be individualized and must be adjusted as cardiovascular fitness and physical work capacity improve. Training adaptation usually requires a minimum of 4 to 6 weeks. The most appropriate modes of exercise for cardiac patients or those interested in cardiovascular function are continuous aerobic activities that utilize upper and lower extremities. Good facilities and equipment are important in well-designed programs, although staff creativity is probably the most important factor of a successful program.

REFERENCES

1. American College of Sports Medicine: Guidelines for Exercise Testing and Prescription. 3rd Ed. Philadelphia, Lea & Febiger, 1986.
2. Getchell, L.H.: Exercise prescription for the healthy adult. J. Cardiopul. Rehab., 6:46, 1986.
3. Franklin, B.A., Hellerstein, H.K., Gordon, S., and
Timmis, G.C.: Exercise prescription for the myocardial infarction patient. J. Cardiopul. Rehabil., 6:62, 1986.
4. Pollock, M.L., Pels, A.E., Foster, C., and Ward, A.: Exercise prescription for rehabilitation of the cardiac patient. In Heart Disease and Rehabilitation. 2nd Ed. Edited by M.L. Pollock and D.H. Schmidt. New York, John Wiley & Sons, 1986.
5. Metier, C.P., Pollock, M.L., and Graves, J.E.: Exercise prescription for the coronary artery bypass graft surgery patient. J. Cardiopul. Rehabil., 6:85, 1986.
6. Franklin, B.A.: Motivating and educating adults to exercise. J. Health Phys. Ed. Rec., 49:13, 1978.
7. Astrand, P.O., and Rodahl, K.: Textbook of Work Physiology. 2nd Ed. New York, McGraw-Hill, 1977.
8. McArdle, W.D., Katch, F.I., and Katch, V.L.: Exercise Physiology: Energy, Nutrition, and Human Performance. 2nd Ed. Philadelphia, Lea & Febiger, 1986.
9. Hellerstein, H.K., et al.: Principles of exercise prescription for normals and cardiac subjects. In Exercise Testing and Exercise Training in Coronary Heart Disease. Edited by J.P. Naughton, H.K. Hellerstein, and I.C. Mohler. Orlando, Fla., Academic Press, 1973.
10. Taylor, H.L., Haskell,W., Fox, S.M., and Blackburn, H.: Exercise tests: A summary of procedures and concepts of stress testing for cardiovascular diagnosis and function evaluation. In Measurement in Exercise Electrocardiography. Edited by H. Blackburn. Springfield, Ill., Charles C Thomas, 1969.
11. Karvonen, M.J., Kentala E., and Mustala, O.: The effects of training on heart rate. A "longitudinal" study. Ann. Med. Exp. Biol. Fenn., 35:307, 1957.
12. Robinson, S.: Experimental studies of physical fitness in relation to age. Arbeitsphysiologie, 10:251, 1938.
13. Zohman, L.R., and Gualitere, W.S.: Exercise by prescription. Cardiac Rehab., 1:9, 1970.
14. American College of Sports Medicine: Guidelines for Exercise Testing and Prescription. 3rd Ed. Philadelphia, Lea & Febiger, 1986.
15. Pollock, M.L., Wilmore, J.H., and Fox, S.M.: Exercise in Health and Disease. 2nd Ed. Philadelphia, W.B. Saunders, 1984.
16. Pollock, M.L.: The quantification of endurance training programs. In Exercise and Sport Sciences Reviews. Vol. 1. Edited by J.H. Wilmore. Orlando, Fla., Academic Press, 1973.
17. Saltin, B., Hartley, L., Kilbom, A., and Astrand, I.: Physical training in sedentary middle-aged and older men. II. Oxygen uptake, heart rate, and blood lactate concentration at submaximal and maximal exercise. Scand. J. Clin. Lab. Invest., 24:323 1969.
18. Sharkey, B.J.: Intensity and duration of training and the development of cardiac respiratory endurance. Med. Sci. Sports, 2:197, 1970.
19. Shephard, R.J.: Intensity, duration and frequency of exercise as determinants of the response to a training regime. Int. Z. Angew, Physiol., 26:272, 1968.

20. Londeree, B.R., and Ames, S.A.: Trend analysis of the %Vo₂ max-HR regression. Med. Sci. Sports, 8:122, 1976.
21. Fardy, P.S., Webb, D.P., and Hellerstein, H.K.: Benefits of arm exercise in cardiac rehabilitation. Physician Sportsmed., 5:33, 1977.
22. Franklin, B., Hodgson, J., and Buskirk, E.R.: Relationship between percent maximal O₂ uptake and percent maximal heart rate in women. Res. Q. Exerc. Sport, 51:616, 1980.
23. Franklin, B.A., Vander, L., Wrisley, D., and Rubenfire, M.: Aerobic requirements of arm ergometry: Implications for exercise testing and training. Physician Sportsmed., 11:81, 1983.
24. Vander, L.B., Franklin, B.A., Wrisley, D., and Rubenfire, M.: Cardiorespiratory responses to arm and leg ergometry in women. Physician Sportsmed., 12:101, 1984.
25. Exercise Testing and Training of Apparently Healthy Individuals: A Handbook for Physicians. New York, American Heart Association, 1972.
26. Fardy, P.S.: Training for aerobic power. In Toward an Understanding of Human Performance. Edited by E.J. Burke. Ithaca, New York, Mouvement Publications, 1977.
27. deVries, H.A.: Physiology of Exercise for Physical Education and Athletics. Dubuque, Iowa, William C. Brown, 1966.
28. Fox, S.M., Naughton, J.P., and Haskell, W.L.: Physical activity and the prevention of coronary heart disease. Ann. Clin. Res., 3:404, 1971.
29. Astrand, P.O.: Physical performance as a function of age. JAMA, 205:105, 1968.
30. Fardy, P.S., and Ilmarinen, J.: Evaluating the effects and feasibility of an at work stairclimbing intervention program for men. Med. Sci. Sports, 7:91, 1975.
31. Saltin, B., et al.: Response to exercise after bed rest and after training. Circulation, 38(suppl. 47):27, 1968.
32. Wilmore, J.H.: Inferiority of the female athlete: Myth or reality? Sports Med. Bull., 10:7, 1975.
33. Fardy, P.S., Hritz, M.G., and Hellerstein, H.K.: Cardiac responses during women's intercollegiate volleyball and physical fitness changes from a season of competition. J. Sports Med. Phys. Fitness, 16:291, 1976.
34. Astrand, I.: Aerobic work capacity in men and women with reference to age. Acta Physiol. Scand., [Suppl]169 49:45, 1960.
35. Franklin, B.A.: The role of electrocardiographic monitoring in cardiac exercise programs. J. Cardiac Rehabil., 3:806, 1983.
36. Williams, M.A., and Fardy, P.S.: Limitations in prescribing exercise. J. Cardiovasc. Pulmon. Tech., 8:33, 1980.
37. Fox, S.M. Naughton, J.P., and Gorman, P.A.: Physical activity and cardiovascular health. III. The exercise prescription: Frequency and type of activity. Mod. Concepts Cardiovasc. Dis., 41:25, 1972.
38. McHenry, P.L., and Morris, S.N.: Exercise electrocardiography—Current state of the art. In Advances in Electrocardiography. Edited by R.C.

Schlant and J.W. Hurst. Orlando, Fla., Grune & Stratton, 1976.
39. Davis, C.T.M., and Knibbs, A.V.: The effects of intensity, duration and frequency of effort on maximum aerobic power output. Int. Z. Angew. Physiol., 29:299, 1971.
40. Sharkey, B.J., and Holleman, J.P.: Cardiorespiratory adaptations to training at specified intensities. Res. Q. Exerc. Sport, 38:398, 1967.
41. Roskamm, H.: Optimum patterns of exercise for healthy adults. Can. Med. Assoc. J., 96:895, 1967.
42. Durnin, J.V.G.A., Brockway, J.M., and Whitcher, H.W.: Effects of a short period of training of varying severity on some measurements of physical fitness. J. Appl. Physiol., 15:161, 1960.
43. Lester, M., Sheffield, L.T., Trammell, P., and Reeves, T.J.: The effect of age and athletic training on the maximal heart rate during muscular exercise. Am. Heart J., 76:370, 1968.
44. Franklin, B.A., et al.: Metabolic cost of extremely slow walking in cardiac patients: Implications for exercise testing and training. Arch. Phys. Med. Rehabil., 64:564, 1983.
45. Pollock, M.L., et al.: Effects of frequency and duration of training on attrition and incidence of injury. Med. Sci. Sports, 9:31, 1977.
46. Meytes, I., et al.: Wenckebach A-V block: A frequent feature following heavy physical training. Am. Heart J., 90:126, 1975.
47. Killip, T.: Time, place, event of sudden death. Circulation, 52(suppl. 3):160, 1975.
48. Wilmore, J.H.: Prescribing exercise for healthy adults. In Adult Fitness and Cardiac Rehabilitation. Edited by P.K. Wilson. Baltimore, University Park Press, 1975.
49. Davis, J.A., and Convertina, V.A.: A comparison of heart rate methods for predicting endurance training intensity. Med. Sci. Sports, 7:295, 1975.
50. The Committee on Exercise: Exercise Testing and Training of Individuals with Heart Disease or at High Risk for Its Development: A Handbook for Physicians. Dallas, American Heart Association, 1975.
51. Fardy, P.S., and Hellerstein, H.K.: Comparison of continuous and intermittent multistage exercise tests. Med. Sci. Sports, 10:7, 1978.
52. Borg, G.A.: Perceived exertion as an indicator of somatic stress. Scand. J. Rehabil. Med., 2:92, 1970.
53. Borg, G.A.: The perceived exertion: A note on "history" and methods. Med. Sci. Sports, 5:90, 1973.
54. Borg, G.A.: Psychophysical bases of perceived exertion. Med. Sci. Sports, 14:377, 1982.
55. Pandolf, K.B.: Differentiated ratings of perceived exertion during physical exercise. Med. Sci. Sports Exerc., 14:397, 1982.
56. Skinner, J.S., and Buskirk, E.R.: The validity and reliability of a rating scale of perceived exertion. Med. Sci. Sports, 5:94, 1973.
57. Noble, B.J.: Clinical applications of perceived exertion. Med. Sci. Sports Exerc., 14:406, 1982.
58. Fardy, P.S.: Effects of soccer training and detraining upon selected cardiac and metabolic measures. Res. Q., 40:502, 1969.

59. Fardy, P.S., et al.: Effects of two years' exercise training in patients with diagnosed coronary artery disease. Med. Sci. Sports, 12:100, 1980.

60. Fox, E.L., et al.: Intensity and distance of interval training programs and changes in aerobic power. Med. Sci. Sports, 5:18, 1973.

61. Crews, T.R., and Roberts, J.A.: Effect of interaction of frequency and intensity of training. Res. Q. Exerc. Sports, 47:48, 1976.

62. Jackson, J.H., Sharkey, B.J., and Johnston, P.: Cardiorespiratory adaptations to training at specified frequencies. Res. Q. Exerc. Sport, 39:295, 1968.

63. Blackburn, H.: Role of exercise in patients with coronary disease. Geriatrics, 26:89, 1971.

64. Ribisl, P.M., and Miller, H.S.: Errors in exercise prescription for cardiac patients in aquatic programs using treadmill data. Circulation, 54(suppl. 2):226, 1976.

65. Atkins, J.M., Matthews, O.A., Blomqvist, C.G., and Mullins, C.B.: Incidence of arrhythmias induced by isometric and dynamic exercise. Br. Heart J., 38:465, 1976.

66. Flessas, A.P., et al.: Effects of isometric exercise on the end-diastolic pressure, volumes, and function of left ventricle. Circulation, 53:839, 1976.

67. Fardy, P.S.: Isometric exercise and the cardiovascular system. Physician Sportsmed., 9:43, 1981.

68. Coplin, J.H.: Isokinetic exercises clinical usage. J. Natl. Athlet. Train. Assoc., 6:222, 1971.

69. Moffroid, M., et al.: A study of isokinetic exercise. Phys. Ther., 49:735, 1969.

70. Thistle, H.G., et al.: Isokinetic contraction: A new concept of resistance exercise. Arch. Phys. Med. Rehabil., 48:279, 1967.

71. Peterson, J.A.: Total conditioning: A case study. Athletic J., 56:40, 1975.

72. Gettman, L.R., Culter, L.A., and Strathman, T.A.: Physiologic changes after 20 weeks of isotonic vs isokinetic circuit training. J. Sports Med. Phys. Fitness, 20:265, 1980.

73. Hellerstein, H.K., and Franklin, B.A.: Exercise testing and prescription. In Rehabilitation of the Coronary Patient. Edited by N.K. Wenger and H.K. Hellerstein. 2nd Ed. New York, John Wiley & Sons, 1984.

74. Fox, E.L., and Mathews, D.K.: Interval Training. Philadelphia, W.B. Saunders, 1974.

75. Cureton, T.K.: The training and seasoning of muscles, tendons and ligaments. J. Assoc. Phys. Med. Rehabil., 16:103, 1962.

76. Clausen, J.P., Trap-Jensen, J., and Lassen, N.A.: The effects of training on the heart rate during arm and leg exercise. Scand. J. Clin. Lab. Invest., 26:295, 1970.

77. Fardy, P.S.: Exercise following a heart attack: Some special considerations. In Research and Practice in Physical Education. Edited by R.E. Stadulis, C.O. Dotson, V.L. Katch, and J. Shick. Champaign, Ill., Human Kinetics, 1976.

78. Freyschuss, U.: Comparison between arm and leg exercise in women and men. Scand. J. Clin. Lab. Invest., 35:795, 1975.

79. Pyörälä, K., et al.: A controlled study of the effects of 18 months physical training on sedentary middle-aged men with high indices of risk relative to coronary heart disease. In Coronary Heart Disease and Physical Fitness. Edited by O.A. Larson and R.O. Malmborg. Copenhagen, Munksgaard, 1971.

80. Wilhelmsen, L. et al.: A controlled trial of physical training after myocardial infarction: Effects on risk factors, nonfatal reinfarction, and death. Prev. Med., 4:491, 1975.

81. Oldridge, N.B.: Compliance and exercise in primary and secondary prevention of coronary heart disease: A review. Prev. Med., 11:56, 1982.

82. White, J.R.: EKG changes using carotid artery for heart rate monitoring. Med. Sci. Sports, 9:88, 1977.

83. Draper, A.J.: Cardioinhibitory carotid sinus syndrome. Ann. Int. Med., 32:700, 1950.

84. Smiddy, J., Lewis, H.D., and Dunn, M.: The effects of carotid massage in older men. J. Gerontol., 27:209, 1972.

85. Zohman, L.R.: Exercise your Way to Fitness and Heart Health. Coventry, Conn., CPC International House, 1974.

86. Karpovich, P.V., and Sinning, W.E.: Physiology of Muscular Activity. Philadelphia, W.B. Saunders, 1971.

87. Control Data 1982 Health Claims Data and 1982 Corporate Wide Employee Health Survey. Minneapolis, Control Data Corporation, 1983.

88. Berry, C.A.: Good Health for Employees and Reduced Health Care Costs for Industry, 1982.

ADMINISTRATIVE CONCERNS

7

ADMINISTRATIVE CONCERNS

This chapter discusses planning, developing, implementing, and managing cardiac rehabilitation and adult fitness programs. The information is designed to benefit those responsible for assessing program feasibility and those in charge of planning and operations. Additional resources are suggested.[1-6]

PROGRAM PLANNING

The first consideration in good management is detailed planning. Two issues must be addressed: (1) Is there a need for cardiac rehabilitation or adult fitness? (2) Is it feasible to offer a program? In order to answer these two questions the following should be considered: population demographics, patient admissions, existing programs in the vicinity, and acceptance by the medical community.

If available national statistics are used,[7] then approximately 2% of the population within a 20- to 30-minute drive of any cardiac rehabilitation program in the U.S.[8-11] would represent the number of patients with myocardial infarct, coronary artery bypass surgery, and stable angina. Consequently, if 100,000 persons live in the area surrounding the proposed center, then an average of 2,000 would be expected to meet the eligibility criteria for cardiac rehabilitation as established by Medicare and most third-party carriers. Of this number 25% to 50% can probably be estimated as viable (author's personal observation). In addition the age and socioeconomics of the

population must be considered. An area consisting largely of senior citizens has a higher percentage of eligible patients than a younger community. Unfortunately, senior citizens are probably more reluctant to drive than younger patients, a fact that also must be taken into consideration. There is also some evidence to indicate that blue collar workers are less likely to enter a program than are white collar workers.[7] Consequently, a thorough understanding of community demographics is very important.

If the program is planned to be in a hospital, then a careful review of medical records is helpful in determining an estimate of eligible patients. Furthermore, the philosophy and goals of the hospital must be clear. Is there an active cardiology program or plans for one? If yes, then long-term cardiac care and follow-up are necessary, and cardiac rehabilitation is desirable. A review of similar services in the area should also be undertaken. This analysis is often ignored, resulting in unnecessary replication of services and increased cost to the consumer.

After the need for a program has been established, it is important that financial goals be defined. If the program is for profit, then the goal is simple. Expenses are estimated, and the minimal patient numbers for the program to be profitable are projected. Financial goals in not-for-profit institutions can be assessed differently. Although the cost-effectiveness of all hospital programs is currently under increased scrutiny, programs that operate at a deficit can still be justified in certain situations. For example, if the program helps to provide a complete cardiology service and benefits the hospital in other ways, then it can be justified. Nevertheless, the program director must approach cardiac rehabilitation as both a needed medical service and a business. Sound management and financial planning are essential. Clearly, financial goals must be understood from the beginning by everyone associated with the program.

The same concerns must be addressed in starting an adult fitness program. Are there sufficient numbers to justify a program, and is there sufficient interest? What are the socioeconomic conditions of the area, and what is the financial goal of the program? Is the program part of a non-profit institution, such as the YMCA, public school or university, or is the facility a for profit health club? Many administrative concerns apply similarly to adult fitness centers and cardiac rehabilitation programs.

The feasibility of starting a program must also take into account the types of services that will be provided. Pulmonary rehabilitation, behavior management, stress management, hypertension control, nutrition, and weight control are services that can usually be incorporated into cardiac rehabilitation without difficulty. Whether these services are included is decided on an individual basis, taking into consideration need, availability and financial return. Since financial viability is closely tied to reimbursement, a clear understanding of medical insurance is necessary. A person should be dedicated to understanding billing procedures and insurance coverage because of the differences among policies and the many changes that the industry is presently undergoing.

PROGRAM OBJECTIVES

After the feasibility and viability of starting a program have been established, it is necessary to develop the program's professional and financial objectives. Professional objectives are clinical, educational, behavioral, and research.

Clinical Objectives

Clinical objectives are affected by the type of programs that are established. For this discussion these programs are classified as follows:

1. *Prevention.* Primary prevention and physical fitness are the principle objectives for nonmonitored, community- and corporate-based fitness programs whose goals are to improve physical condition and prevent or delay the onset of coronary disease. These programs ostensibly are for healthy individuals, those with coronary disease risk factors, and patients with diagnosed coronary disease who have not had an infarct or surgery.

2. *Rehabilitation.* For patients with diagnosed coronary disease, who have had a myocardial infarction (MI), coronary angioplasty or coronary artery bypass surgery, or who have angina and/or substantially elevated risk factors, the focus of the program shifts to rehabilitation (secondary prevention). Cardiac rehabilitation refers to the process of returning an individual with known coronary artery disease (CAD) to a life-style of optimal health and well-being.

3. *Arrhythmia Detection.* Patients with frequent arrhythmias but no other evidence of CAD can benefit from being monitored during periods of rest, increased physical activity, and recovery. Monitored exercise classes can also be useful for adjusting antiarrhythmic medications. Electrocardiogram (ECG) monitoring during several successive exercise sessions often is better than during stress testing.[12-17] Monitoring can also be performed during home exercise

programs that incorporate transtelephonic electrocardiography. Telephonic monitoring can provide increased convenience and comfort for the patient as compared with attending regularly scheduled classes at a designated center.

4. *Research.* Whether research is to be a primary or secondary objective needs to be addressed and decided during the planning stage, since the decision affects expenses and personnel assignments. Unless grants can be obtained, conducting research can be a costly undertaking for which there may be no immediate pay back. However, even though immediate monetary benefits are not realized, research can be justified on the basis of public relations value. If the hospital community perceives that its health and well-being are enhanced, then research can benefit the hospital, even if expenses are increased.

Even if active research is not an objective of the program, there still should be a plan for systematic data collection and analysis. The merits of a program can best be illustrated when sufficient data are available to demonstrate its benefits.

Educational and Behavioral Objectives

Although individually prescribed and monitored exercise is the primary emphasis of cardiac rehabilitation, a comprehensive program needs to be multidisciplinary and include patient education and behavior modification. Educational programs need to be available to patients, spouses, and significant others. The need for these other programs and the fact that they should assume an integral role in a total program must be established at the onset. Since most educational and behavioral programs are not reimbursable, their priority must be well established. These programs utilize specifically trained instructors with the appropriate educational background.

Equipment and materials necessary to conduct group and individual classes are also required. It is unfortunate that patient education and behavior modification are not reimbursable, because they are a costly and yet necessary part of long-term patient management.

Education programs are also recommended for the professional staff so that they have a better understanding and appreciation of cardiac rehabilitation. Periodic programs with continuing education units should be planned for the medical staff, nurses, and other health-related professionals. These programs include hospital or clinic grand rounds, seminars, conferences, medical society meetings, and presentations to local and state medical associations, nurse associations, and public health and vocational rehabilitation agencies. In fact any group of professionals who are regularly involved and interested in cardiac rehabilitation and fitness should be considered for such programs. For the hospital-based program, it is important to provide informative seminars to the medical and nursing staffs. In-service sessions, continuing education accredited conferences and even informal group meetings are recommended.

Community service and community education objectives should also be included as important features in a comprehensive program. Because cardiac rehabilitation is a service and a business, the long-term and indirect financial consequences must be assessed when considering these objectives. How much do community service and education benefit other programs in the hospital? Do the benefits of public relations as a result of community service enhance the image of the hospital? It is important to consider these questions in order to provide and develop long-term plans.

If it is within the philosophy of the hospital to promote good health as well as to treat acute illness, it is likely that community service and education will be encouraged. In the eyes of the community, the hospital is in a natural position to provide these services. However, it must be realized that meaningful community programs are costly. This needs to be considered in the early stage of financial planning. Intangible, indirect, and potential revenues for the future have to be balanced against current operational costs, patient census, and overall financial stability. Examples of community service and education are media releases, education programs, speakers bureau, dissemination of educational materials, health fairs, school programs, education, and service programs for health organizations and agencies.

Health education and fitness programs should also be available to hospital employees. In fact it is a good idea to target this group first among those to whom the program will be offered. This can be accomplished through periodic formal or informal meetings and classes, regular announcements or newsletters, and health-oriented bulletin boards that are visible and easily accessible to all employees. In order to encourage participation in these programs, it is suggested that the cost to the employee be kept at a minimum. A small fee is recommended, so that the employee is at least a partial contributor. Time constraints of hospital employees must be taken into consideration when scheduling programs.

Financial Objectives

The financial objectives of the cardiac rehabilitation or adult fitness center must be established during the planning stage. Although more and more physician-directed freestanding centers have been established, the majority of cardiac rehabilitation programs at present are hospital based. If the program is hospital based, the issue of for-profit or not-for-profit is decided by the hospital's ownership and administration. This decision influences the financial objectives of cardiac rehabilitation. Traditionally, hospital-based programs have not

been created to make a large profit, but rather to provide a good service that would eventually pay for itself. Most of these programs have operated at a financial loss. In today's health-care market, deficit-operating programs are not as acceptable as they were a few years ago. Cost/benefit ratio and cost-effectiveness are being closely monitored, and programs that are operating at a loss are likely to be scrutinized more closely and placed under more pressure to show fiscal viability.

Freestanding, physician-directed centers have become increasingly popular in recent years, because they provide a needed service and can be profitable if run efficiently. In accordance with Medicare regulations, freestanding facilities must be physician-directed clinics.[18] The most common way to develop a program is to have a group of cardiologists establish a center to meet the needs of their patients and other patients that might be incidentally referred. In a large cardiology practice, the program will likely be profitable.

In a different business arrangement, one that can be equally successful monetarily, individual physicians or businessmen would own the center. In this situation the program would be marketed to the entire medical community. In either case federal regulations that outline the requirements for such centers have been clearly defined.[18–21] More information on program finance is presented in Chapter 8.

PROGRAM DESCRIPTION

Traditionally, cardiac rehabilitation is comprised of three or four phases. Phase I represents the in-hospital, inpatient part of the program. Emphasis is on education for the patient and family, low-level physical activity, and establishing a positive attitude in the patient. Of these goals the last is probably the most important. It prepares and motivates the patient for phase II and the lifetime commitment that has to be made.

Phase II is an outpatient program that is usually conducted in a hospital center or physician-directed clinic. The patient is advanced through a progressive, monitored exercise program for a period up to 24 weeks, although the usual length of reimbursement is limited to 12 weeks. The goals of phase II are to enhance the patient physically and psychosocially and to provide sufficient direction for a safe and beneficial long-term program.

The long-term, nonmonitored or intermittently monitored program is designated as phase III or sometimes as phases III and IV. In phase IV, cardiac rehabilitation or adult fitness, the goals are continued improvement followed by maintenance. The atmosphere is generally less structured, and an attempt is made to incorporate activities that are beneficial as well as fun. The aim is to establish a program that promotes long-term interest and commitment. If enjoyable activities are not provided, then there is less likelihood of long-term compliance.

Management of emergencies is an integral part of all programs. A plan should be devised that outlines procedures and objectives of cardiopulmonary resuscitation, physician orders until the arrival of emergency personnel, staff assignments and responsibilities, patient transfer, and notification of the referring physician. Emergency plans are described elsewhere.[22]

ALTERNATIVE PROGRAMS IN CARDIAC REHABILITATION

Even though third-party reimbursement generally allows for 12 weeks of monitored phase II cardiac rehabilitation, there are frequent occasions when 12 weeks is neither feasible nor necessary. Alternative programs are needed to meet patient needs under those circumstances. Greater emphasis may have to be placed on home exercising after appropriate guidelines have been developed in a monitored program. In some cases it may be necessary to reduce

the length of the outpatient program to as few as 2 weeks. This is the minimal length of time recommended to allow the staff sufficient time to observe the patient during exercise and to develop guidelines that are safe and beneficial. The use of transtelephonic electrocardiography is becoming more widespread as a means of better ensuring patient safety and compliance with home exercise. Home programs and transtelephonic electrocardiography are discussed again in Chapter 13.

ANCILLARY PROGRAMS

Exercise by itself is not a panacea. Even though physical activity is the focal point of cardiac rehabilitation and adult fitness, ancillary programs are also essential for a comprehensive program. Examples of these services include nutrition management, weight control, stress management, group and individual counseling, smoking cessation, and other activities designed to educate and modify patient life-style. For a more detailed presentation of patient education and behavior modification refer to Chapters 12 and 15.

MARKETING

One of the most important requirements of a successful cardiac rehabilitation program is good marketing. In a hospital-based program, the medical staff has already been identified and receives first consideration. Afterward, physicians who are not on the medical staff of the hospital should also be contacted. Actual marketing should begin during the planning stage. Physicians should be consulted for their input into the program, and a medical advisory board should be formed as a part of an ongoing effort to solicit medical advice.

Marketing needs are different in a freestanding, physician-owned and -directed clinic. If rehabilitation is part of an active cardiology practice, then marketing is mostly to that group of doctors and those primary care physicians who normally refer to that practice. While this may seem obvious, even physicians who own their facility are often unaware of important details and need to be marketed regularly. The primary-care physicians must be kept well informed about the progress and follow-up of their patients. Services normally ascribed to the primary-care physician should not be usurped by the cardiologist.

If the rehabilitation center is owned by individual physicians, a group of doctors who are not cardiologists, or persons outside the medical community, then all physicians within the geographic area that the program serves must be solicited. Under these circumstances an individual who is experienced in marketing to doctors is suggested as part of the staff.

Certain marketing strategies are recommended regardless of whether the program is hospital based or freestanding.

1. Individual members of the medical community must be informed of the program's existence. Announcements should be mailed to all physicians in the community, and at the appropriate time an invitation should be extended to attend the program's open house.

2. Referring physicians must be kept informed as to how their patients are doing. Progress reports should be provided regularly. Examples of these reports are in Chapter 14.

3. Emphasize that the essence of the program is to complement the care of the referring physician by offering a quality program that is a needed service. Pay particular attention to assure physicians that the doctor–physician relationship, which they have cultivated, is not going to be compromised. In the case of any emergency or clinical problem, be certain that the referring physician is notified as soon as possible.

4. Have available documented scientific evidence of the efficacy of cardiac rehabilitation and risk-factor management in reducing morbidity and mortality as well as improving physical and psychological well-being.

Although the medical community is the primary target of marketing for rehabilitation programs, the general public should also be included. Word of mouth can be an excellent source of patient referral. Community marketing is especially necessary in promoting adult fitness. Competition in the fitness industry is tremendous. Therefore, a well-prepared marketing scheme is vital.

An advisory board of influential citizens from the community can be valuable for good public relations for both cardiac rehabilitation and adult fitness programs. In addition, it is always good to work closely with community service organizations, health agencies, educational institutions, and large employers. Community resources should be known and utilized to their fullest. Concentrate on the local market before seeking more widespread exposure.

Adult fitness centers should utilize newsworthy events to attract media coverage. Although the media is not likely to provide free advertising to for-profit facilities, they are sure to cover important happenings in these centers. Therefore, it is suggested that a plan be devised to keep the name of the center regularly in the news. The extent and type of marketing is influenced by the socioeconomic level of the community and the clientele of the center. Employing a professional marketing firm may be valuable, particularly in those locations where that approach is expected. However, professional marketing is expensive and often needs direction from the program director and governing board.

FACILITIES

The facilities required for a cardiac rehabilitation program depend on which phase is being discussed. In phase I most exercises are performed at the bedside and in adjacent corridors and stairwells, although there are some programs with an area designated exclusively for inpatient group exercise. These facilities are planned and used for patients who can be exercised more aggressively. Examples of this type of facility are presented in Chapter 11.

Phase I facilities should also include a room for patient education that is pleasant in appearance, conducive for learning, and large enough to comfortably accommodate several patients and family members. Appropriate audiovisual equipment should be available, along with a chalkboard and other educational materials.

A traditional phase II program has very specific space requirements. There is an exercise room large enough to accommodate four to eight patients at a time. The size and shape of the area is designed for close patient supervision and to maintain direct eye contact at all times. Although a large room might seem impressive to the casual observer, increased floor space raises cost and decreases the close supervision and personal contact that are so important. The exercise room should provide approximately 100 square feet per patient. Ample space for dressing and showering should also be available. In addition, a phase II program has to have sufficient office space for the staff to conduct business. A separate area for stress testing and a conference room that will seat 15 to 20 persons is recommended. In a freestanding facility, particular attention should be given to a good location. Examples of floor plans are found in Chapter 11.

Phase III, IV, and adult fitness programs require considerably more space than does phase II. Although phase III sometimes is merely a continuation of phase II, a larger area to accommodate a greater variety of physical activities is more desirable. Therefore, fun, diversification of activities, and group dynamics are emphasized. Consequently, phases III & IV cardiac rehabilitation are often conducted in a large gymnasium such as at a YMCA, Jewish Community Center (JCC), school, or community center. Exercise facilities should include one or more large rooms, swimming pool, and a nice outdoor area in which to exercise when the weather permits. Examples of these facilities and a detailed discussion of facility planning are presented in Chapter 11.

EQUIPMENT

The equipment needed for cardiac rehabilitation also depends on which phase of the program is being discussed. A phase I program can be operated with little equipment, most of which is for patient education and behavior modification. Exercise and monitoring equipment necessary for phase I includes sphygmomanometers, stethoscopes, and light weights. In some programs exercise bicycles are used and are transported into patient rooms for prescribed activity. When the program is conducted at bedside, telemetry may be used to monitor patient responses. If central station telemetry is unavailable, small portable devices should be considered to ensure safety and document ECG rhythm strips. In those institutions with monitored phase I programs, the equipment that is needed is comparable to phase II. In either case equipment is required for exercise, patient monitoring, and emergencies.

The exercise equipment required for long-term cardiac rehabilitation and adult fitness programs is generally more extensive than that required for phases I and II. A typical equipment list includes exercise devices for aerobic activities and low-level group activities and games, as well as monitoring and emergency equipment. Equipment and their costs are further discussed in Chapters 8 and 11.

PERSONNEL

Personnel are discussed in more detail in Chapter 10. As a general rule, the size and makeup of the staff are determined by the scope of the program. A comprehensive cardiac rehabilitation program is multidisciplinary and should include the following staff: physicians, nurses, exercise specialists, educators, nutritionists, psychologists, physical and occupational therapists, administrators, marketers, and support staff. Not all of these positions are necessarily full-time. Some staff members may be hired on a part-time basis and others as consultants.

The schedule for adding staff is influenced by a number of factors. It is unusual to start a program with a complete complement of professional personnel. More likely, programs and staff are introduced as resources become available and patient needs are identified.

In adult fitness programs most personnel have a health, physical education, or recreation background. A business manager, marketing person, and support staff are also necessary in most instances. Special classes are generally offered according to need. These classes, such as aerobic dance, stress management, selected sport skills, are often taught by part-time instructors.

BILLING AND REIMBURSEMENT

Projections of expenses and revenues are an important part of program planning. Expenses are usually estimated more easily than revenues, since the latter is dependent on the number of patient referrals, which generally is an unknown at the start. Expenditures also may vary according to the number of referrals, although many costs are fixed or relatively predictable.

Regardless of whether the cardiac rehabilitation program is hospital based or freestanding, someone who is experienced with billing procedures and understands how to deal with commercial third-party carriers as well as Medicare and Medicaid, and the diagnosis-related group (DRG) system needs to serve as financial administrator. At the onset it may be advisable to employ an outside agency for this service. A good billing service is familiar with procedures and possesses the computer hardware and software to do the job efficiently. The cost of this service is typically between 5% and 10% of collections.

In addition to understanding the nuances of reimbursement, the billing person must be familiar with diagnostic codes and billing codes.[23,24] Since these frequently change, it is essential to keep abreast of current information and trends. Finances are covered in detail in Chapter 8.

PATIENT ACCESSION INTO CARDIAC REHABILITATION

Thus far, the focus of the chapter has been planning. The next section deals with administrative considerations with entering patients into the program and following them through the system.

Eligibility Criteria

Cardiac rehabilitation is considered acceptable and appropriate therapy for patients who have been referred by their attending physician and have a clear medical need. The following diagnoses are generally those defined as indicating medical need and eligible for reimbursement from third-party carriers.[18–21]

1. A documented diagnosis of acute MI, usually within the preceding 12 months
2. History of coronary artery bypass surgery, usually within the preceding 12 months
3. History of coronary angioplasty
4. Stable angina pectoris
5. Significant risk factors for coronary heart disease (CHD)

Eligibility of patients with elevated risk factors is assessed on a case by case basis and usually requires documentation from the referring physician and perhaps from the medical director of the program.

According to published Medicare guidelines, patients who are eligible for cardiac rehabilitation are allowed 12 weeks of a supervised and monitored program. Continuation beyond that is allowed up to a total of 24 weeks if sufficient justification can be made by the referring doctor.[18–21]

PATIENT REFERRAL AND ORIENTATION

A patient can only enter a cardiac rehabilitation program with a physician's referral. The referral should provide the patient diagnosis and some basic medical information. A written referral is required. In the case of a question of program suitability, the medical director usually makes the final decision.

A separate referral is required for phase II and III. Following the referral to phase II, eligible patients and family members are invited to attend an orientation. The purpose of the orientation is to introduce the staff, discuss objectives, procedures and financial obligations, show the facility and equipment, and provide an opportunity for questions and answers. Interested patients are then started in the program.

Patient Evaluation

The written referral must be obtained before being evaluated. The evaluation consists of a comprehensive physical examination and lab work, functional exercise stress test, selected fitness tests and body measurements, and a medical and life-style history. Some of these tests may not be necessary if they have been done recently. Furthermore, it is suggested that the referring physician be responsible for the physical exam, thus enabling the doctor to take an active role in the program and derive some financial benefit. The stress test is usually within the domain of the cardiologist or internist, although some general practitioners are beginning to do stress tests in their offices.

The exercise prescription is fashioned from information derived from the evaluation. Follow-up evaluations are scheduled to assess the benefits of the program and to update the exercise prescription. Evaluation procedures, exercise stress testing, and exercise prescription are presented in detail in Chapters 4, 5, and 6. These are very similar for both cardiac rehabilitation and adult fitness.

PROGRAM DESCRIPTION

As previously mentioned, the initial training program in cardiac rehabilitation is phase II, which is started after the exercise prescription has been established.[17] The exercise program is usually between 70% and 85% of maximal heart rate, three times a week for approximately 40 minutes per session. Electrocardiogram monitoring is generally continuous, athough this is not the case in every program. Blood pressures are also monitored before, during, and after exercise. Records of ECG rhythm strips, heart rates, blood pressures, and adverse signs or symptoms are regularly provided to the primary care physician in order to maintain a continuity of care.

The training program consists of upper and lower body exercises, which are designed to improve cardiovascular function, muscular endurance, strength, flexibility, psychosocial factors, and the patient's overall clinical status. Following exercise, the patient may be instructed in relaxation techniques and participate in educational activities. A detailed discussion of the phase II exercise training program is provided in Chapters 6 and 13.

Phase II leads into the long-term programs, phase III, IV, and adult fitness. The activities of these programs are similar, although phase III is usually supervised by a physician or nurse. Intermittent monitoring and emergency equipment is recommended and is usually on hand for phase III, which is primarily for cardiac patients. Phase IV "maintenance" or adult fitness may be an extension of phase III or a completely separate program. Since this program is designed for those at least ostensibly healthy, clinical precautions observed in phase III are generally not provided. A comprehensive program description is illustrated in Figure 7–1.

PATIENT FOLLOW-UP

The patient and family have to understand that cardiac rehabilitation is really about changing life-style and that its success depends on a lifetime commitment. With this objective as the focal point of the program, a plan for follow-up can be established that provides continual motivation and reinforcement, although eventually the patient needs to accept greater personal responsibility. Patient follow-up is discussed in more detail in Chapters 9 and 14.

DEVELOPMENT OF SUPPORT SYSTEMS

An important part of follow-up in cardiac rehabilitation, particularly after the conclusion of phase II, is to establish patient support systems. Examples include coronary clubs, periodic social gatherings, monthly newsletters and other informative materials. These programs are especially valuable to further long-term goals.

MEDICOLEGAL CONSIDERATIONS

The incidence of serious or fatal complications in cardiac rehabilitation and adult fitness programs has been reported elsewhere.[25–28] Although the risk of life-threatening cardiovascular complications is small, it does raise the question of program safety and liability. It is recommended, therefore, that medicolegal and safety factors be clearly understood by the staff.[29–31] The program and professional staff must be covered by liability insurance. Hospital programs usually have an umbrella policy, while freestanding and fitness facilities

have to "shop around" for the best insurance coverage and premium. In any case the program administrator should be familiar with city, state, and federal regulations that impact on the conduct of the program. Standards for conduct of programs.[32–34] have been developed by the American Medical Association, American Heart Association, American College of Sports Medicine, and the American Association of Cardiovascular and Pulmonary Rehabilitation. These are well thought out criteria that should be used by the program director in the planning and operation of the center. Patient records need to be maintained carefully, and policies and procedures must be clearly and concisely documented. Finally, contingency plans for dealing with emergencies need to be developed and regularly practiced. The program director needs to have utmost confidence that everything has been done to promote safety.

CONCLUSIONS

Although a good administrator may delegate responsibility for some of the issues presented in this chapter, it is important to realize that a comprehensive program requires considerable administrative skill and knowledge. In review the key considerations follow:

1. Ascertain the feasibility of a program.
2. Define the objectives.
3. Have a good understanding of the finances of the project.
4. Be able to describe each phase.
5. Understand marketing techniques.
6. Understand facility development and planning.
7. Be familiar with equipment.
8. Understand what personnel are needed and develop good channels of communication with all personnel.
9. Understand the nuances of billing and reimbursement.
10. Know the patient flow through the program.

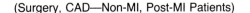

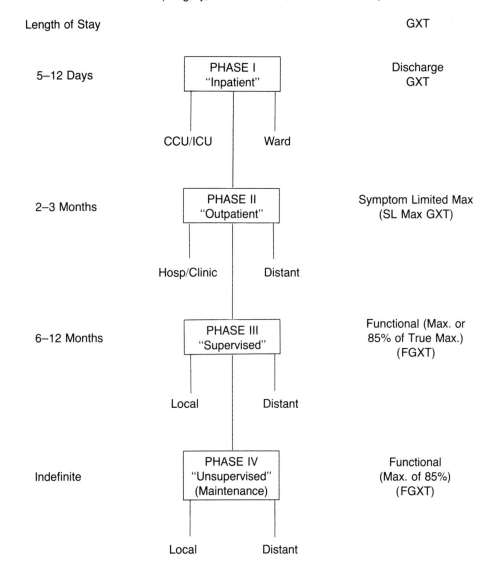

GXT = Graded exercise testing; FGXT = Functional graded exercise testing.

Fig. 7–1. Cardiac rehabilitation program, Gundersen Clinic, Ltd. & La Crosse Exercise Program (UW-L), La Crosse, Wisconsin.

11. Have a knowledge of medicolegal considerations.
12. Develop clearly written policy and procedure manuals.

REFERENCES

1. Wilson, P.K., Fardy, P.S., and Froelicher, V.F.: Cardiac Rehabilitation, Adult Fitness and Exercise Testing. Philadelphia, Lea & Febiger, 1981.
2. Pollock, M.L., and Schmidt, D.H. (eds.): Heart Disease and Rehabilitation. 2nd Ed. New York, John Wiley & Sons, 1986.
3. Hall, L.K. (ed.): Cardiac Rehabilitation: Exercise Testing and Prescription. Jamaica, N.Y., Spectrum, 1984.
4. Fox, S.M., III (ed.): Coronary Heart Disease: Prevention, Detection, Rehabilitation with Emphasis on Exercise Testing. Denver, International Medical Corp., 1974.
5. Fardy, P.S., Bennett, J.L., Reitz, N.L., and Williams, M.A.: Cardiac Rehabilitation: Implications for the Nurse and Other Health Professionals. St. Louis, C.V. Mosby, 1980.
6. Wilson, P.K., Gushiken, T.T.: Policies and Procedures of a Cardiac Rehabilitation Program: Immediate to Longterm Care. Philadelphia, Lea & Febiger, 1978.
7. Heart Facts. Dallas, American Heart Association, 1986.
8. Andrew, G.M., and Parker, J.O.: Factors related to drop-out of post myocardial infarction patients from exercise programs. Med. Sci. Sports, 11:376, 1979.
9. Oldridge, N.B.: Compliance and exercise in primary and secondary prevention of coronary heart disease: A review. Prev. Med., 11:56, 1982.
10. Franklin, B.A.: Exercise program compliance: Improvement strategies. In Behavioral Intervention in Obesity. Edited by J. Storlie, and H.A. Jordan. Spectrum, 1984.
11. Teraslinna, P., Partanen, T., Koskela, A., and Oja, P.: Characteristics affecting willingness of executives to participate in an activity program aimed at coronary heart disease prevention. J. Sports Med. Phys. Fitness, 9:224, 1969.
12. Kosowsky, B.D., Guiney, T.: Occurrence of ventricular arrhythmias with exercise as compared to monitoring. Circulation, 44:826, 1971.
13. Vitasalo, M.T., and Halonen, P.I.: Ventricular arrhythmias during exercise testing, jogging and sedentary life. Chest, 75:21, 1979.
14. Simoons, M., Lap, C., and Pool, J.: Heart rate levels and ventricular ectopic activity during cardiac rehabilitation. Am. Heart J., 100:9, 1980.
15. Dolatowski, R.P., et al.: Dysrhythmia detection in myocardial revascularization surgery patients. Med. Sci. Sports. Exerc., 15:281, 1983.
16. Fardy, P.S., Williams, M.: Monitoring cardiac patients: How much is enough? Physician Sports Med., 10:146, 1982.
17. Fardy, P.S.: Cardiac rehabilitation for the outpatient: A hospital based program. In Heart Disease and Rehabilitation. 2nd Ed. Edited by M.L. Pollock and D.H. Schmidt. New York, John Wiley & Sons, 1986.
18. Medicare Bulletin. Medicare Part B. Blue Cross and Blue Shield of Indiana, Jan. 1983.
19. Medicare Bulletin. Utilization Review. Capitol Blue Cross, Harrisburg, Penn., Nov. 1981.
20. Medicare Notes. Information of Special Interest to Florida Physicians. Blue Cross and Blue Shield of Florida, Sept. 1983.
21. Medicare Hospital Manual. Department of Health and Human Services, Health Care Financing Administration, Transmittal No. 312, HCFA Pub. No. 10, Sept. 1982.
22. Reitz, N.L.: Preventing emergencies. In Cardiac Rehabilitation: Implications for the Nurse and Other Health Professionals. Edited by P.S. Fardy, J.L. Bennett, N.L. Reitz, and M.A. Williams. St. Louis, C.V. Mosby, 1980.
23. Fanta, C.M., et al.: Physicians Current Procedural Terminology. 4th Ed. Chicago, American Medical Association, 1985.
24. International Classification of Diseases. 9th Revision. Clinical Modification. Vols. 1 and 2. Ann Arbor, Mich., Commission on Professional and Hospital Activities, March 1980.
25. Thompson, P.D.: The cardiovascular risks of cardiac rehabilitation. J. Cardiopul. Rehabil., 5:321, 1985.
26. Haskell, W.L.: Cardiovascular complications during exercise training of cardiac patients. Circulation, 57:920, 1978.
27. Hossack, K.F., and Hartwig, R.: Cardiac arrest with supervised cardiac rehabilitation. J. Cardiac Rehabil., 2:402, 1982.
28. Fletcher, G.F., and Cantwell, J.D.: Ventricular fibrillation in a medically supervised cardiac exercise program. JAMA, 238:2627, 1977.
29. Pyfer, H.R.: Safety, precautions, and procedures in cardiac exercise rehabilitation programs. In Heart Disease and Rehabilitation. 2nd Ed. Edited by M.L. Pollock and D.H. Schmidt. New York, John Wiley & Sons, 1986.
30. Sagall, E.L.: Legal implications of cardiac rehabilitation programs. In Heart Disease and Rehabilitation. 2nd Ed. Edited by M.L. Pollock and D.H. Schmidt. New York, John Wiley & Sons, 1986.
31. Abbott, R.A.: Medicolegal considerations in professional services. In Cardiac Rehabilitation: Exercise Testing and Prescription. Edited by L.K. Hall. Jamaica, N.Y., Spectrum, 1984.
32. American College of Sports Medicine: Guidelines for Exercise Testing and Prescription. 3rd Ed. Philadelphia, Lea & Febiger, 1986.
33. Guidelines for Cardiac Rehabilitation Centers. Los Angeles, American Heart Association, Greater Los Angeles Affiliate, 1982.
34. Exercise Standards Book. Dallas, American Heart Association, 1979.

8

BUDGET AND FINANCE

The implications of finances to the staff and the directors of adult fitness and cardiac rehabilitation programs will have a significant impact on their daily activities. The time of programs with little or no financial constraints is disappearing, as hospital programs and freestanding facilities must carefully consider the services they offer, based on a careful evaluation of revenues and expenditures. The entire staff, either directly or indirectly, is involved in the budget process and must proceed with program development on the basis of sound budgetary principles. This chapter reviews reimbursement, budgetary, and other financial considerations related to adult fitness and cardiac rehabilitation programs. The chapter concludes with a discussion of profit-making techniques and fund raising.

REIMBURSEMENT

The issue of reimbursement for cardiac rehabilitation services is controversial. In 1985 the National Blue Cross/Blue Shield Association recommended that reimbursement be limited to three visits rather than the 36 visits recommended by the Medicare guidelines of 1982.[1,2] In an attempt to resolve the controversy, in 1985 the U.S. Health Care Finance Administration asked the Public Health Service to "assess the safety and effectiveness of cardiac rehabilitation" as well as examine "criteria for selection of patients, the content as well as duration of course of therapy, the medical necessity of continuous ECG [electrocar-

diographic] telemetric monitoring, and the measurement of improvement in the cardiac status of patients receiving cardiac rehabilitation services."[3,4] The results of this evaluation should have a significant effect on the future of cardiac rehabilitation beyond the issue of reimbursement.

Trends in Criteria

Although there is considerable inconsistency around the country, some coverage is being provided for various portions of phase I and II cardiac rehabilitation. Figure 8–1 indicates the likelihood of insurance coverage for exercise testing and various phases of cardiac rehabilitation.[5] Insurance companies with a history of providing coverage for some cardiac rehabilitation services are listed in Table 8–1.

Some states have established criteria for certification of rehabilitation programs that result in reimbursement. In North Carolina, for example, the criteria for full certification are listed in Table 8–2. Table 8–3 lists the recommended criteria for reimbursement established by the Wisconsin Affiliate of the American Heart Association. The New York County Medical Society has established "uniform safeguards" for cardiac rehabilitation, which are described in Table 8–4.[6]

Figure 8–2 illustrates the dilemma faced when considering insurance coverage for any medical procedure. Society determines the need for appropriate medical services; the expense of benefits must then be bal-

SERVICES	COVERAGE Yes Possibly Unlikely No

GRADED EXERCISE TESTING (GXT)
  Diagnostic GXT (DGXT) _____ X
  Functional GXT (FGXT) _____ X

CARDIAC REHABILITATION
  Phase I "In Patient"
    Rehabilitation (Exercise Therapy, Education) _____ X
    Discharge GXT, w/exercise prescription _____ X

  Phase II "At Home, Clinic"
    Bicycle Rental (Home) _____ X
    Prescription Checks (Clinic) _____ X
    Ex. Therapy (Clinic) _____ X
    FGXT _____ X

  Phase III/IV "Supervised/Maintenance"
    Ex. Therapy (1st 6 months, M.D. Supervision) _____ X
    Ex. Therapy (2nd 6 months, non-M.D. Supervision; Maintenance) _____ X
    FGXT, Initial and Immediate Follow-up M.D. Supervision _____ X
    FGXT, Later Follow-up non-M.D. Supervision (Maintenance) _____ X

Fig. 8–1. Insurance coverage for cardiac rehabilitation and graded exercise testing (GXT).

anced by the revenue of premiums. The challenge is to establish cardiac rehabilitation as a necessary component of a nationwide quality care system and then control costs so that they are covered by reasonable insurance premiums. A key to this effort will be to control the profit of both the provider of the service and the involved insurance company.

The Diagnosis-Related Groups System

The diagnosis related groups (DRG) system is currently utilized in most locales for hospitalized Medicare patients. In some areas, however, the system has been applied to outpatient services and, in a few cases, to physician fees.[7] Historically, the system began as an effort to control hospital costs.[8,9] Many feel this system or a modified system, although it may be opposed, will soon be adopted for all medical services throughout the nation.

Table 8–5 lists the terminology necessary to understand the DRG system. The 23 Major Diagnostic Categories are listed in Table 8–6. Once a patient's diagnosis falls within the major diagnostic categories, further classification based on approximately 470 subcategories will be determined by the particular characteristics of the patient's illness and management. As an example, Figure 8–3 illustrates one portion of the "tree" for the Major Diagnostic Category 05, "Diseases and Disorders of the Circulatory System." If a patient survives an acute myocardial infarction (MI), illustrated in Figure 8–4, the DRG number is 115. If cardiovascular complications then develop and the patient survives without having catheterization, the DRG category becomes 121. Table 8–7 lists all the diagnoses within DRG 121, each of which have a cost of service recommended and an amount specified, which would be reimbursed through Medicare.

Table 8–8 lists the 10 most commonly assigned DRG codes.[7] Six of these are related to the cardiovascular system. The amount of payment to an institution for providing services under the DRG system is calculated by multiplying the DRG rate for each particular code times the institution's markup. This markup is determined by the institution's overhead, percentage of

Table 8–1. List of Insurance Carriers With a History of Honoring Cardiovascular Rehabilitation Claims

Admar	Lincoln National Life Insurance Co.
Aetna Life & Casualty (Federal Employees)	Local 420 (Sheet Metal Workers)
Allstate Insurance Company	Local 652 (Labors Health & Welfare)
American Baptist Churches	Lockheed
American General Life Insurance Co.	Lumber Mills & Cabinets
American Heritage Insurance Co.	Lumbermen's Mutual Insurance Co.
American National Life	Massachusetts Casualty Company
American Postal Workers Union	Massachusetts Mutual Life Insurance Co.
American States Life Insurance Co.	Medicare (Hospital Based)
Associated Dry Goods	Metropolitan Life Insurance Co.
Astech	Mary Knoll Fathers
Baltimore Life Insurance Co.	Montgomery Ward Group
Bankers Life Insurance Co.	Mutual of New York
Bankers Life & Casualty	Mutual Benefit Life Insurance Co.
Benefit Trust Life	Mutual of Omaha
Berkshire Life Insurance Co.	National Association of Letter Carriers
CNA Insurance	Nationwide Mutual
California Savings & Loans League Imperial Insurance	New England Life
California Western States Life	New England Mutual
Catholic Diocese of Richmond Health Insurance Plan	New York Life Insurance Co.
Carpenters Health & Welfare	Northern California Retail Clerks
Columbus Mutual	Northwestern National Life Insurance Co.
Confederation Life Insurance Co.	Occidental Life
Connecticut General Life Insurance Co.	Occidental Life of California
Continental Assurance Company	Ohio Conference of Driver Salesmen and Industry Welfare Fund
Continental Insurance Co. of Chicago	Operating Engineers Trust Fund
Continental Life & Accident	Pacific Mutual Life Insurance Co.
Cosmopolitan Insurance Co.	Pacific National Life
County of Automechanics Trade	Penn Automotive Association
Crown Life Insurance Co.	Penn Mutual Life Insurance Co.
Dairy Industry Trust Fund—Darigold	Pennsylvania National Insurance
Educator's Mutual Life Insurance Co.	Pilot Life Insurance Co.
Empire State Mutual Insurance Co.	Providence Indemnity
Employer's Insurance of Wausau	Provident Mutual Insurance of Philadelphia
Equitable Life Assurance Society in the U.S.	Provident Life and Accident
Fireman's Fund American	Prudential Insurance Co. of America
First Far West	Prudential Indemnity Insurance Co.
First Federal Trust	Phoenix Mutual Life Insurance Co.
Founders Life Insurance Co.	Republic National Life
General American Life Insurance Co.	Republic Vanguard
Great West Life Insurance Co.	Safeco Insurance Company
Globe Life Insurance Co.—under review	Seaboard Life Insurance Co.
Government Employees Hospital Association	Sears Roebuck & Company
Gulf Life Insurance Co.	Security Beneficial Life
Hartford Life Insurance Co.	Sentry Insurance
Health Guard (HMO)	Southwest Administrators
Health & Welfare Group Insurance	Southwest Administrators (United Airlines)
Home Life Insurance Co.	State Farm Insurance Co.
Home Security Insurance Co.	State Mutual Life Insurance of America
IBM	Teamsters Mutual
Independent Life & Accident	Tower Life Insurance Company
Innerstate	Travelers Insurance Company
Insurance Company of North America	Underwriters National Insurance Co.
Integon (Winston & Salem, N.C.)	Union Central Life Insurance Co.
International Garment Workers Union	Union Labor Life Insurance Co.
Hartford Insurance Company	Union Mutual
John Hancock Mutual	United Federation of Postal Workers
Kemper Insurance Group	United Life & Accident
Liberty Mutual Life Insurance Co.	United of Omaha
Liberty National	United Pacific
Life of Virginia	Virginia Retail Clerks, Kroger
	Washington National Life

From Timmons, D.R.: Cardiovascular rehabilitation program development and organizational concerns. *In* Cardiac Rehabilitation: Exercise Testing and Prescription. Edited by L.K. Hall. Jamaica, N.Y., Spectrum, 1984. Courtesy of Cardiac Treatment Centers, Harrisburg, PA.

Table 8–2. North Carolina Cardiac Rehabilitation Plan: Criteria for Full Certification[a]

Identification of staff and their qualifications
Facilities and equipment
Personnel for testing/training
Entrance criteria
Assessment procedures
Prescriptive/therapeutic procedures
Exit procedures

[a]Used with permission of Mr. Paul E. Hirschaner, North Carolina Vocational Rehabilitation Department.

Table 8–3. Criteria for Insurance Coverage*

Referral by primary physician, written
Individual *classifications* for patients
Defined *medical supervision*
Individualized program
Defined end points

*Used with permission of State Committee on Exercise and Rehabilitation, American Heart Association, Wisconsin Affiliate.

profit, and other considerations. Accordingly, the less the markup the lower the pay rate to an institution and the more business for that institution compared to institutions with higher markups. Health maintenance organizations (HMOs) and other prepaid medical plans will usually send their patients to an institution that has the assurance of quality service at the lowest cost.

Inherent within the DRG system is a set amount to be paid, regardless of the length of stay in the hospital. As a result "length of stays" for all conditions has decreased significantly in recent years. The risk is that patients will be discharged before the appropriate time. This is of particular concern to phase I cardiac rehabilitation patients.

Cardiac rehabilitation, on the other hand, may be advantageous to the DRG system if it enables patients recovering from MI or heart surgery to be discharged earlier than the number of days specified by the DRG codes. Phase I cardiac rehabilitation services must be efficiently provided by the staff in order to maximize the benefits to both patients and hospital. In a similar fashion phase II cardiac rehabilitation programs and adult fitness programs are advantageous to prepaid health plans and HMOs if the resulting health benefits of these services reduce the need for subsequent hospitalizations and expensive therapies.

DEVELOPING A BUDGET: REVENUES

In developing a budget for a new program or updating a budget for an existing program, one must examine and project

Table 8–4. Position Statement on Cardiovascular Exercise Training Programs

For the protection of those patients who have elected to avail themselves of the training provided by such facilities, the Society recommends that these facilities provide the following uniform safeguards:

  a) That acceptance for participation in these programs should be limited to suitable patients who have been referred by a qualified physician.

  b) That a qualified cardiologist or internist be available at all times to supervise the exercise and testing and to provide emergency medical care in case of need.

  c) That drugs, facilities, and equipment necessary for cardiorespiratory resuscitation be available on the premises.

  d) That persons responsible for patient care and guidance be trained in cardiopulmonary resuscitation (CPR).

  e) That interval reports should be sent to the referring physician on the patient's status and progress.

  f) That the program be in accord with appropriate medical guidelines as to type of exercise, frequency, duration, and intensity.

  g) That there be continuous monitoring during the entire exercise period in patients felt to be vulnerable to cardiac arrhythmias.

  h) That informed consent be given in writing to both the attending physician and the facility before a patient participates in exercise programs.

From Position Statement on Cardiovascular Exercise Training Programs. New York County Medical Society, New York, 1983.

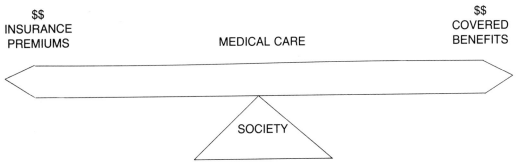

Fig. 8–2. The dilemma of insurance coverage for medical procedures.

revenues and expenditures. The following is a discussion of specific procedures to consider in this process.

Projected revenues provide the basis of the budget in that they influence specific services offered by the program. It is advisable to conservatively estimate revenues rather than trying to balance the budget exactly on projections. Program revenue may be a fixed amount or may fluctuate, depending on interest in the program, time of year, and services offered. If the revenues are fixed for a designated period of time, then expenditures can be established to more precisely equal program income,

Table 8–5.   Terminology

DRG—Diagnosis-Related Group (467 subcategories)
PPS—Prospective Payment System
PPO—Preferred Provider Organization
HMO—Health Maintenance Organization
PRO—Peer Review Organizations (PSROs)
HCFA—Health Care Financing Administration
HHS—Health and Human Services Department
MDC—Major Diagnostic Categories (23)
IDC-9-cm—International Classification of Diseases, 9th Revision, Clinical Modifications
Tree Diagram—Diagram for each MDC
Grouper—Computer software program (Health Systems International, New Haven, CT)
Trim Points—Minimum and maximum length of stay for each DRG
Outliers—Additional payment for unusually long hospital stays (less or more trim points)
LOS—Length of stay
Winner Codes—Codes that usually are a profit for the hospital
Loser Codes—Codes that usually are a loss for the hospital
Pay rate—What is paid
Discharge—On leaving hospital and results in payment of full DRG rate
Appeals—To Provider Reimbursement Review Board

Table 8–6.   Major Diagnostic Categories (MDCs)

1: Diseases and Disorders of the Nervous System
2: Diseases and Disorders of the Eye
3: Diseases and Disorders of the Ear, Nose, and Throat
4: Diseases and Disorders of the Respiratory System
5: Diseases and Disorders of the Circulatory System
6: Diseases and Disorders of the Digestive System
7: Diseases and Disorders of the Hepatobiliary System and Pancreas
8: Diseases of the Musculoskeletal System and Connective Tissue
9: Diseases of the Skin, Subcutaneous Tissue, and Breast
10: Endocrine, Nutritional, and Metabolic Diseases
11: Diseases and Disorders of the Kidney and Urinary Tract
12: Diseases and Disorders of the Male Reproductive System
13: Diseases and Disorders of the Female Reproductive System
14: Pregnancy, Childbirth, and the Puerperium
15: Normal Newborns and Other Neonates with Certain Conditions Originating in the Perinatal Period
16: Diseases and Disorders of the Blood and Blood-forming Organs and Immunity
17: Myeloproliferative Disorders and Poorly Differentiated Malignancy, Other Neoplasms NEC (not elsewhere classified)
18: Infectious and Parasitic Diseases (Systemic)
19: Mental Disorders
20: Substance Use Disorders and Substance-induced Organic Disorders
21: Injury, Poisoning, and Toxic Effects of Drugs
22: Burns
23: Selected Factors Influencing Health Status and Contact with Health Services

From Smith, C.E.: DRG's, Making them work for you. Nursing, Jan.:34, 1984.

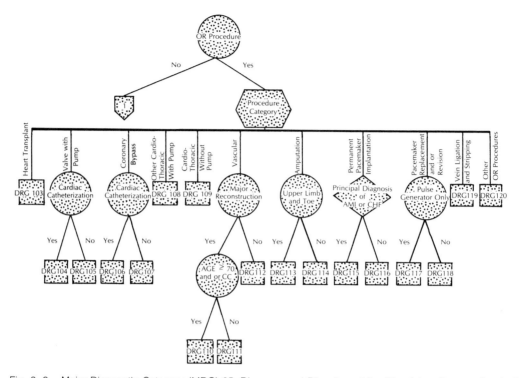

Fig. 8–3. Major Diagnostic Category (MDC) 05: Diseases and Disorders of the Circulatory System. Surgical partitioning. AMI (acute myocardial infarction), CHF (congestive heart failure), CC (comorbidity and/or complication).

although they may need to be adjusted again later. If revenues vary monthly, however, it is necessary to adjust expenditures to a percentage of the revenue. All programs, unfortunately, will have unexpected expenses. Accordingly, a conservative approach to expenditures helps to accommodate most unexpected expenses or a sudden decline in revenues.

Revenues of a phase II cardiac rehabilitation program will likely be variable, depending on the number of referred patients and the number of actual visits. If referrals and visits are greater than projected, then additional funds will be available for the next budget period, and the projected revenues and expenditures for the next budget period are adjusted accordingly. Adult fitness programs, in contrast, are more likely to have a stable budget, because the participants' fees are usually set for a fixed time period. In this case expenditures can more closely equal revenues, because a fixed revenue will be received regardless of the number of participant visits. In planning a budget it is advisable to keep expenditures at 75% to 85% of the projected revenues for each budget period.

Cardiac Rehabilitation

Phase I cardiac rehabilitation services include exercise therapy and education sessions. The usual charge for these services is $30 to $40 per session, depending to some extent on who is providing the services. Programs where physical therapists supervise the exercise sessions are usually more expensive than those where similar services are provided by the floor nurse. The formal program may be initiated while the patient is still in the intensive care unit or after transfer to the ward. Patients usually have one to two exercise sessions and

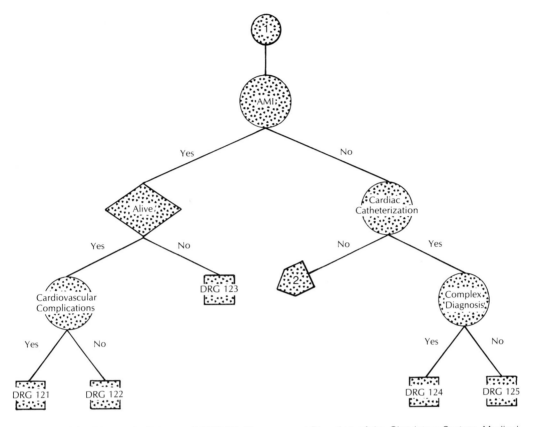

Fig. 8–4.   Major Diagnostic Category (MDC) 05: Diseases and Disorders of the Circulatory System. Medical partitioning. AMI (acute myocardial infarction).

one to two educational sessions per day. The total cost per patient can be estimated from the average length of stay in the hospital.

The services provided by a phase II cardiac rehabilitation program are usually more diverse and extend over a longer period of time than those of phase I. The usual phase II program lasts 12 weeks and involves three sessions per week for a total of 36 sessions. Charges for phase II services vary considerably within North America and generally range from $30 per session to as high as $80 per session. Although most patients require continuous ECG monitoring during phase II exercise activities, some patients will not require monitoring toward the end of their program and therefore reduce the cost per session. There may be an additional charge for ed-

ucation and behavior modification programs provided during phase II.

Charges for phase III cardiac rehabilitation services are usually much lower than for phase II, because the exercise classes are usually larger with less direct supervision, and continual ECG monitoring is generally not indicated. Like phase II, however, patients are usually charged per visit rather than for a projected, fixed period of participation. Revenues for the education and behavior modification services during phase III vary with the extent of the services. Projected revenues during phase III, therefore, can be calculated by considering the charge per session (including exercise, education, and behavior modification), number of sessions to complete the program, and the approximate number of patients expected to participate.

Table 8–7. MDC 05 Definitions of DRGs

DRG 121, MDC 05M, Circulatory Disorders W AMI & C.V. Comp. Disch. Alive

Any Diagnosis

40201	Mal Hypert Hrt Dis W CHF	42731	Atrial Fibrillation
40211	Benign Hyp Hrt Dis W CHF	42732	Atrial Flutter
40291	Hyperten Heart Dis W CHF	42741	Ventricular Fibrillation
4110	Post MI Syndrome	42742	Ventricular Flutter
41410	Aneurysm, Heart (Wall)	4275	Cardiac Arrest
41411	Coronary Vessel Aneurysm	4280	Congestive Heart Failure
41419	Aneurysm of Heart Nec	4281	Left Heart Failure
4151	Pulmon Embolism/Infarct	4289	Heart Failure Nos
4260	Atriovent Block Complete	4295	Chordae Tendinae Rupture
42610	Atriovent Block Nos	4296	Papillary Muscle Rupture
42612	Atrioven Block-Mobitz II	42981	Papillary Muscle Dis Nec
42613	AV Block-2nd Degree Nec	4410	Dissecting Aneurysm
4263	Left BB Block Nec	4589	Hypotension Nos
42651	Rt BBB/Lft Post Fasc Blk	5845	Lower Nephron Nephrosis
42652	Rt BBB/Lft Ant Fasc Blk	5846	AC Renal Fail, Cort Necr
42653	Bilat BB Block Nec	5847	AC Ren Fail, Medull Necr
42654	Trifascicular Block	5848	AC Renal Failure Nec
4270	Parox Atrial Tachycardia	5849	Acute Renal Failure Nos
4271	Parox Ventric Tachycard	78550	Shock Nos
4272	Parox Tachycardia Nos	78551	Cardiogenic Shock

Any Diagnosis

4100	AMI Anterolateral Wall	4105	AMI Lateral Wall Nec
4101	AMI Anterior Wall Nec	4106	True Posterior Infarct
4102	AMI Inferolateral Wall	4107	Subendocardial Infarct
4103	AMI Inferoposterior Wall	4108	Myocardial Infarct Nec
4104	AMI Inferior Wall Nec	4109	Myocardial Infarct Nos

DRG 122, MDC 05M, Circulatory Disorders W AMI W/O C.V. Comp. Disch. Alive

Any Diagnosis

4100	AMI Anterolateral Wall	4105	AMI Lateral Wall Nec
4101	AMI Anterior Wall Nec	4106	True Posterior Infarct
4102	AMI Inferolateral Wall	4107	Subendocardial Infarct
4103	AMI Inferoposterior Wall	4108	Myocardial Infarct Nec
4104	AMI Inferior Wall Nec	4109	Myocardial Infarct Nos

Table 8–8. The 10 Most Commonly Assigned DRG Code Numbers, According to the Federal Department of Health and Human Services

1. DRG 127/Heart failure and shock
2. DRG 039/Lens procedures
3. DRG 182/Esophagitis, gastroenteritis, and miscellaneous digestive disorders
4. DRG 014/Specific cerebrovascular disorder (except transient ischemic attack)
5. DRG 089/Simple pneumonia and pleurisy
6. DRG 140/Angina pectoris
7. DRG 088/Chronic obstructive pulmonary disease
8. DRG 138/Cardiac dysrhythmias and conductive disorders
9. DRG 243/Medical back problems
10. DRG 096/Bronchitis and asthma

From Smith, C.E.: DRGs, making them work for you. Nursing, Jan.:34, 1985.

In summary Figure 8–5 illustrates the approximate cost of phase I, II, and III cardiac rehabilitation services for a patient participating over a 9-month period. The total amount includes the charges for exercise testing, ambulatory monitoring, exercise classes, and education. Although these costs vary considerably around the country, they serve to illustrate the relatively low cost of rehabilitation compared to the usual high costs of hospitalization for acute cardiac conditions.

Adult Fitness

Adult fitness and nonphysician-supervised phase III and IV cardiac rehabilitation programs usually have fixed revenues

SERVICE	ITEM TIME	TOTAL TIME	ITEM COST	TOTAL COST
Phase I-Inpatient	10 days	10 days		
14 step, $40.00 per day			$ 560.00	
Ambulatory monitoring			100.00	
LL GXT			200.00	
Total			$ 860.00	$ 860.00
Phase II-Outpatient (Clinic/Home)	2½ months	3 months		
3 per week, 10 weeks, $40.00 per session (30)			$1200.00	
SLMax.GXT			250.00	
Total			$1450.00	$2310.00
Phase III-Supervised	6 months	9 months		
3 per week, 24 weeks, $10.00 per session (72)			$ 720.00	
SLMax.GXT			250.00	
Pt. Education			100.00	
Total			$1070.00	
GRAND TOTAL		9 months		$4240.00
Phase IV-Unsupervised (Maintenance) Exercise Therapy, Pt. Ed., GXT. Etc.		Indefinite	?	?

Fig. 8–5.   Approximate cost of cardiac rehabilitation.

for a specific length of time, monthly, quarterly, biannually, or annually. Often the cost for participation in the program is the membership fee for joining the organization. The type of membership also varies; some membership plans allow use of the facility only during the hours of the program, and others allow complete use of the facility whenever it is open. Because of the fixed revenues of these membership-type programs, it is easier to maintain a balanced budget.

Another method of fees in adult fitness and phase III and IV programs is to have a decreasing charge for a 3- to 5-month period until a minimum fee is reached. This fee is normally only for the exercise sessions and excludes laboratory procedures. As with phase I and II programs, the education and behavior modification services usually have additional fees and are based on either a fixed fee for an entire series of sessions or on a per session basis.

Exercise Testing

Another important source of revenue, which is applicable to all phases of cardiac

rehabilitation and adult fitness, is that derived from exercise testing and other laboratory procedures. The fee for exercise testing may vary, depending on the purpose of the test and whether or not the test is supervised and interpreted by a physician. In situations where testing is performed on individuals with documented heart disease or at high risk for heart disease, physician supervision is essential. Fees for this procedure vary from approximately $150 to $300 per test. The maximum income from an exercise laboratory can be estimated from the cost per test and assuming one test per hour per station, 8 working hours/day, and 5 days/week.

The question of whether exercise testing should be conducted only in a clinical setting or as a service of phases III and IV and adult fitness programs has been much debated. Some physicians feel that all exercise testing in this high-risk group of individuals should be in a clinic or hospital setting. Others feel that some phase III, IV, and adult fitness facilities are equipped and staffed to do exercise testing safely. In general, however, it is prudent for all diagnostic and early post MI exercise testing to be carried out under physician supervision in a hospital or clinic setting, while functional testing might be conducted in a phase III/IV or adult fitness facility, assuming experienced staffing.

Other Sources of Revenue

In addition to sources of revenue derived from cardiac rehabilitation services, education and behavior modification classes, and exercise testing and related laboratory fees, there are other forms of income that may be of considerable importance to a program. Fund raising and donations can contribute substantial amounts of money to support a developing program, although each mature program is expected to pay its own way. Research grants are another important source of funds and can be used to support personnel and acquire additional equipment. Some programs raise additional funds by selling exercise equipment, clothing, and literature to the public.

DEVELOPING A BUDGET: EXPENDITURES

Like revenues, expenditures also vary according to the number of participants and specific services of a program. Because of start-up expenses such as purchase of equipment, renovation, or construction, expenditures are usually greater during the first year of a program and decrease in succeeding years. After the first year the expenditures are specific to the operational costs. The following discussion considers the typical expenditures in developing a program as well as the operational costs of cardiac rehabilitation and adult fitness programs.

Initial Expenditures

The initial costs of a program often involve renovation or construction and the purchase of equipment. Renovation or construction costs depend on the scope of the program and the size of the facility. As an example of minimal expense, a small room can be renovated and used as an outpatient phase II cardiac rehabilitation center. In contrast an entire building with classrooms, laboratory space, exercise areas including an indoor swimming pool, and locker and shower facilities can be constructed at considerable expense. The planned facility is dependent on initial funding and financial resources available for developmental costs. The income of a cardiac rehabilitation or adult fitness program is rarely sufficient to meet the costs of constructing a new facility. Income may be sufficient, on the other hand, to meet the costs of renovating an existing area.

Operational Costs

Operational expenditures can also vary considerably. The least expensive program to operate is phase I cardiac rehabilitation. Typical expenditures for this program are for personnel, supplies, and possibly an overhead or indirect charge for security, telephone, maintenance, and janitorial services. Personnel are discussed further in Chapter 10. The supplies for phase I programs are primarily materials for ECG-monitored exercise and educational materials. Overhead and service charges depend on local circumstances within the particular hospital.

Expenditures of an outpatient phase II facility are much greater. Personnel expenses include salaries for the program director, nurses, exercise technicians, exercise specialists, education staff, and secretarial staff. Supplies include materials for ECG monitoring and education materials. In addition there are overhead charges relating to the use of the outpatient facility that depend on local circumstances. Similar operational items may be required for phase III and adult fitness programs, although the expenditures are usually much less because personnel can be part-time and there is less need for ECG monitoring.

Personnel

Employee compensation is a major portion of a program's expenditures and has been discussed by many authors.[10-13] Tables 8–9 and 8–10 list yearly salaries and hourly wages for adult fitness personnel. Salaries appear to be reasonably consistent for these positions. In contrast, payment for cardiac rehabilitation personnel may vary among regions and programs. Nursing and physical therapy personnel may be paid more than health educators or exercise instructors, although salaries depend on the responsibilities of each position. The fringe benefits provided to personnel also vary widely, depending on the job classification. Fringe benefits can be as low as 5% for a part-time employee and as high as 25% for a highly classified, full-time individual.

Additional Expenses

There are numerous additional expenditures in cardiac rehabilitation and adult fitness programs that may or may not be considered as annual expenses, depending on the individual program priorities. These include costs of liability insurance, expenses for professional advancement such as travel, memberships to professional organizations, books and journal subscriptions, and expenditures for office supplies. The expense for professional advancement depends on the size and philosophy of the program. It is generally felt that these costs will eventually bring an equal or greater return to the program as staff members expand their concepts, understandings, interests, and talents from their educational pursuits.

The overhead charged to cardiac rehabilitation can be as much as 30% to 40% of the total operating costs, especially if the program is hospital based. For most adult fitness facilities, however, the overhead is usually 10% to 20% of operating budget. Overhead is an indirect charge, a service or building usage charge that is usually necessary for a hospital or other facility to continue to offer varied and diversified programs. The charge should be specifically for the services offered by the sponsoring agency. Overhead services include maintenance, repair, security, accounting, telephone, mail service, heating and air conditioning, water and electricity. In some hospitals the indirect cost of space is averaged throughout the hospital. Under these circumstances a cardiac rehabilitation program could have a much higher overhead because of the space involved. Over-

Table 8–9. Compensation of Club Managers and Professionals

	Tennis Facilities	Racquetball Facilities	All Multi-Recreation
Club manager			
Average annual compensation	$31,446	$30,016	$34,478
Composition			
Salary and bonuses	29,752	28,007	32,692
Paid expenses and other	1,694	2,009	1,786
Head tennis professional			
Average annual compensation	27,331		28,610
Head racquetball professional			
Average annual compensation		12,200	
Head swimming (teaching) professional			14,857
Fitness center manager/director			17,385

All of the figures cited are from the International Racquet Sports Association's 1984 Industry Data Survey. From Employee compensation. Club Industry, July/Aug.:65, 1985.

Table 8–10.   Employees Average Hourly Wages

Employee Category	Average Hourly Wage		
	Tennis Facilities	Racquetball Facilities	All Multi-Recreation
Assistant club manager	$ 7.82	$ 8.31	$ 8.11
Controller/head bookkeeper	7.34	8.88	7.39
Assistant bookkeeper	5.16	6.12	5.81
Office and clerical	4.74	5.71	5.11
Front desk	4.26	4.19	4.41
Program/social director	6.28	6.63	6.63
Sales staff	5.97	5.98	7.10
Pro shop	4.44	4.72	4.73
Food and beverage	4.25	4.65	4.49
Maintenance	5.26	9.57	5.38
Pool attendants	4.14	3.50	4.12
Head dance/exercise instructor	10.33	11.48	11.81
Other dance/exercise instructors	7.77	8.83	8.62
Nursery attendants	4.03	3.97	4.13
Locker room attendants		4.47	4.09

From Employee compensation. Club Industry, July/Aug.:65, 1985.

head costs must be provided and included as an expenditure in the budget.

The program budget must reflect the philosophy of the institution and staff and the purposes for which the program was established. Expenditures should not exceed current and future goals of the program or exceed revenues unless previously anticipated and planned. Often, an institution is willing to accept a loss at the beginning until an adequate patient load is achieved and the program becomes self-sustaining. Long-range planning must be continually considered in the budgetary process. Growth patterns and program trends must be taken into consideration when planning equipment purchases, facilities, staff, and services.

ADMINISTRATIVE CONSIDERATIONS

There are various methods of billing a participant in an adult fitness or cardiac rehabilitation program. The individual can be billed for each exercise therapy session, behavior modification class, or educational offering with an itemization of the service provided. A second billing procedure is for the person to be billed for an entire program (e.g., for all services of a phase I program or an entire phase II program) with an itemization of the services provided. A third method of billing is to bill for a period of time that the service is received, monthly, quarterly, semiannually, or annually. There are advantages and disadvantages for each of these three methods of billing, and accordingly, each program must determine its own optimal billing strategies. For services where a patient may receive third-party insurance coverage, it is recommended that the bill be itemized by date of service and the exact procedure performed. The billing procedure selected for a program must be appropriate for the particular setting and type of program. Generally, phase I, II, and III cardiac rehabilitation services are itemized and billed for services or program, while phase IV and adult fitness programs bill for a period of participation in the program or the entire program.

Delinquent Accounts

Most programs are faced with the problem of a small number of participants who do not pay a portion of the entire amount of their bill. Various options are available when this occurs. Initially, a decision must be made by the program's advisory board whether an effort will be made to obtain these uncollected funds. The following options are available: (1) make no effort to obtain the funds; (2) make an effort to collect the funds, but if repeated contacts are unsuccessful take no legal action and discontinue efforts to seek the funds; and (3) make every effort to obtain the funds, including referring the account to a bill collector agency and eventually, if necessary, to a small-claims court for legal action. The decision regarding the degree to which a program will actively attempt to collect unpaid accounts is based on the amount of funds not collected, both from individual accounts and the total amount from all accounts in which funds are outstanding. For the individual accounts in which a small amount is due, it is usually best to make an initial effort to obtain the amount, but if unsuccessful, not to pressure the matter. The publicity resulting from legal action, the time spent preparing the case, and the paper work involved in the action are not worth the amount received. However, an effort should still be made to secure the amount owed through a series of letters and possibly a telephone call. Figure 8–6 is an example of an initial letter requesting payment of overdue amounts. If payment does not occur, subsequent letters requesting payment should be worded more strongly and may be followed by a telephone call.

If the total amount owed to the program exceeds 2% to 5% of the total budget, an evaluation should be made of the billing and fee-collecting system and whether an aggressive attempt should be made to obtain uncollected funds. Normally a collection percentage rate of 95% to 97% is considered excellent, while a collection percentage below 90% to 95% should result in a reevaluation of the billing procedures. Many large hospital and clinic programs enjoy the privilege of having all billing handled by an accounting or billing department, while the majority of small clinic or hospital cardiac rehabilitation programs and most adult fitness programs must do their own collection of fees.

Assistance Fund

Irrespective of the effectiveness and efficiency of a billing system, there are people who cannot afford the cost of services provided. An arrangement should be available that allows these individuals to participate and receive program services at a reduced

---

Date:

Dear _____:

In checking our records for the Cardiac Rehabilitation Program, we find that you have been billed for the past several months with no resulting payment. Your present balance is _____. In that the operation of our Cardiac Rehabilitation program depends heavily on payment of amounts due from patients, the failure on your part to pay the billed amount is placing participation by others in jeopardy. Would you, therefore, compensate the program for the amount involved as soon as possible.

As I am sure you realize, the requested amount should be sent in check form to the Business Office. Please feel free to contact me if you have any questions on this matter.

Sincerely,

Program Director

Fig. 8–6. Delinquent fee letter No. 1.

fee. An assistance fund or some mechanism to provide reasonable financial relief to those deserving a fee adjustment should be routinely available. There should be a formal procedure in applying for such assistance, and criteria must be established regarding the amount of financial assistance, the exact services, and the exact period of time. Figure 8–7 illustrates an application form that can be utilized in establishing the financial justification of a request for financial assistance. The application form should require the individual to be specific in revealing personal financial information. Use of such an application form discourages those who do not really need assistance from applying. Such persons are usually reluctant to reveal their actual financial situation and subsequently do not follow through with the procedure.

One should always be on the lookout for those who might be in need of financial assistance. Individuals who have been active in the program and then give indication of dropping out are often those who need financial assistance but are embarrassed to ask for it. In addition referring physicians should be made aware of the existence of an assistance fund and the procedure followed to provide program services at a reduced fee for deserving patients. No one should be without the services of any phase of a cardiac rehabilitation program because of the expenses involved.

Insurance Coverage

A major concern of a program is not only insurance reimbursement for services rendered but also insurance coverage for the program.[14,15] All adult fitness and cardiac rehabilitation programs must be fully insured for staff liability, facility failure, and other concerns. Freestanding cardiac rehabilitation programs and adult fitness programs are finding it increasingly difficult to get insurance coverage. Programs located in a clinic or hospital are usually not a problem since these facilities are nor-

mally insured for services far beyond the risk of phase I or II cardiac rehabilitation. In contrast, phase III/IV and adult fitness programs in a community setting such as a high school, college, or university can often be a problem because coverage can be very expensive. As a solution many phase III/IV and adult fitness programs have combined their services with the phase I and II programs located in hospitals or clinics in order to receive adequate insurance coverage. Normally, the freestanding facility may need to be rented at a nominal fee and the staff paid a nominal amount by the clinic or hospital. The investigation of insurance coverage should be carefully considered. Often two policies are necessary, as one may exclude many items.

PROFIT CENTERS

Most adult fitness and some cardiac rehabilitation programs are finding that establishing "profit centers" as a relief to budget problems is a financially rewarding consideration.[15–18] A profit center is defined as an activity or item that primarily results in a profit where the revenue far exceeds the expenditures. The opportunities for adult fitness programs are almost limitless. Equipment and supplies sold through a pro shop have a significant markup. Other successful services that provide additional revenues include the health food bar and travel agency. Sun-tanning units also have potential for high profits. Although criticized by many as a frill and potentially injurious, profits from tanning may be substantial. Regardless of the facility, participants should at least pay for its use. The dues, court time, or user fees for each part of the facility should not only be paid for by the users but each should show a profit.

Profit centers for cardiac rehabilitation are a bit more unusual but do exist. The purchase of shirts and other clothing, rental or sale of equipment, and the purchase of educational materials are common

Name _____ Date _____
          Last   First   Initial

Address _____
        Street   City   State   Zip

Age _____ Birth Date _____ Home Phone _____

Marital Status: S   M   D   W   Number & Ages of Children _____

Occupation (Present or Most Recent) _____

Employment Status (Please Circle): (1) Full time (2) Part Time (hours per

week) _____ (3) Unemployed—Medical Reasons (4) Unemployed—Other

(5) Retired (If retired, how much are you receiving from pension or

retirement funds?) _____

Employer _____ Business Phone _____

Address _____

Monthly Salary _____

Other Income _____ Source _____

Spouse's Employer _____

Address _____

Monthly Salary _____

Bank _____ Checking _____
                                     Loan _____
                                     Savings _____

Do you have insurance coverage for: Exercise Sessions _____
                                 Lab Evaluations _____

Expenses and other financial circumstances that create this need (write on back of

sheet if needed) _____

_____

Please indicate how much you can afford to pay of the program costs:

Exercise Sessions are approximately $30.00 (Beginning Group) or $18.00

(Advanced Group) per month. I can afford paying _____ per month.

Laboratory Evaluations cost $150.00. I can afford to pay _____

of this amount.

        Signature of Applicant: _____

Fig. 8–7. Assistance fund application.

sources of additional revenues for programs. Some programs have shown profit in the sale of basic cardiac life-support classes, other educational offerings, and exercise prescription cards. Regardless of the item or service, the establishing of profit centers for cardiac rehabilitation makes financial sense.

FUND RAISING

A program should make an aggressive attempt to solicit financial support in the form of donations and contributions.[19–22] In a hospital-based program, this should not conflict with general hospital fund-raising efforts. The impact of prevention, intervention, and rehabilitation programs on an individual, a family, and an entire community is great, and obtaining significant financial assistance in the form of donations, wills, and bequests can be meaningful to these programs. The key to community fund raising is to involve program participants. Past and present participants are important not only for the donation of funds but also for direction to other sources of funds. In addition fund-raising efforts should be directed at members of professional groups in the community such as dentists, physicians, and lawyers. Efforts should also be directed toward selected businesses and industries in the community. In every case, whether contacting a member of a professional group, a business, an industry, or a past or present participant, the contact to the potential contributor should be by personal telephone call, visit, or letter. As indicated, the contact may be made by an active or past participant in the program who has some connection with the group or individual being contacted. For example, participating dentists in the program can be formed into a "dental task force," and that group can then contact various members of the dental profession in the area. Finally, fund raising is an ongoing and never-ending project. Every opportunity should be made to pub-licize the program, and every effort should be extended to make the public and selected individuals within the community aware of the financial needs of the program. Many contributors are more inclined to give in the spring of the year than at other times because of the April 15 income tax deadline. For some, December is the best time to contribute, because of the oncoming end of the calendar year and the tax benefits of the contributed funds for that year. Because of the new tax law, this process should be reviewed in order to maximize deduction potential. Finally, for some, January is the best time to contribute because of bonuses from the previous year. If properly organized and effectively conducted, a significant portion of the budget can be offset by contributed funds. A continual, everyday effort should be directed toward the solicitation of donated funds.

CONCLUSIONS

The business of cardiac rehabilitation and adult fitness is extremely important. The program director and staff must have an ongoing appreciation of financial considerations. Reimbursement issues will continue to develop that require understanding by the staff. The budget itself requires intensive planning, preparation, and continual daily surveillance. If administered properly, budget matters can become routine. The ultimate success of a program depends on a well-developed and well-administered budget. If developed properly, efficiently, and effectively administered and periodically reviewed, the budget becomes the cornerstone of a successful program. Administrative considerations such as billing, delinquent accounts, assistance programs, and insurance policies must be addressed. Finally, establishing profit centers and a well-planned fund-raising process add greatly to the program's revenues.

REFERENCES

1. Cardiac rehab faces challenge. Optimal Health, Jan./Feb.:40, 1986.

2. Medicare Intermediary Manual. Part 3. Claims Process. Transmittal No. 998. Department of Health and Human Services, Health Care Financing Administration, Sept. 1982.

3. PHS Announces Assessment of Cardiac Rehab Services. Med. Rehabil. Rev., 2(33):4, 1985.

4. Medical technology: Scientific evaluations, cardiac rehabilitation services. Federal Register. Public Health Service. Vol. 50, No. 158, 32911, August 15, 1985.

5. Timmons, D.R.: Cardiovascular rehabilitation program development and organizational concerns. In Cardiac Rehabilitation: Exercise Testing and Prescription. Edited by L.K. Hall. Jamaica, N.Y., Spectrum, 1984.

6. Position Statement on Cardiovascular Exercise Training Programs. New York County Medical Society, New York, May 9, 1983.

7. Smith, C.E.: DRGs, making them work for you. Nursing, Jan.:34, 1985.

8. DRGs, cost containment, and our vocation. Hosp. Pract., Jan. 15:12, 1985.

9. Shaffer, F.A.: DRG's: History and overview. Nursing and Health Care, Sept.: 388, 1983.

10. Employee compensation. Club Industry, July/Aug.:65, 1985.

11. Burlin, R.: Cost center reporting. Club Industry, Oct.:43, 1985.

12. Boggs, R.: Aerobics. Club Industry. Sept.:24, 1985.

13. Berra, K., and Fry, G.: YMCArdiac therapy. San Francisco, National Council of YMCAs, 1981.

14. Caro, R.: Insurance policies: A buyer's guide. Club Industry, Sept.:44, 1985.

15. Denley, J.: Two ways to reduce your insurance costs. Club Industry, Feb.:61, 1986.

16. Leve, M.: Increasing profit potential in your club's profit centers. Athletic Business, Dec.:44, 1984.

17. McCarthy, J.: Profitable clubs and how they do it. Athletic Business, March:26, 1986.

18. Ten commandments of profitability. Fitness Management, Sept./Oct.:38, 1985.

19. Bronzan, R.T.: Fund raising today demands better ideas. Athletic Purchasing and Facilities. May:12, 1984.

20. Palmisano, M.: Fund raising's first rule: Get organized. Athletic Business, May:20, 1984.

21. McKenzie, B.: Fifteen projects. Athletic Business, March:44, 1986.

22. Palmisano, M.: Fund raising ideas that really work. Athletic Business, Nov.:34, 1984.

COMPUTER UTILIZATION AND DATA PROCESSING

Since the 1940s when the massive EN-IAC initiated the computer age, there has been a remarkable transformation of our society, largely due to the impact of computers on both professional and personal lives. From this sparse beginning to the 1980s, computer products and services have evolved far beyond what anyone would have guessed. Today, millions of computers have been purchased by the American public for both home and business applications, and it is estimated that by 1990 over 65% of professional, managerial, and administrative personnel will be computer literate.[1]

The application of computer techniques to sports medicine, adult fitness, cardiac rehabilitation, and exercise testing is especially impressive and is the focus of this chapter. Fry and Berra[2] described the use of computers in their YMCArdiac programs as early as 1973.[2] In 1981 Moore[3] discussed the value of computer analyses to sports medicine applications (Fig. 9–1). The implications of studies of biomechanics to coaches and athletes are very significant and likely to have a major impact on performance. Computer applications to large exercise programs were discussed by Jensen in 1984.[1] Numerous articles have appeared in recent years, detailing the use of computers to the health-spa industry and corporate fitness programs.[4–9] Computers are frequently used by participants in exercise programs who wish to track their progress over time. Computer analyses of exercise laboratory data, including electrocardiograms (ECGs), respiratory gases, and other physiologic data, have been described for many years and have significantly improved patient evaluations.[10–16] Finally, the computer is invaluable to the administration of exercise treatment programs. Budgeting, billing, payroll, inventory, and word processing are but a few of the areas where the computer has had an impact.[17–19]

Accordingly, an understanding of computer technologies is fast becoming a requirement for adult fitness, cardiac rehabilitation, and exercise test personnel. Program administrators should motivate the staff to become computer literate and provide the necessary support to accomplish that task. Computer literacy continues to be a focus of concern in our society,[17] and program directors need to appreciate that there may be an initial reluctance of staff to become familiar with computer concepts. A brief glossary of computer terminology is given in Appendix 9–1.[20]

This chapter discusses computer applications to adult fitness, cardiac rehabilitation, and exercise testing that are important for health professionals working in these areas. Specific topics that are considered include program administration, exercise laboratory procedures, training applications, and education.

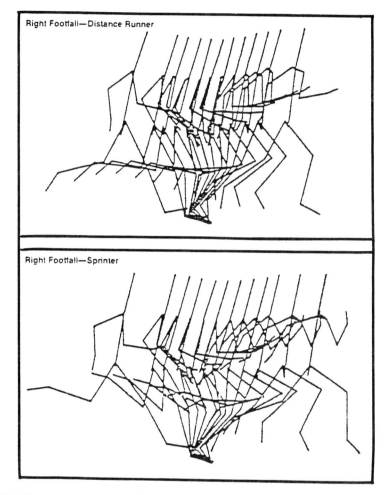

Right Footfall—Distance Runner

Right Footfall—Sprinter

Fig. 9–1. "A digitizer-generated comparison of the strides of a distance runner and a sprinter." Courtesy of Barry T. Bates, PhD., University of Oregon, Eugene. Moore, M.: The computerization of sports medicine. Physician Sportsmed., 9:118, 1981.

ADMINISTRATION

The application of computers to program administration is most likely the easiest of all program activities to implement. The following administrative areas can be computerized for a more efficient and cost-effective operation: (1) secretarial and clerical activities, (2) program enrollment, (3) records and forms, (4) scheduling, (5) financial matters, (6) marketing, and (7) summary reports.

Secretarial and Clerical Activities

The secretarial and clerical duties that are immediately benefited by computeri-

zation are record keeping, storage of files, and word processing. The most difficult task in implementing a computerized office system, however, may well be personnel resistance.[20,21] Often, older personnel have only used conventional typewriters and traditional filing methods for their entire careers and are reluctant to convert to a computerized system. Younger employees are more likely to be trained in computerized methods. If a new office system is being implemented, employees should be informed of the purchased equipment and given a time schedule and recommended approach to learning the system. In many cases sending personnel on released time to a workshop has proven beneficial. Once the staff have acquired the new skills and totally learned the new system, they usually become enthusiastic users of the system and convinced of its value.

Enrollment

Another administrative area enhanced by computerization is enrollment and tracking of participants.[22] Immediate access to participant files with demographic information such as age, sex, area of residence, occupation, and other information can be of great value. Specific services to meet the needs of individuals can more easily be provided if this information is readily available. Many programs have incorporated an automated front desk check-in system to screen for expired memberships, unpaid fees, current laboratory data, and other pertinent information. This type of check-in system is also of great value in assessing the usage of the facility. Individuals who are not using the facility can then be called and urged to become more active. Information on time of usage can also be of benefit in developing a staffing schedule. Finally, a computerized check-in service can be used to generate a guest list for future marketing efforts. When a participant brings a guest, the individual is asked to fill out the necessary information, which is then used in marketing the program to that person through personal letters, telephone calls, and other methods.

Records and Forms

The most obvious administrative benefit of a computerized management system is record keeping. Storage space and accessibility to files is always a problem when using traditional methods but one that is easily solved by computerization. Computer storage allows immediate access of data, enables almost total removal of files and boxes of old data, and solves the general problem of lack of office space. The

updating of files is more efficient with a word processing system. Information is simply entered on the terminal, and the file is immediately updated. There is not the necessity of physically pulling a file, entering the information—which might require redoing that page or section—and then replacing the file. The word processing system allows for rapid data entry, storage, and options for printing or not printing.

Scheduling

The scheduling requirements of a program can be greatly enhanced by the utilization of a computer.[23,24] The combination of participants, staff, facilities, and available slots lends itself to computerization of all scheduling needs. Participant data needed for scheduling include facilities used and time of usage; staff information includes participant needs, particular skills of the staff, and preferred staffing hours. Once this information is processed, a staffing schedule can be developed that best meets the needs of the participants.

Financial Considerations

Computerization of program data has great implications for financial management including budgeting, revenue and expenses, and billing.[22] Administratively, a computerized system expedites routine procedures while reducing the chance of error. Quick visual review of computer printouts and spreadsheets provides immediate information on the program's financial status and a visual check for errors. The financial savings of a computerized system as opposed to paying an individual to do the "books" can be significant. Billing can be reduced from days to hours of work with fewer errors and immediate access to financial data once the information is entered. A spreadsheet process that details revenues and expenditures improves the operation of the program.[25] Payroll packages that include state and federal tax amounts and all necessary financial fringe benefits are also available.[22]

Marketing

Program marketing, an essential aspect of all successful programs, can be improved by computer techniques. As an example a mailing list of potential participants can be generated from telephone inquiries, leads from people who have visited the program, past participants, and other sources. Personal letters can be sent to these individuals with follow-up telephone calls. Efforts to enroll new members are easier to organize using computerized data. The computerized list of participants can also facilitate fund raising using personal letters, telephone calls, and in many cases, personal visits.

Program Summary Reports

The computerized status report or program summary is of considerable value to program operation. Figures 9–2 and 9–3 illustrate two such reports utilized for cardiac rehabilitation programs. Figure 9–2 details all the necessary information for an immediate status report on the program. The data include grand totals and current totals such as referrals, patient classification, drop outs with the reasons, and attendance. A low attendance might indicate a lack of motivation or program shortcomings. Also on the report is the "total exercise hours," which can be related to mortality and morbidity as an indication of program safety. The report illustrated in Figure 9–3 is more specific to mortality and morbidity of both current and past participants. Both of these reports provide staff with the necessary information to assess program status.

LABORATORY SERVICES

The evaluation of individuals for adult fitness and cardiac rehabilitation programs can be significantly enhanced by comput-

erization. The areas of computer applications include processing of health history and life-style questionnaires, analyses of exercise test data, and generation of exercise prescriptions. Questionnaire techniques are discussed in Chapter 4, which also shows an example of a comprehensive self-administered medical questionnaire (see Fig. 4–1).

Exercise Test and Prescription Applications

Computer processing of exercise testing and prescription data are becoming increasingly popular in cardiac rehabilitation and adult fitness programs. Although these services can be provided by commercial sources, it is recommended that program personnel develop their own expertise. All systems considered should be compatible with the computer equipment that is used for the administrative needs of the program.

Figure 9–4 illustrates a data form for exercise testing, which includes heart rate (HR), blood pressure (BP), metabolic parameters, and ECG data. This type of form requires that data be entered while the test is being performed and has the advantage of providing the laboratory staff with information during exercise to facilitate decision making. The data are easily entered into a computer system, as most systems allow automatic and immediate data entry.

Figure 9–5 is an example of a computer-generated exercise test report used at the Mayo Clinic in Rochester, Minnesota. The report provides heart rate and blood pressure data during exercise and recovery according to a programmed test protocol. Functional capacity and maximal heart rate are shown along with signs, symptoms, and reasons for test termination. Many laboratories also utilize the computer for ECG analyses both for conventional ST segment measurements as well as for more sophisticated ECG parameters (Chapter 5).

Exercise prescriptions and coronary risk

Grand Totals	Present Totals	Referrals*	Dropped**	Length in Program (months)
Total involved since inception (June, 1971)	Enrolled –111	B. A. (6)	C. B. (10)	0– 3, 8%
	M-W-F –40	L. A. (1)	R. O. (12)	4– 6, 4%
	T-TH –71	R. B. (1)	E. O. (8)	7–12, 24%
Referred–440	Male –95	E. D. (1)	G. O. (10)	13–24, 20%
Accepted–412	Female –16			25–36, 44%
Total GXTs–1181	Conducted GXTs–7	*G. S. (1) re-entered		
Total exercise hours–45,335	Exercise hours–1172	*L. S. (1) re-entered		
	% of attendance–71.20%	*E. D. (1) re-referred		
		*A. F. (1) re-referral		

Total Patients	Cardiac Prone	Post Infarct	Patient Status Post-operative	Rheumatic H.D.	ASHD Non-MI	Other
111	48	29	12	2	8	12
Male Patients 95	39	28	12	2	6	8
Female Patients 16	9	1	0	0	2	4

*Classification of Patients

1. Cardiac prone
2. Postmyocardial infarction
3. Postoperative
4. Rheumatic heart disease
5. ASHD-Non-myocardial infarction
6. Other

**Reasons for Dropping

1. Business conflict
2. Moved out of area
3. Dissatisfaction with progress
4. Re-referred to personal physician
5. Deceased
6. Loss of interest
7. Graduated
8. Medical reasons
9. Distance
10. Personal
11. Vacation
12. Nonattendance
13. Transfer to AFP

Fig. 9–2.   La Crosse Exercise Program, Cardiac Rehabilitation Unit, monthly summary, September, 1979. (GXT, graded exercise testing.)

CAPRI

CARDIO PULMONARY
RESEARCH INSTITUTE

ENROLLMENT AND CLINICAL EXPERIENCE SUMMARY

May 1968 through ___June 1979___

ENROLLMENT

___1876___ Enrolled since inception (___1527___ men - ___349___ women)

  ___1438___ CHD   ___77___ %

     ___974___ MI s   ___52___ %

     ___464___ Angina/Ischemia   ___25___ %

   ___61___ Pulmonary   ___3___ %

  ___377___ Other   ___20___ %

  ___1876___ Total   ___100___ %

___594___ Enrolled as of ___July 1, 1979___ .

Average attendance for ___June 1979___   ___79___ %

CLINICAL EXPERIENCE OF CAPRI IN RELATION TO:

A. Active Participants

	Initial 12 weeks		After 12 weeks		Total	
	not in class	in class	not in class	in class	not in class	in class
MI (deaths)	19 (4)	1 (0)	41 (13)	2 (0)	60 (17)	3 (0)
Deaths from all causes	11	0	43	0	54	0
Circulatory Arrest (resuscitated)	3 (0)	1 (1)	21 (2)	19 (19)	24 (2)	20 (20)

B. Past Participants (Not enrolled in supervised rehabilitation at time of incident)

MI (deaths)	53 (22)
Deaths from all causes	106
Circulatory Arrests - none successfully resuscitated	27

C. Other Relevant Events, Overall (A & B)

	Active Participation	Past Participants
Angiography (Deaths)	440 (1) 2	25 (0)
Surgery (Deaths)	259 (1) 2	17 (6)

D. Cumulative Experience To Date (May 1968 through ___June 1979___)

1. Supervised Hours of Exercise Training   269,188
2. Supervised Maximal Exercise Tolerance Tests   4,665
3. Deaths During Exercise Training and Testing   0

914 EAST JEFFERSON · SEATTLE, WASHINGTON 98122 · (206) 323-7550
Non-Profit Organization

Fig. 9–3. CAPRI-Cardio Pulmonary Research Institute, Seattle, enrollment and clinical experience summary. Used with permission of Richard C. Frederick, CAPRI, Seattle, WA.

GUNDERSEN CLINIC, LTD.   DATE: _____
GXT REPORT

Patient: _____Physician: _____

Clinic No: _____Cardiologist: _____

Patient Ht: _____cm.   Wgt:_____kg.   Age: _____yrs.

Resting (Supine) HR: _____   BP: _____

Predicted Max HR: _____   90% _____   70% _____

Predicted Max BP: Systolic _____   Diastolic _____

Attained Max Hr _____   SBP _____   DBP _____

Predicted RPP Max _____Attained RPP Max _____

Predicted $\dot{V}O_2$ Max _____L/min _____ml/kg/mir

Attained $\dot{V}O_2$ _____L/min _____ml/kg/mir

Functional Aerobic Impairment (FAI): _____

FAI (   )+ Att. $\dot{V}O_2$ (   ) = 100% $\dot{V}O_2$ Max (Bruce nomogram)

Energy Expenditure (   ) K.Cal   (   ) METS

Functional Class (AHA): (   )   Fitness Level (   )

Reason for Stopping: _____

Resting (standing) ECG _____

Post Hypervent. ECG _____

1. EXERCISE ECG:

2. POST EXERCISE ECG:

3. CONCLUSION:

Fig. 9–4.   GXT Summary Form, Gundersen Clinic, Ltd., La Crosse Wisconsin. Used with permission of Joseph W. Edgett, Jr., M.D., Gundersen Clinic, Lts., La Crosse, WI.

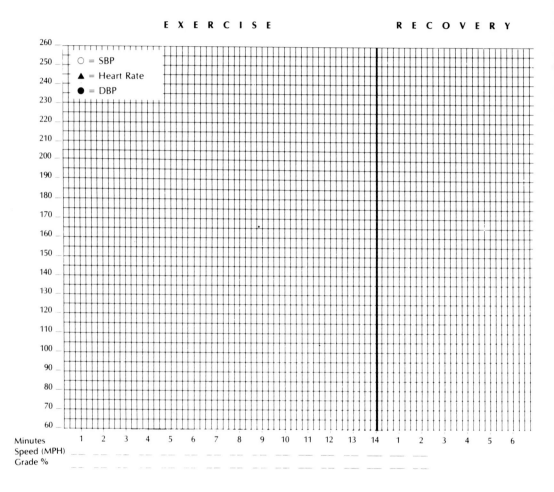

Fig. 9–4. Cont'd.

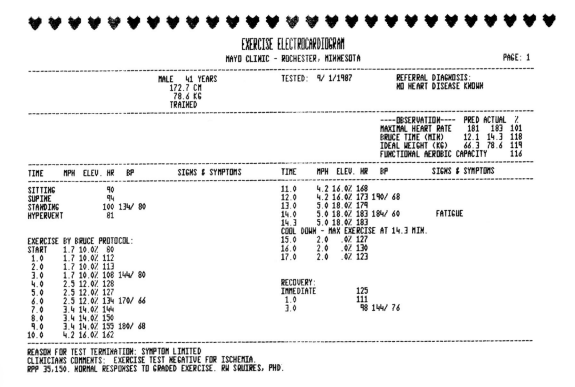

EXERCISE ELECTROCARDIOGRAM
MAYO CLINIC - ROCHESTER, MINNESOTA
PAGE: 1

MALE 41 YEARS	TESTED: 9/ 1/1987	REFERRAL DIAGNOSIS:	
172.7 CM		NO HEART DISEASE KNOWN	
78.6 KG			
TRAINED			

	----OBSERVATION----	PRED	ACTUAL	%
MAXIMAL HEART RATE		181	183	101
BRUCE TIME (MIN)		12.1	14.3	118
IDEAL WEIGHT (KG)		66.3	78.6	119
FUNCTIONAL AEROBIC CAPACITY				116

TIME	MPH ELEV. HR	BP	SIGNS & SYMPTOMS	TIME	MPH ELEV. HR	BP	SIGNS & SYMPTOMS
SITTING	90			11.0	4.2 16.0% 168		
SUPINE	94			12.0	4.2 16.0% 173	190/ 68	
STANDING	100 134/ 80			13.0	5.0 18.0% 179		
HYPERVENT	81			14.0	5.0 18.0% 183	184/ 60	FATIGUE
				14.3	5.0 18.0% 183		
				COOL DOWN - MAX EXERCISE AT 14.3 MIN.			
EXERCISE BY BRUCE PROTOCOL:				15.0	2.0 .0% 127		
START	1.7 10.0% 80			16.0	2.0 .0% 130		
1.0	1.7 10.0% 112			17.0	2.0 .0% 123		
2.0	1.7 10.0% 113						
3.0	1.7 10.0% 108 144/ 80						
4.0	2.5 12.0% 128			RECOVERY:			
5.0	2.5 12.0% 127			IMMEDIATE	125		
6.0	2.5 12.0% 134 170/ 66			1.0	111		
7.0	3.4 14.0% 144			3.0	98 144/ 76		
8.0	3.4 14.0% 150						
9.0	3.4 14.0% 155 180/ 68						
10.0	4.2 16.0% 162						

REASON FOR TEST TERMINATION: SYMPTOM LIMITED
CLINICIANS COMMENTS: EXERCISE TEST NEGATIVE FOR ISCHEMIA.
RPP 35,150. NORMAL RESPONSES TO GRADED EXERCISE. RW SQUIRES, PHD.

Fig. 9–5. Computer-generated exercise test report used at the Mayo Clinic, Rochester, Minnesota.

CARDIOVASCULAR HEALTH CLINIC
Mayo Clinic, Rochester, Minnesota

CARDIOVASCULAR RISK PROFILE   MALES: 30–39 YEARS OF AGE

Name _____ Age _____ Sex _____

Clinic number _____ Date _____

MODIFIABLE

Percentile Ranking	Treadmill Time* (min)	% Body Fat	Cholesterol mg %	Triglyceride mg %	Resting Blood Pressure Systolic/Diastolic		Smoking Habit	Tension Anxiety
V E R Y L O W 1	14.0	7	157	47	105	68	None	None
5		11	166	54	109	70		
10	13.0	13	173	60				
15		15	178	65				
20	12.0	16						
L O W 25	11.0	17	183	70	117	77	Pipe	Slight
30		18	187	74			Cigar	
35	10.5	19	192	79			Past only	
40		20	196	83				
45	10.0	21	200	88				
M O D E R A T E 50	9.5	22	204	92	125	83	1–20	Mod.
55		23	208	97				
60	9.0	24	212	102				
65		25	216	108				
H I G H 70	8.5	26	221	114	134	90	20–40	High
75		27	226	122				
80	8.0	28	233	131				
85		30	240	142				
V E R Y H I G H 90	7.5	32	250	158	146	99	40+	Very High
95	6.5	36	264	182	154	105		
99	5.0	46						

------- M--E---D---I---A---N -------

RISK

NON-MODIFIABLE

Personal History of Heart Attack:
( ) None
( ) Over 5 years ago
( ) 2–5 years ago
( ) 1–2 years ago
( ) 0–1 years ago

Family History of Heart Attack:
( ) None
( ) Yes, over 50 years
( ) Yes, 50 years or under

Resting ECG— Exercise ECG—
( ) Normal (Negative) ( )
( ) Equivocal (Borderline) ( )
( ) Abnormal (Positive) ( )

Age Factor:
( ) Under 30 years of age
( ) 30–39 years of age
( ) 40–49 years of age
( ) 50–59 years of age
( ) 60+ years of age

Diabetes:
( ) None
( ) + Family history
( ) Late onset
( ) Early onset

Total Cardiovascular Risk
☐ Very Low
☐ Low
☐ Moderate
☐ High

*Bruce Protocol

SCORE _____ _____ _____

TOTAL _____

Fig. 9–6.   Cardiovascular risk profile used at the Mayo Clinic.

profiles are equally enhanced by computerization.[26] Figure 9–6 illustrates a cardiovascular risk profile utilized at the Mayo Clinic, which relates exercise test data to other coronary risk parameters in order to compare each patient with others of the same age and sex. From these computerized data comprehensive life-style and exercise prescriptions can be generated for each individual patient. Often the recommendations are printed out in a conversational or letter format from the clinic staff to the patient with copies sent to the referring physician.

The most common ancillary procedures related to exercise testing are strength and flexibility testing and body composition. These studies also can be better understood by patients using computer-generated reports. As an example, Appendix 9–2 illustrates a report of body composition analysis generated at the Cleveland Clinic Foundation for a 30-year-old woman. In this example, the data are from skinfold measurements, and the report details the results along with recommended actions.

APPLICATIONS TO EXERCISE TRAINING

The computer has had a significant effect on the adult fitness and cardiac rehabilitation participants' involvement in exercise programs. The benefits are not only due to analyses of laboratory data resulting in computerized exercise prescriptions but also to analysis of the actual exercise sessions and the reporting process of exercise participation. This section discusses computer applications to exercise training with particular emphasis on generation of exercise session progress reports.

"High-Tech" Exercise

Technology is having a significant impact on exercise training.[27] Heart rate monitors that can be worn like a watch provide continuous heart rate data during exercise and sound an alarm when the rate

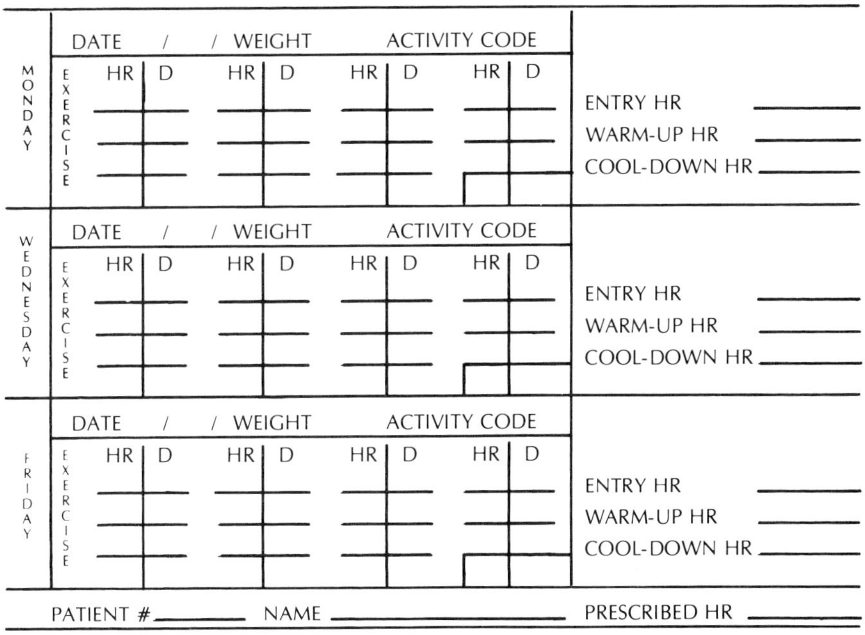

Fig. 9–7. La Crosse Exercise Program. Exercise session progress report, data card.

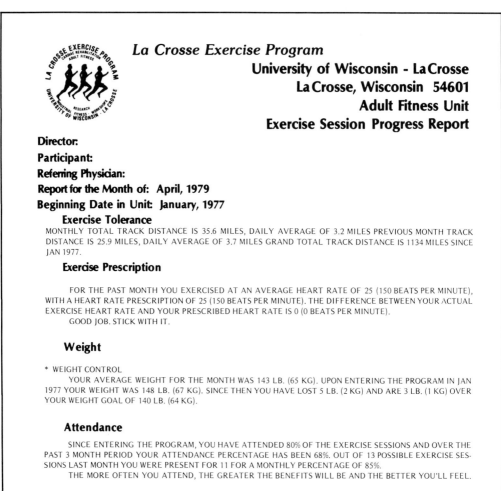

La Crosse Exercise Program
University of Wisconsin - La Crosse
La Crosse, Wisconsin 54601
Adult Fitness Unit
Exercise Session Progress Report

Director:

Participant:

Referring Physician:

Report for the Month of: April, 1979

Beginning Date in Unit: January, 1977

Exercise Tolerance

MONTHLY TOTAL TRACK DISTANCE IS 35.6 MILES, DAILY AVERAGE OF 3.2 MILES PREVIOUS MONTH TRACK DISTANCE IS 25.9 MILES, DAILY AVERAGE OF 3.7 MILES GRAND TOTAL TRACK DISTANCE IS 1134 MILES SINCE JAN 1977.

Exercise Prescription

FOR THE PAST MONTH YOU EXERCISED AT AN AVERAGE HEART RATE OF 25 (150 BEATS PER MINUTE), WITH A HEART RATE PRESCRIPTION OF 25 (150 BEATS PER MINUTE). THE DIFFERENCE BETWEEN YOUR ACTUAL EXERCISE HEART RATE AND YOUR PRESCRIBED HEART RATE IS 0 (0 BEATS PER MINUTE).
GOOD JOB. STICK WITH IT.

Weight

* WEIGHT CONTROL
YOUR AVERAGE WEIGHT FOR THE MONTH WAS 143 LB. (65 KG). UPON ENTERING THE PROGRAM IN JAN 1977 YOUR WEIGHT WAS 148 LB. (67 KG). SINCE THEN YOU HAVE LOST 5 LB. (2 KG) AND ARE 3 LB. (1 KG) OVER YOUR WEIGHT GOAL OF 140 LB. (64 KG).

Attendance

SINCE ENTERING THE PROGRAM, YOU HAVE ATTENDED 80% OF THE EXERCISE SESSIONS AND OVER THE PAST 3 MONTH PERIOD YOUR ATTENDANCE PERCENTAGE HAS BEEN 68%. OUT OF 13 POSSIBLE EXERCISE SESSIONS LAST MONTH YOU WERE PRESENT FOR 11 FOR A MONTHLY PERCENTAGE OF 85%.
THE MORE OFTEN YOU ATTEND, THE GREATER THE BENEFITS WILL BE AND THE BETTER YOU'LL FEEL.

THE INFORMATION CONTAINED IN THIS REPORT IS FOR YOUR BENEFIT. ANY QUESTIONS REGARDING IT SHOULD BE REFERRED TO YOUR EXERCISE LEADER.

Fig. 9–8.   Exercise therapy session progress report—to primary physician, La Crosse Exercise Program (Adult Fitness Unit).

July 1979 Progress Report for _____

Referring Physician _____

EXERCISE
Monthly total track distance is (25.0 miles,) daily average of (2.2) miles. Previous month track distance is (30.8 miles,) daily average of 2.4 miles. Grand total track distance is (496 miles) since Oct. 1978.

For the past month you exercised at an average heart rate of (22) (132 beats per minute) with a heart rate prescription of (24) (144 beats per minute). The difference between your actual exercise heart rate and your prescribed heart rate is (2) (12 beats per minute).
*(Good job. Stick with it.)

WEIGHT CONTROL
Your average weight for the month was (212 lb (96 kg).) Upon entering the program in Oct 1978 your weight was (222 lb (101 kg).) Since then you have lost (10 lb (5 kg)) and are (22 lb (10 kg)) from your weight goal of (190 lb (86 kg).)

*ATTENDANCE
Since entering the program, you have attended, (100%) of the exercise sessions and over the past 3-month period your attendance percentage has been (100%) Out of 12 possible exercise sessions last month you were present for 12 for a monthly percentage of (100%)
* *(Keep up the good work.)
The information contained in this report is for your benefit. Any questions regarding it should be referred to your exercise leader.

Fig. 9–9. La Crosse Exercise Program. Exercise session progress report, sample.

TO: All La Crosse Exercise Program Participants

By now you should have received your first exercise session progress report. The following is an explanation of the various numbers and phrases which will perhaps clarify the report. The numbers and phrases correspond to the circled numbers and phrases on the attached progress report.

1. 25.0—The distance (track, pool, etc.) for the month just completed.
2. 2.2—The number of times the participant attended the exercise sessions divided into the monthly distance.
3. 30.8—The previous month's distance.
4. 496—The grand total of miles run by the participant since entering the program.
5. 22—The average heart rate for the month just completed (taken for 10 seconds).
6. 132—The heart beats per minute for the monthly average heart rate.
7. 24—The heart rate prescription.
8. 2—The difference between the actual exercise heart rate and the prescribed heart rate.
∗—The participant should always try to maintain the prescribed heart rate, observing carefully not to exceed the prescriptive level.
9. 212 LB. (96 KG)—The average weight of the participant for the month just completed. (LB = pounds; KG = kilograms.)
10. 222 LB. (101 KG)—The initial weight of the participant observed upon entering the program.
11. 10 LB. (5 KG)—The amount of weight the participant has lost since entering the program.
12. 22 LB. (10 KG)—The amount of weight the participant needs to lose in order to reach his/her weight goal.
13. 190 LB. (86 KG)—The weight goal desired by the participant.
14. 100%—The attendance percentage of the participant since entering the program.
15. 100%—The attendance percentage of the participant for the previous three months.
16. 100%—The attendance percentage of the participant for the month just completed.
∗ ∗—A note commenting on the attendance for the month just completed.

Fig. 9–10.   La Crosse Exercise Program. Exercise session progress report, explanation.

Your printout gives a day by day listing of your exercise.

It gives distances in miles and yards, also quantities.

Everything is converted into Aerobic Points.

Times are shown so you can watch your improvement.

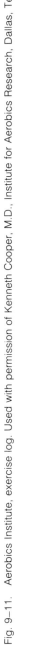

DATE	ACTIVITY	DISTANCE/QUANTITY	DURATION	AEROBIC POINTS	ERROR CODES		DATE	ACTIVITY	DISTANCE/QUANTITY	DURATION	AEROBIC POINTS	ERROR CODES
Mar 1	Jogging/Running	2.00 MI	16:00	11.00			Mar 1	Calisthenics		30:00	.75	
Mar 2	Jogging/Running	3.00 MI	25:00	16.40			Mar 2	Rope Skipping	90.00 SM	15:00	6.25	
Mar 3	Rope Skipping	90.00 SM	20:00	9.00			Mar 4	Swimming	600.00 YD	11:00	6.82	
Mar 5	Jogging/Running	5.00 MI	43:00	27.26			Mar 6	Stationary Running	100.00 SM	15:00	10.00	
Mar 7	Walking	2.00 MI	30:00	5.00			Mar 7	Cycling	5.00 MI	17:00	7.32	
Mar 8	Treadmill	3.30 10	30:00	3.91			Mar 8	Stationary Cycling	170.00 35	25:00	11.56	
Mar 9	Jogging/Running	2.00 MI	15:35	11.27			Mar 9	Tennis (Doubles)	3.00 SE	1:20:00	2.00	
Mar 10	Calisthenics		30:00	.75			Mar 10	Jogging/Running	4.00 MI	33:00	22.39	
Mar 11	Handball		1:30:00	13.50			Mar 12	Stationary Running	100.00 SM	15:00	10.00	
Mar 12	Rope Skipping	90.00 SM	15:00	6.25			Mar 13	Jogging/Running	3.00 MI	23:30	17.32	
Mar 14	Treadmill	3.30 10	10:00	3.91			Mar 14	Basketball		1:45:00	15.75	
Mar 15	Calisthenics		30:00	.75			Mar 15	Jogging/Running	3.00 MI	24:00	17.00	
Mar 16	Jogging/Running	6.00 MI	50:00	33.80			Mar 17	Stationary Running	100.00 SM	15:00	10.00	
Mar 17	Swimming	600.00 YD	12:00	6.25			Mar 18	Calisthenics		30:00	.75	
Mar 18	Tennis (Singles)	2.00 SE	1:00:00	4.00			Mar 19	Jogging/Running	4.00 MI	32:30	22.69	
Mar 20	Treadmill	3.30 10	30:00	3.91			Mar 21	Walking	2.00 MI	29:00	5.28	
Mar 21	Tennis (Doubles)	3.00 SE	1:20:00	2.00			Mar 22	Stationary Running	100.00 SM	15:00	10.00	
Mar 22	Treadmill	3.30 10	30:00	3.91			Mar 23	Jogging/Running	5.00 MI	42:00	27.81	
Mar 24	Jogging/Running	3.00 MI	23:00	17.65			Mar 24	Volleyball		1:00:00	4.00	
Mar 25	Walking	2.00 MI	31:00	4.74			Mar 25	Stationary Cycling	170.00 30	45:00	15.42	
Mar 26	Stationary Cycling		20:00	9.25			Mar 27	Jogging/Running	6.00 MI	50:00	33.80	
Mar 28	Volleyball		1:00:00	4.00			Mar 28	Jogging/Running	3.00 MI	23:30	17.32	
Mar 29	Skiing		1:00:00	6.00			Mar 29	Skiing		1:00:00	6.00	
Mar 30	Jogging/Running	5.00 MI	43:00	27.26			Mar 30	Calisthenics		30:00	.75	

MONTHLY and ACCUMULATIVE TOTALS

	A. Pts.	Mileage	Cycling	Swim	St. Run	St. Cyc.	Ten. S.	Ten. D.	Treadml.	Calisth.	Rope Sk.	Skiing	Volleyb.	Handbal.	Baskebl.
Start Mar. '77	512.8	257.3	82.8	1.3	1:00:	1:30:	1:00:	2:40:	2:00:	2:30:	50:	2:00:	2:00:	1:30:	1:45:
Totals	115.8/W	60.0	5.0	.7											
		317.3	87.8	2.0											

0000000

AIRS, ANDY
12100 PRESTON ROAD
DALLAS   TX 75230

AEROBICS
EXERCISE
LOG

This bar lists your weekly Aerobic Points as well as your overall points.

Here's where you'll find your total mileage.

Your printout can chart 14 of the 28 activities.

Actual size 8 1/2 x 11 in.

Fig. 9–11.   Aerobics Institute, exercise log. Used with permission of Kenneth Cooper, M.D., Institute for Aerobics Research, Dallas, Texas.

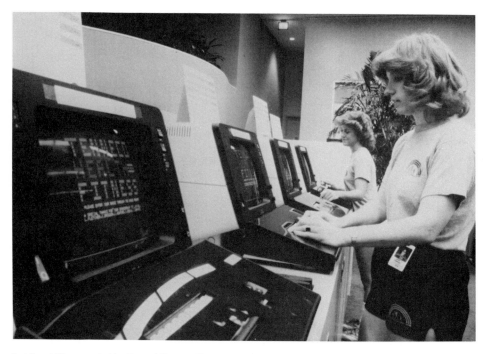

Fig. 9–12. At Tenneco's Health and Fitness Center, members log their activities following exercise and receive immediate feedback—information that is not only useful but is also motivational. From Baum, W.B., and Baum, M.: A corporate health and fitness program: Motivation and management by computers. JOPERD, April, 1984.

exceeds the prescribed training range. Electronic stationary bicycles are available that inform the rider of speed, distance, exercise time, calories consumed, pulse rates, and work rates. Most recently, a running shoe has been developed with a computer chip in the heel, which records, during the exercise session and which afterward, using a personal computer, provides a printout detailing the duration, distance, calories burned, and a graphic comparison to past data. Probably no area of exercise equipment has been more affected by computers than resistance equipment.[28] Software is now available that allows the lifter to program a workout that provides both strength and cardiovascular benefits.

Undoubtedly, more computerized exercise equipment will be developed for adult fitness and cardiac rehabilitation programs in the years to come. Although much of this equipment will pass as fads, many items will be of value to participants. For

these reasons it is recommended that program staff maintain an awareness of new equipment and objectively determine their value to program participants.

Exercise Session Progress Reports

There are a number of opportunities for computer analysis during exercise training programs.[26,29,30] Computerized exercise progress reports are not only motivational to the participants but also allow for updating exercise prescriptions, plotting exercise activity trends, auditing facility utilization, and various research applications. Figure 9–7 illustrates the exercise session data form, which provides the basis for an automated progress report. This is a manual entry system with the resulting report shown in Figure 9–8. Figure 9–9 is a number-coded report, with the codes explained in Figure 9–10. As illustrated, this report is specific to the exercise prescription and includes distance and intensity, weight, and

TENNECO HEALTH & FITNESS   **ACTIVITY REPORT**

EMPLOYEE			MONTH	YEAR	DEP. CODE	SOC. SEC. NO.
			MARCH	1984	CC	439 74 8476

w. B. BAUN
BLDG. TEC ROOM 826

MONTHLY BODY WEIGHT		MONTHLY CALORIES BURNED	
Prior 73KG 161LBS	Prior	13425 Calories =	3.836 LBS
Current 73KG 161LBS	Current	14425 Calories =	4.121 LBS

MESSAGE: APRIL IS AEROBUCK PICK UP MONTH
THURSDAY, APRIL 19, 11AM-1PM, TEC8 LOUNGE
SHOW EMPLOYEE BADGE TO COLLECT AEROBUCKS

DATE	EXER CODE	INTEN LEVEL	MILES RESIST.	ACTIVITY TIME MINUTES SECONDS	LOC CODE	ACTIVITY	CALORIES BURNED
03-19-84	04	H		60	1	FITNESS CLASSES	664
03-20-84	06	H		40	1	HANDBALL	590
03-21-84	06	H		90	1	HANDBALL	1328
03-21-84	04	H		30	1	FITNESS CLASSES	332
03-23-84	04	M		30	1	FITNESS CLASSES	253
03-23-84	04	H		40	1	FITNESS CLASSES	443
03-24-84	02		4.0	30	2	JOGGING	491
03-26-84	04	H		30	1	FITNESS CLASSES	332
03-28-84	04	H		30	1	FITNESS CLASSES	329
03-29-84	04	H		30	1	FITNESS CLASSES	329
03-29-34	04	H		30	1	FITNESS CLASSES	329
03-30-84	02		4.0	30	2	JOGGING	487
03-31-84	02		6.0	48	2	JOGGING	732

SUMMARY

ACTIVITY	PRIOR			CURRENT			YEAR-TO-DATE		
	SESS	CALORIES	MILEAGE	SESS	CALORIES	MILEAGE	SESSIONS	CALORIES	MILEAGE
FITNESS CLASSES	22	7569		19	6731		57	19799	
HANDBALL	6	3529		5	3712		19	12587	
JOGGING	4	1888	15.0	5	2699	22.0	15	6707	53.5
WALKING	1	321	3.0	3	1045	10.0	4	1366	13.0
NAUTILUS WGT LIFTING	1	118		2	238		5	596	
OTHER							1	100	
TOTAL ▶	34	13425	18.0	34	14425	32.0	101	41155	66.5

373

TEN 5354 8/81

Fig. 9–13.   Computerized exercise log. From Baum, W.B., and Landgreen, M.A.: Tenneco health and fitness: A corporate program committed to evaluation. JOPERD, Oct., 1983.

is specific to the exercise prescription and includes distance and intensity, weight, and attendance data. This report is also the basis of the billing system and the production of the monthly unit summary used by the LaCrosse (Wisconsin) Exercise and Health Program.

Figure 9–11 illustrates the computerized exercise log used at the Institute for Aerobics Research in Dallas, Texas. The report presents information on activity, distance, duration, and aerobic points with monthly and accumulative totals. Figures 9–12 and 9–13 are from the Tenneco Health and Fitness Center in Houston, Texas.[6,7] Figure 9–12 illustrates the data entry process with the final report shown in Figure 9–13. Termed "exercise logging" by the Tenneco staff, this system allows the participants to record their activities immediately following exercise. The computer then provides the user with an exercise session report including calories burned for that day as well as total calories used over a given period of time.

The success of computerization depends on the ease and accuracy of data entry. A system that is not "user friendly" will not be utilized by most participants; however, a system that permits mistakes will not provide meaningful analyses to the participants or the program staff. A computerized data management system must be refined for efficiency and effectiveness of operation prior to implementation and then thoroughly explained to the potential user. The staff must also be familiar with the system, be able to answer questions of the program participants, and provide the necessary input for maintaining and improving the system.

PATIENT EDUCATION APPLICATIONS

The educational component of adult fitness and cardiac rehabilitation programs can also be strengthened by computers. The need for appropriate life-style changes is enhanced by identifying current risk factors, especially if the data can be presented in an easily understood format with appropriate recommendations for change. Laboratory data are most meaningful when personalized. Figure 9–14 illustrates a report that identifies the risk of developing coronary heart disease (CHD) from very low to very high, relative to current data as well as previously collected data. This information is detailed for 15 coronary risk factors and 5 additional fitness factors. The educational effect of showing these risk factors, recommending behavioral changes, and retesting to show improvement can be very significant. Figure 9–15 illustrates another example of a coronary risk profile from laboratory tests provided by the Cooper Clinic of Dallas, Texas.

Nutritional assessment has been significantly aided by the computer. Twenty-four hour diet recall followed by nutritional counseling has become an integral part of adult fitness and cardiac rehabilitation programs. Appendix 9–3 is an example of a computerized nutritional analysis based on the U.S. Department of Agriculture's Recommended Daily Allowance for each nutrient. The computer program determines what the individual is currently consuming and then, in conversational format, recommends appropriate actions for change.

CONCLUSIONS

In implementing a computer system, it is most important to work with individuals or firms specializing in computer start-up assistance. Numerous references are available on steps to follow in planning for computerization.[31-36] All operational aspects of a program will benefit from a well-designed computerized data management system. Although implementation may be difficult and expensive, if the correct system is selected and the necessary assistance provided to the staff, the system will be accepted and the cost justified.

S.S. NO.

DATE

TEST
DATA
ANALYSIS
FOR

LOCATION

GROUP

FITNESS MONITORING
SUMMARY REPORT

A. CORONARY HEART DISEASE RISK FACTOR ANALYSIS	CORONARY HEART DISEASE RISK CATEGORY					CURRENT TEST		MOST RECENT TEST		EVALUATION OF CHANGE	
NAME OF TEST	VERY LOW	LOW	MOD. ERATE	HIGH	VERY HIGH	TEST RESULTS	RISK POINTS	TEST RESULTS	RISK POINTS	RISK POINT CHANGE	% CHANGE
1 CARDIOVASCULAR FITNESS		+				44	0.8	32	4.2		
2 SYSTOLIC BLOOD PRESSURE		+				124	0.8	142	4.0		
3 DIASTOLIC BLOOD PRESSURE	+					80	0.0	86	1.0		
4 BODY FAT PERCENTAGE YOUR IDEAL BODY WEIGHT 161	+					16.2	0.0	33	3.2		
5 L.D.L. CHOLESTEROL	+					196	0.0	270	3.5		
6 H.D.L. CHOLESTEROL				+		38.9	2.2	37.8	2.4		
7 TRIGLYCERIDES	+					101	0.0	181	1.1		
8 GLUCOSE				+		130	2.0	130	1.0		
9 RESTING ELECTROCARDIOGRAM	+					1	0.0	1	0.0		
10 STRESS ELECTROCARDIOGRAM	+					1	0.0	1	0.0		
11 SMOKING		+				2	1.0	2	1.0		
12 TENSION & STRESS		+				2	1.0	2	1.0		
13 PERSONAL HISTORY OF HEART ATTACK	+					1	0.0	1	0.0		
14 FAMILY HISTORY OF HEART ATTACK			+			3	2.0	3	2.0		
15 AGE FACTOR				+		40	2.0	39	1.9		
16											
TOTAL RISK POINTS →							9.8		18.3		

B. SUPPLEMENTARY TESTS	TEST RESULTS					CURRENT TEST		MOST RECENT TEST		EVALUATION OF CHANGE	
NAME OF TEST	VERY HIGH	HIGH	MOD. ERATE	LOW	VERY LOW	TEST RESULTS	% TILE	TEST RESULTS	% TILE	CHANGE	% TILE
17 PULMONARY FUNCTION - VITAL CAPACITY	+					5.24	133	4.8	99		
EXPIRATORY VOLUME 1 SEC		+				4.15	131	3.71	89		
18 STRENGTH UPPER BODY			+			213	51	162	9		
LOWER BODY		+				19	30	14	21		
ABDOMINAL	+					25	90	16	50		
GRIP	+					122	90	112	75		
19 REACTION TIME	+					163	87	189	68		
20 FLEXIBILITY HIP & TRUNK		+				+5	70	+1	63		
SHOULDER GIRDLE			+			99	43	104	35		
21 POSTURE						89	95	83	91		
22 (FEF-75%=1.4L.=54%ile) (FEF-75-85%=.76L.=69%ile)											
OVERALL PERCENTILE →											

COMMENTS:

PATIENT - 1

Fig. 9–14. Exercise report showing risk of developing CHD.

COOPER CLINIC/ Dallas, Texas

Coronary Risk Profile

NAME:

Males: * <30 Years of Age

PERCENTILE RANKINGS	BALKE TREADMILL TIME (min.)	TOTAL CHOLESTEROL/ HDL RATIO	TRIGLYCERIDE (mg. %)	GLUCOSE (mg. %)	% BODY FAT	RESTING BLOOD PRESSURE SYSTOLIC (mm HG)	DIASTOLIC (mm HG)
YOUR VALUES							
99	31:04	2.3	32.0	73.0	2.4	91.6	57.6
97	29:00	2.5	39.4	79.0	4.2	98.0	60.0
95	28:00	2.6	45.0	80.5	5.3	100.0	62.0
90	26:20	2.9	50.0	84.0	7.2	104.0	66.0
85	25:00	3.1	56.0	86.0	8.4	108.0	68.0
80	23:22	3.2	60.0	88.0	9.4	110.0	70.0
75	23:00	3.4	65.0	89.0	10.8	110.0	70.0
70	22:00	3.5	69.0	90.0	11.9	114.0	72.0
65	21:10	3.6	73.0	92.0	12.9	115.0	74.0
60	20:45	3.8	78.8	93.0	14.1	118.0	75.0
55	20:00	3.9	83.0	94.0	15.1	118.0	76.0
50	19:52	4.1	88.0	95.0	16.0	120.0	78.0
45	19:00	4.2	94.0	96.0	16.8	120.0	80.0
40	18:05	4.3	101.0	97.0	17.5	122.0	80.0
35	18:00	4.5	109.6	99.0	18.4	124.0	80.0
30	17:00	4.7	120.9	100.0	19.6	125.0	80.0
25	16:23	4.9	131.0	102.0	20.7	128.0	82.0
20	15:03	5.2	145.0	104.0	22.2	130.0	84.0
15	15:00	5.6	167.9	105.0	23.6	132.0	86.0
10	13:45	6.0	190.0	109.0	25.9	138.0	90.0
5	11:35	6.9	240.7	112.0	29.1	142.0	92.0
3	10:30	7.2	283.9	115.5	31.0	145.7	96.0
1	8:35	8.6	414.5	123.5	35.7	154.0	100.0
N	1831	920	1546	1549	1526	1877	1877

PERSONAL HIST
ATTACK O

0 □ NONE
2 □ OVER 5 YE/
4 □ 2 - 5 YEAR!
5 □ 1 - < 2 YE/
8 □ 0 - < 1 YE

SMOKING HABITS

THE COOPER CLINIC

Dallas, Texas

Definition of Fitness Categories for Males*

Your Treadmill Performance _____ Your Age _____

AGE FACTOR

0 □ UNDER 30 YEARS OF AGE
― 39 YEARS OF AGE

FAMILY
CORONAR'

0 □ NONE O
2 □ YES, AC
4 □ YES, UI

FITNESS CATEGORY	Age Group (years)				
	< 30	30 - 39	40 - 49	50 - 59	60 +
VERY POOR	< 14:59	< 13:29	< 11:59	< 9:59	< 6:59
POOR	15:00 - 17:59	13:30 - 15:59	12:00 - 14:39	10:00 - 12:24	7:00 - 10:04
FAIR	18:00 - 21:09	16:00 - 19:59	14:40 - 17:59	12:25 - 15:59	10:05 - 13:42
GOOD	21:10 - 24:59	20:00 - 23:29	18:00 - 21:58	16:00 - 19:29	13:43 - 17:14
EXCELLENT	25:00 - 27:59	23:30 - 26:29	21:59 - 24:59	19:30 - 22:59	17:15 - 20:59
SUPERIOR	28:00 +	26:30 +	25:00 +	23:00 +	21:00 +

KNOWN COF
W/O HEAF

0 □ NONI
2 □ OVEI
4 □ 2 - 5
5 □ 1 - < 2 YEARS AGO
6 □ 0 - < 1 YEAR AGO

*Based on the Cooper Clinic modified Balke treadmill protocol: 3.3 mph (90m/min), 0% for 1st min, 2% for 2nd min, + 1% for each additional min. to 25%, then + .2 mph until exhaustion.

© Institute for A...

Fig. 9–15. Coronary Risk Profile, Aerobics Institute, Dallas, Texas.

REFERENCES

1. Jensen, M.A.: Computer applications—An introduction. Leisure today. JOPERD, April:30, 1984.
2. Berra, K., and Fry, G.: Computerization. *In* YMCArdiac Therapy. San Francisco, National Council of YMCAs, 1981, p. 11–17.
3. Moore, M.: The computerization of sports medicine. Physician Sports Med., 9:118, 1981.
4. Computer: A resource for fitness. Fitness Management, Sept./Oct.:14, 1985.
5. High-Tech equipment research project. Fitness Management, Sept./Oct.:24, 1985.
6. Baum, W.B., and Landgreen, M.A.: Tenneco health and fitness: A corporate program committed to evaluation. JOPERD, Oct.: 1983.
7. Baum, W.B., and Baum, M.: A corporate health and fitness program: Motivation and management by computers. JOPERD, April: 1984.
8. Computer systems: Does your club need one? IRSA Club Business, Aug.:29, 1985.
9. Morgan, S.: Keeping track of progress. Corporate Fitness and Recreation, Dec./Jan.:35, 1986.
10. Jones, N.L., Campbell, E.J., Edwards, R.H., and Robertson, O.O.: Computers in Exercise Testing, Clinic Exercise Testing. Philadelphia, W.B. Saunders, 1975.
11. Seigel, W.: A computer-assisted system for clinical use in maximal exercise testing. Cleve. Clin. Q., 43:143, 1976.
12. Kissen, A.T., and McGuire, D.W.: New approach for on-line continuous determination of oxygen consumption in human subjects. Aerospace Med., 38:686, 1967.
13. Pearce, D.H., et al.: Computer-based system for analysis of respiratory responses to exercises. J. Appl. Physiol., 42:968, 1977.
14. Wilmore, J.H., and Costill, D.L.: Semi-automated systems approach to the assessment of oxygen uptake during exercise. J. Appl. Physiol., 36:618, 1974.
15. Wilmore, J.H., Davis, J.A., and Norton, A.C.: An automated system for assessing metabolic and respiratory function during exercise. J. Appl. Physiol., 40:619, 1976.
16. Kyle, M.C., et al.: A new microcomputer based ECG analysis system. Clin. Cardiol., 6:447, 1983.
17. Mayhew, J.L., and Rankin, B.A.: Data management. JOPERD, Nov./Dec.:22, 1983.
18. Watkins, D.L.: Computers can streamline your program operations. Athletic Purchasing and Facilities, Jan.:26, 1984.
19. Zimmerman, F., and Reactor, A.: Computer for the Physician's Office, Medical Computing Series. Vol. 2. Forest Grove, Ore., Research Studies Press, 1978.
20. Farrell, P.: Computer literacy: What does it mean. JOPERD, Apr.:54, 1984.
21. Ewert, A.: Employee resistance to computer technology. JOPERD, Apr.:4, 1984.
22. Computer systems: Does your club need one? IRSA Club Business, Aug.:29, 1985.
23. Danziger, G.: Scheduling with computers: Reducing complexities to manageable problems. Athletic Business, Dec.:78, 1984.
24. Danziger, G.: Scheduling with computers: Refining the system for speed and efficiency. Athletic Business, Jan.:58, 1985.
25. Stuyt, J.: The spreadsheet, two applications. JOPERD, Apr.:25, 1984.
26. Bain, A.: Computerized fitness evaluations: Outlining the options. IRSA Club Business, Nov.:39, 1984.
27. Jerome, J.: The high tech workout training by computer. Outside, Jan./Feb.:25, 1984.
28. Computer-age weight lifting: Trainer created software to match his program. Athletic Business, March:52, 1984.
29. Morgan, S.: Keeping track of programs. Corporate Fitness and Recreation. Dec./Jan.:35, 1986.
30. Lacy, E., and Marshall, B.: Fitnessgram. JOPERD, Jan.:18, 1984.
31. Andresen, M.J., and Zach, H.L.: Working with a computer consultant. IRSA Club Business, Aug.:25, 1985.
32. Bain, A.: Choosing a computer system. IRSA Club Business, Aug.:23, 1985.
33. Cheng, V.S.: Don't leave computers to the experts. Athletic Business, Sept.:52, 1985.
34. Mohoney, K.: Computers. Club Industry, Jan.:13, 1986.
35. Richard, J.G., and Engelhorn, R.: Selecting a microcomputer. JOPERD, Nov./Dec.:19, 1983.
36. Tontomonia, T.L.: Choosing a computer that fits your needs. Athletic Business, Oct.:32, 1984.

Appendix 9-1.

Glossary

Access Time. (1) The time interval between the instant at which data are called up and delivery begins. (2) The time interval between the instant at which data are requested to be stored and storage is started.

Application Program. A program designed to do a specific task such as data base, file, etc.

ASCII. (American Standard Code for Information Interchange) The code used to represent letters, numbers, and other characters in most data transmissions.

Backup. Provision for duplicating data and programs as protection against damage or loss, or a copy so made.

BASIC. (Beginners All-Purpose Symbolic Instruction Code) A common computer language that is easy to learn but not suitable for complex programming.

Batch-Processing. Sometimes referred to as sequential processing, the process requires that one go through the entire file from the beginning to the end. This particular process is justified on the basis of the speed with which it can be done when compared to random-access processing.

Baud Rate. The standard measure of data transmission speed. For example, one baud equals one-half dot cycle per second in Morse code, one bit per second in a train of binary signals, and one 3-bit value per second in a train of signals each of which can assume one of eight different states.

Bit. The simplest unit of data, having only two values (yes/no, on/off, 0/1).

Benchmark. A point of reference from which measurement can be made.

BPI. Bits per inch.

BPS. Bits per second. In serial transmission, the instantaneous bit speed with which a device or channel transmit a character.

Buffer. A storage area that is temporarily reserved for use in performing an input/output operation, into which data is read or from which data is written. Also known as I/O area.

Bug. A mistake or malfunction.

Byte. Eight bits. This unit is used for most data storage and instructions on microcomputers.

Character Printer. A printer, like a typewriter, which prints fully formed characters.

COBOL. COmmon Business-Oriented Language. A business data processing language.

Compatibility. The ability to run applications programmed for one computer on another computer.

Compiler. A program which converts another program (such as an application program written in a high-level language into machine code for use on a given computer). Compiled programs run fast and occupy little memory.

Computer. A general purpose symbol manipulator which comes in a variety of models. The computer is made up of

(1) *Input units*—which feed data into the system.

(2) *Central processor*—which controls the processing function, and essentially is a big filing cabinet which is completely indexed and capable of storing large amounts of data.

(3) *Output units*—which serve the functions of creating records and reports, and create new media which can be used to satisfy further automated processing needs.

Computer Advantages. There are essentially four reasons why a computer is thought to be advantageous.

(1) *Speed.* The computer is so fast that it saves a tremendous amount of time as well as making it possible to tackle problems that would take too much time to perform manually. For example, all the adding you can do in 100 days can be done in 10 seconds by a computer.

(2) *Accuracy.* The computer can perform unerringly as many times as required.

(3) *It imposes discipline.* For the computer to solve a problem, YOU must first understand the problem and then program the computer to give you the right answer. Regardless of whether or not your final decision is to use a computer, this means that you will be thoroughly familiar with the problem and understand it to a depth seldom understood before.

(4) *Versatility.* Some people think of a computer as an adding machine. Actually, the computer can add, subtract, multiply, divide, sort, compare, or merge with other information.

Computer Disadvantages. These would include such things as initial expense, the cost and difficulty of programming, the channeling of work, and conversion to an electronic system.

CP/M. (Control Program/Microcomputer) A disk operating system used on many different microcomputers and supported by a wide variety of programs.

CPS. Characters per second.

CPU. Central Processing Unit.

Data. Includes the figures, words, or charts that describe some situations.

Data Bank. This is a stored volume of data which is available for retrieval as required. Changes occur only when the data is updated.

Date Base. An inherent part of the operating system. The data contained in the files is constantly updated and changed as inputs are entered into the system.

Data File. A collection of related data rec-

ords organized in a specific way, such as an inventory file or a personnel file.

Disks. Magnetic data-recording devices onto which programs and other information can be inputted and stored.

(1) *Floppy Disks* are low-cost, removable disks within protective plastic envelopes. The most common are the 5¼ inch mini-diskette and the 8-inch diskette.

(2) *Hard Disks* are of solid magnetic material, hold and cost more than floppies, and work more rapidly than the floppy disks. Most hard disks are of the removable cartridge or nonremovable winchester types.

Documentation Manual. The instructions written to accompany software—primarily a teaching manual.

DOS. (Disk Operating System) A program which controls the computer's transfer of data to and from a hard or floppy disk; frequently combined with the main operating system.

Down Time. A situation whereby the equipment is inoperable until such time as the breakdown, repairs or preventative maintenance has been completed.

Dump. To copy the contents of all or part of a storage, usually from an external storage.

Field. One item within a computer record. In a payroll record, for example, an employee's name would be one field, his pay rate another.

File. A set of related records treated as a unit. For example, one line of an inventory would form an item; a category within the inventory may form a record; the complete inventory would form a file; the collection of inventory control files may form a library; and the libraries used by an organization are known as its data base.

File Maintenance. The activity of keeping a file up to date by adding, changing or deleting data.

Firmware. Programs in ROM memory, so-called because they combine properties of hardware and software.

Flowchart. A graphic representation of the data processing system which shows the flow of data from the source document through the final reports.

Format. The arrangement of data.

FORTRAN. (FORmula TRANslator) A common language designed for scientific applications.

Hard Copy. A printed copy of machine output in a form which is visual and readable; for example, printed reports, lists, documents, or summaries.

Hardware. Another term for the electrical, electronic, and mechanical equipment used for processing data. The computer is an example of hardware.

Input. The raw facts (data) to be processed.

Inquiry and Transaction Processing. A type of teleprocessing application in which inquiries and records of transactions received from several terminals are used to interrogate or update one or more master files maintained by the central system.

Instruction. A single command to the computer system telling it what to do and where to do it.

Interactive. An application whereby the programmed entry elicits a response from the operator. An interactive system may also be conversational, implying a continuous dialog between the user and the system.

K . . . Bytes. Used in referring to storage capacity.

Keypad. A supplementary set of keys added to the regular keyboard. This addition is usually numerical and arranged in the same configuration as a calculator.

Language. A system for writing computer programs in a somewhat human-oriented, rather than strictly computer-oriented form, and having highly specific, inflexible vocabularies of commands and rules of syntax.

LOGO. A powerful educational language for teaching children the concepts of computer usage.

Mass Storage Device. A device with large storage capacity such as a magnetic disk or magnetic drum.

Memory. Computers vary in memory or storage capacity, and in type of memory. Memory can be used to store data or to store instructions.

Merge. To combine items from two or more similarly ordered sets into one set and arranged in the same order.

Microcomputer. Any computer built around a microprocessor.

Microprocessor. An integrated-circuit "chip," containing the basic logical circuits of a computer.

Modem. (MOdulator/DEModulator) A device to convert computer data into audible tones and back again, for transmission over telephone lines.

Password. A unique string of characters that a program, computer operator, or user must supply to meet security requirements before gaining access to data.

Peripheral Devices. Auxiliary pieces of equipment such as printers, modems, etc. These devices expand and enhance the computer's capabilities.

Pilot. A useful computer language for parents and educators to instruct children on a wide variety of subject matters.

Printer. An output device used to report the results of data processing in a readable form. Most common printers are daisy-wheel, dot-matrix, and thermal.

Program. A series of instructions.

Random-Access Processing. For this process, all records concerning a particular computer application are held in a large-capacity storage unit. The transactions are fed to a computer at random as they occur rather than being put in a predetermined sequence.

Remote Inputs. These devices are installed at the source of the workload and can receive data, transmit it to the central facility, and once the process has been completed, print out the finished product.

Record. The number of characters, either alpha or numerics, or a combination which contain specific data.

ROM. (Read-Only-Memory) A memory whose contents do not change when power is turned off.

Response Time. The time between the submission of an item of work to a computing system and the return of results.

RPG. Report Program Generator.

Sector. A section of a disk.

Software. The collection of programs and routines associated with a computer.
 (1) *Canned* software is written to meet general purpose programs, and is sold to those who are interested in buying it.
 (2) *Custom* software is written specifically for an application.

Speeds.
 (1) *Microsecond:* One-millionth of a second.
 (2) *Millisecond:* One-thousandth of a second.
 (3) *Nanosecond:* One-thousand-millionth of a second.

Telecommunications. Data transmission between a computer system and remotely located devices via a unit that performs the necessary format conversion and controls the rate of transmission.

Teleprocessing. The processing of data that is received from or sent to remote locations by way of telecommunication lines.

Terminal. A computer peripheral usually equipped with a keyboard and some kind of display.

Throughput. The total volume of work performed by a computing system over a given period of time.

Time-Sharing. A system through which many users can execute programs concurrently.

Turnaround Time. The amount of time between submission of a job to a computing center and the return of results.

Update. To modify a master file with current information according to a specified procedure.

User. Anyone who needs the services of a computing system.

Word. A character string or a bit string considered as an entity.

This glossary is reprinted with permission from the Journal of Physical Education, Recreation, and Dance, April, 1984, p. 30. The Journal is a publication of the American Alliance for Health, Physical Education, Recreation, and Dance, 1900 Association Drive, Reston, Virginia 22091.

Appendix 9–2.

Body Composition Assessment

SPORTS MEDICINE SECTION—CLEVELAND CLINIC FOUNDATION
Name: Age: 30   Date: 24-FEB-87
Height (inches): 60.1   Weight (pounds): 101.4

The body can be divided into two compartments: the fat mass (FM) compartment and the lean body mass (LBM) compartment. Excess percent of body weight as fat has been tied to such things as coronary heart disease, high blood fats, obesity, impaired cardiovascular function, and physical inactivity. The lean body mass is composed of bone, internal organ, and muscle weight. Changes in the lean body mass will usually be reflective of changes in the muscle mass, as organ and bone weight change very little.

We have two methods of assessing body composition. The first method involves measuring the thickness of the skin and layer of fat immediately beneath the skin (subcutaneous fat) at various sites on the body (e.g., thigh, abdominal skinfolds). A relatively accurate estimation of percent body fat is attained through skinfolds, since we know that the body deposits approximately 50% of its fat subcutaneously. A body density of 1.063 g/cc was calculated using some of your skinfold measurements, which indicates that 15.7% of your body weight is fat.

Another point of interest is to note whether your sum of skinfold measurements is greater or less than 110 mm. See Table I below. A sum over 110 mm tends to reflect an excess of body fat, whereas a sum under 110 mm indicates a more acceptable level of fat.

Table I—Skinfold measurements and sum of skinfolds.

Subscapular:	11		Suprailiac:	7
Triceps:	11		Umbilicus:	8
Midaxillary:	12		Thigh:	18
			Sum of Skinfolds:	65

Our more accurate method of assessment involves underwater weighing. This involves a comparison of a person's dry weight and underwater weight. The underwater weight is taken after complete submersion and maximal exhalation (this latter qualification introduces a source of error, as there are some people who are uncomfortable underwater and either can't or won't exhale maximally). This added buoyancy artificially raises the percent of fat measured. Of two people with equal air weights, the fatter individual will weigh less underwater, since fat is less dense than water. Corrections are made for residual volume (amount of air left in the lungs after a complete expiration). What is actually measured is body density, which is then converted to percent of fat. The underwater weighing indicates that 24.8% of your 101 pounds is fat. This means 25 pounds is being carried as fat and 76 pounds as lean body mass. Figure Ia. below graphically displays your body composition.

242

Figure I

a. Your current body composition.

b. What would your body composition be if you gained or lost weight as fat?

200	FM = 25					
150						
100	LBM = 76	FM = 5	FM = 10	FM = 15	FM = 20	FM = 25
50						
0						
% BF	24.8%	5%	10%	15%	20%	25%
Wt. (lbs)	101	80	85	90	95	102

NOTE: You do not have a severe weight problem, but it may be to your advantage to lose a few pounds.

It is generally recommended that females be below 28% fat and males under 20% fat. Essential (minimal) fat is around 5% for both males and females, with an extra 5% sex-specific fat in women. It is, therefore, NEVER recommended that males reduce below 5% of fat or women below 10% (most women encounter menstrual changes as the percent of fat drops below the 12%–14% area).

Weight loss is a balance of the number of calories you consume through food and drink and calories you expend in your daily activities (plus calories expended to maintain basal and resting metabolism). If you are maintaining your present weight, your average daily caloric consumption is approximately equal to your caloric expenditure. If you consume more calories than you burn during the day, your body stores the excess calories as fat. To lose fat weight, one can increase their daily activity level and/or slightly decrease their daily food intake (or change from high-caloric foods to low-caloric foods). If it is advantageous for you to lose a few pounds of fat, and you are interested in doing so, we suggest a combination of a small alteration in the diet (one that you can realistically make into a permanent life-style change), and begin participating regularly in activities you thoroughly enjoy (swimming, bicycling, walking, etc.).

For example, if you wished to lose 1 lb of fat in a week, you could:

a. DECREASE your caloric intake (diet) by 3,500 calories; that is 500 calories per day (500 × 7 = 3,500 less calories consumed).

b. INCREASE your caloric output (exercise) by 3,500 calories; that is 5 miles per day per week (5 miles × 100 calories per mile × 7 days = 3,500 calories expended).

c. Decrease your caloric intake by 300 calories per day AND walk or jog 2 miles per day. That would be 300 × 7 = 2,100 fewer calories taken in and 2 miles × 100 calories per mile × 7 days = 1,400 calories expended. Add that up, and it's 3,500 fewer calories in that week.

Since there are a lot of calories in 1 pound of fat (3,500 calories), weight gains (fat weight) are usually long, gradual occurrences, hence, fat weight loss is also a long, gradual process. A rapid body weight loss (more than 1%–2% of body weight) results in an immediate water loss and significant LBM weight loss (primarily muscle mass loss). Recognizing these principles allows you to be confident that weight you lose gradually is fat.

See Table II for an idea of how many calories you burn when you walk or jog 1 mile.

Table II—Calories Used Per Mile of Walking or Running, Based on Your Approximate Weight

Weight (pounds)	Pace (min per mile)							
	5:20	6:00	6:40	7:20	8:00	8:40	9:20	10:00
120	83	83	81	80	79	78	77	76
130	90	89	88	87	85	84	83	82
140	97	95	94	93	92	91	89	88
150	103	102	101	99	98	97	95	94
160	110	109	107	106	104	103	101	100
170	117	115	113	112	111	109	107	106
180	123	121	120	119	117	115	114	112
190	130	128	127	125	123	121	120	119
200	137	135	133	131	129	128	126	124
210	143	141	139	137	136	134	132	130
220	150	148	146	144	142	140	138	136
	10:40	11:20	12:00	12:40	13:20	14:00	14:40	
120	75	74	73	72	71	70	69	
130	81	80	79	78	77	76	75	
140	87	86	85	84	83	82	81	
150	93	92	91	90	89	88	87	
160	99	98	97	96	95	94	93	
170	105	104	103	102	101	100	99	
180	111	110	109	108	107	106	105	
190	117	116	115	114	113	112	111	
200	123	122	121	120	119	118	117	
210	129	128	127	126	125	124	123	
220	135	134	133	132	131	130	129	

From Cleveland Clinic Foundation, Sports Medicine Section, Cleveland, Ohio.

Appendix 9–3.

Computerized Nutritional Analysis Based on U.S. Department of Agriculture's Recommended Daily Allowance for Each Nutrient

NUTRIENTS OF FOODS ENTERED

Day 1

Item Entered	# Ser	kcal	Prot (g)	TFat (g)	Carb (g)	Fibr (g)	Calc (mg)	Iron (mg)	Pota (mg)	Sodi (mg)	Vi-C (mg)	V-B1 (mg)	V-B2 (mg)	Niac (mg)	Vi-A (iu)	SFat (g)	UFat (g)	Chol (mg)	Meal
Corn—kernels—frozen	1	130	5	1	31	—	5	1.3	304	2	8	0.15	0.1	2.5	580	—	—	—	S
Cereal—oatmeal—inst.	1.5	156	6	3	27	0	244.5	9.5	150	429	—	0.8	0.44	8.2	2,271	—	—	—	B
Orange juice—concen.	1	112	2	0	27	0	22	0.2	474	2	97	0.2	0.05	0.5	194	0	0	0	B
Bran muffin	2	210	6	8	34	—	114	3	344	358	0	0.14	0.2	3.4	180	2.4	1.6	—	S
Cornbread—home	1	161	6	6	23	—	94	0.9	122	490	1	0.1	0.15	0.5	120	1.4	1.3	—	L
Corn—kernels—frozen	1	130	5	1	31	0	5	1.3	304	2	8	0.15	0.1	2.5	580	—	—	—	L
Cereal—wheat—puffed	0.75	33	1.5	0	7.5	0	2.25	0.4	31.5	0	—	0.02	0.02	1	0	—	—	0	S
Salad—mixed veg.	2	0	0	0	0	0	0	0	0	0	0	0	0	0	0	0	0	0	D
Strawberries—raw	0.5	22.5	0.5	0.5	5.5	0.5	10.5	0.3	123.5	1	42.5	0.02	0.05	0.2	20.5	0	0.1	0	D
Melon—honeydew	0.25	11.25	0.25	0	3	0.25	2	0	87.5	3.25	8	0.02	0.01	0.2	13	0	0	0	D
Bagel—water	1.5	247.5	9	1.5	45	0	12	1.8	63	420	0	0.23	0.17	2.1	0	0.3	0.9	0	D
Ginger ale	1	115	0	0	29	—	—	—	0	0	0	0	0	0	0	0	0	—	D
Banana—raw	1	105	1	1	27	1	7	0.4	451	1	10	0.05	0.11	0.6	92	0.2	0.1	0	D
Thous. Island—low-cal	1	24	0	2	2	0	2	0.1	17	153	—	—	—	—	49	0.2	0.9	2	D
Fruit salad—can—water	0.5	37	0.5	0	9.5	1	8.5	0.4	95.5	3.5	2.5	0.02	0.03	0.5	539	0	0	0	S
Bagel—water	1	165	6	1	30	0	8	1.2	42	280	0	0.15	0.11	1.4	0	0.2	0.6	0	S
Total of Day 1		1,659	49	25	332	3	537	21	2,609	2,145	177	2.1	1.5	24	4,639	5	6	2	

Activity k/cal expended for day 1 = 2,728

Day 2

Item Entered	# Ser	kcal	Prot (g)	TFat (g)	Carb (g)	Fibr (g)	Calc (mg)	Iron (mg)	Pota (mg)	Sodi (mg)	Vi-C (mg)	V-B1 (mg)	V-B2 (mg)	Niac (mg)	Vi-A (iu)	SFat (g)	UFat (g)	Chol (mg)	Meal
Nutri grain—wheat	2	204	4	0	48	2	16	1.6	154	386	30	0.74	0.85	10	2,504	—	—	—	B
Banana—raw	1	105	1	0	27	1	7	0.4	451	1	10	0.05	0.11	0.6	92	0.2	0.1	0	B
Milk—skim—prot forti	1	100	10	1	14	0	352	0.2	446	144	3	0.11	0.48	0.2	500	0.4	0	5	B
Bagel—water	1	165	6	1	30	0	8	1.2	42	280	0	0.15	0.11	1.4	0	0.2	0.6	0	L
Apple—raw—unpeeled	1	81	0	0	21	1	10	0.3	159	1	8	0.02	0.02	0.1	74	0.1	0.1	0	L
Vegetables—mix—froze	1	116	6	0	24	—	46	2.4	348	96	15	0.22	0.13	2	9,010	0	0	0	L
Diet soda	1	—	0	0	—	—	—	—	—	—	0	0	0	0	0	0	0	0	L
Chicken a la king	1	470	27	34	12	0	127	2.5	404	760	12	0.1	0.42	5.4	1,130	12.7	3.3	64	D
Potato—baked—peeled	1	145	4	0	33	—	14	1.1	782	6	31	0.15	0.07	2.7	0	0	—	0	D
Sesame seeds	0.5	23.5	1	2	0.5	0	5	0.3	16.5	1.5	—	0.03	0	0.2	2.5	0	—	0	D
Soup—tomato	0.75	63.75	1.5	1.5	12.75	0	9	1.3	198	653.2	49.5	0.07	0.04	1.1	516	0.3	0.7	0	D
Nutri grain—wheat	1.5	153	3	0	36	1.5	12	1.2	115.5	289.5	22.5	0.55	0.64	7.5	1,878	0	0	0	S
Milk—skim—prot forti	0.5	50	5	0.5	7	0	176	0.1	223	72	1.5	0.06	0.24	0.1	250	0.2	0	2.5	S
Breadstick—w/o salt	4	152	4	0	32	—	12	0.4	36	280	0	0.02	0.03	0.4	1	0.2	0.4	0	D
Raisins—seedless	1	28	0	0	7	0	5	0.2	70	1	0	0.02	0.01	0.1	1	0	0	0	S
Total of Day 2		2,186	85	44	364	6	815	16	3,529	3,531	183	2.6	3.4	35	15,958	15	6	72	

Activity k/cal expended for day 2 = 2,938

Summary of 2 Days

Item	kcal	Prot (g)	TFat (g)	Carb (g)	Fibr (g)	Calc (mg)	Iron (mg)	Pota (mg)	Sodi (mg)	Vi-C (mg)	V-B1 (mg)	V-B2 (mg)	Niac (mg)	Vi-A (iu)	SFat (g)	UFat (g)	Chol (mg)
Nutrient avg of 2 days	1,923	67	35	348	4	676	18	3,069	2,838	180	2.3	2.5	29	10,298	10	6	37
Recommended	2,833	101	94	388	50	800	10	3,750	2,200	60	1.4	1.6	18	5,000	31	62	300
% of recommended	68	66	37	90	8	85	180	82	129	300	164	156	161	206	32	10	12

Average k/cal expended for 2 days = 2,833

%   OF RECOMMENDED

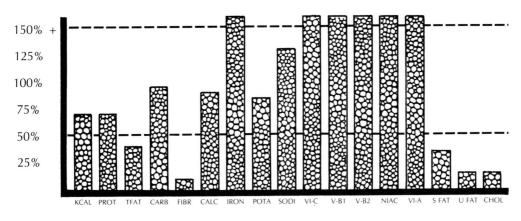

| | KCAL | PROT | TFAT | CARB | FIBR | CALC | IRON | POTA | SODI | VI-C | V-B1 | V-B2 | NIAC | VI-A | S FAT | U FAT | CHOL |

Comments

Nutrients in which your diet is 50% below recommended and some foods high in these nutrients

Total fat:	Animal fats	Plant fats	Fatty meats	Vegetable oils
Fiber:	Bran	Whole wheat bread	Vegetables	Fruits
Saturated fat:	Fatty meats	Coconut oil	Lard	Dairy products
Unsaturated fat:	Vegetable oils	Safflower oil	Corn oil	Fatty fish
Cholesterol:	Egg yolk	Liver	Whole dairy prod.	Shellfish

Nutrients in which your diet is 50% above recommended and your corresponding high food sources

Iron:	Cereal—oatmeal—inst.	Bran muffin	Chicken a la king	Vegetables—mix—froze
Vitamin C:	Orange juice—concen.	Soup—tomato	Strawberries—raw	Potato—baked—peeled
Vitamin B_1:	Cereal—oatmeal—inst.	Nutri grain—wheat	Nutri grain—wheat	Bagel—water
Vitamin B_2:	Nutri grain—wheat	Nutri grain—wheat	Milk—skim—prot forti	Cereal—oatmeal—inst.
Niacin:	Nutri grain—wheat	Cereal—oatmeal—inst.	Nutri grain—wheat	Chicken a la king
Vitamin A:	Vegetables—mix—froze	Nutri grain—wheat	Cereal—oatmeal—inst.	Nutri grain—wheat

CALORIES FROM ACTIVITY AND FOOD

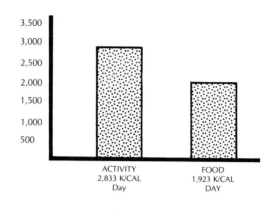

Comments

The k/calories of the food that you ate are less than the k/calories of your daily activities.

If you continue the same diet and activity habits, you should lose approximately 8 lbs per month. However, this may vary due to different weekly variations.

Your current body weight is within 5% of your ideal body weight.

If you do not wish to lose weight, then you should increase your food intake.

% OF CALORIES FROM NUTRIENTS

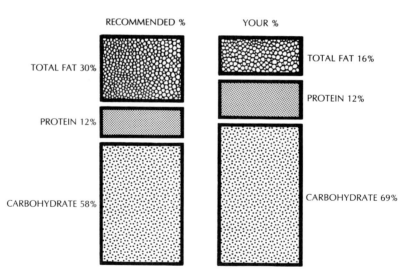

Comments

According to your current diet, 16% of the calories that you ate came from fat. This is 46% below the value of 30% suggested by many authorities. It is beneficial to have values 30% and below.

The percentage of protein in your diet is 25% above the suggested value of 12%. A high percentage of protein is usually associated with a high percentage of fat.

The calories from carbohydrates should make up 58% of your diet. Your diet is made up of 69% carbohydrates. This is 18% above the recommended value.

% OF CALORIES FROM EACH MEAL

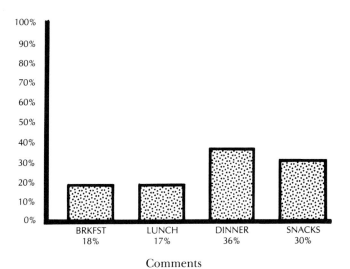

Comments

The IDEAL percentage of calories from each meal is controversial. However, it makes good nutritional sense to receive a good supply of calories through the day at each meal and possibly through snacking.

Your major meals of breakfast, lunch, dinner, and snacks are not well balanced throughout the day.
—Your
   DINNER
   is high in caloric content compared to the other meals.

Snacks make up 30% of the calories from your diet. If you do snack, the snack should be a nutritious one. Not candies, sweets, and sugars but fruits, vegetables, and grain products.

10

PERSONNEL

The success of any exercise testing, adult fitness, or cardiac rehabilitation program depends on the expertise and other personal characteristics of the individuals directing the program and providing the various services. The selection of personnel, therefore, requires a great deal of consideration, and the eventual performance of the staff depends on the management techniques and skills of the program director. This chapter discusses the issues that need to be considered in the administration of personnel working in the exercise-related professions.

MANAGEMENT TECHNIQUES

Although each program director has an individual personality and style of operation, certain characteristics are typical of all successful managers. Among these are knowledge, confidence, fairness, flexibility, and the ability to delegate responsibility with authority.

Knowledge

The program director must be knowledgeable about and well acquainted with all aspects of the program. Although it is not necessary to be an expert in every facet of the program, the director should have access to other individuals with appropriate expertise in those areas. The staff's confidence in administrative decisions is greatly enhanced when the director is knowledgeable. In addition, a director who

knows what is right and what works can simplify and save time in the decision-making process.

Confidence

In addition to being knowledgeable, the program director must also have confidence in all areas of management. This confidence must be apparent to the staff in the decisions that are made and the actions that are taken. Often, a decision may not immediately seem to be correct and at times may even prove to be incorrect. In these circumstances the director must be able to admit mistakes when they are made. This is the true test of the confidence of the program director.

Fairness

Another important attribute of a good administrator is fairness. Inexperienced program directors often display favoritism to some employees and ignore the accomplishments of others. The director must be fair and equally attentive to all staff members regardless of personal feelings. The ultimate evaluation of the merits and worth of an employee must be based on productivity and performance, not on favoritism or friendship. Every employee should feel special.

Flexibility

There may be several ways to accomplish the same task. In these circumstances flexibility is an important trait among administrators. Experienced program directors realize that they do not always know the best way to complete a particular task. Flexibility allows them to shift gears in the middle of a task and select an alternative method.

Delegating Responsibility

One of the most important characteristics of a good administrator is the ability to delegate responsibility and authority. Inexperienced administrators often delegate but are hesitant to give the necessary authority to complete the task. One must delegate, provide direction, and then allow the individual to work on the task without interference. A good administrator does not hesitate to delegate responsibility and authority and when doing so should expect and accept mistakes. Ultimately, the program director is responsible for task performance and the overall conduct of the program.

Additional Management Concerns

One of the most difficult and stressful management skills concerns the approach to incompetent employees. Employees must be made aware of their responsibilities. If the employee is unable to accomplish a particular job description, then either the job is too complex or the individual is not capable. The program director should carefully review the job description and resolve the problem. If incompetence is the case, the responsibilities of the position must be documented in writing, and the individual informed that a performance review is being undertaken. A reasonable time period must then be established, after which the individual's performance is evaluated again. If the employee is still performing unsatisfactorily, then that person must either be reassigned to another position or released. The retention of incompetent employees can be detrimental to other employees as well as to

the entire program. A second mistake often made with an incompetent employee is to reassign some responsibilities to another person. This results in a good employee having to complete the tasks of two people and often has a negative impact on the morale of the entire staff.

Although dealing with incompetent employees is difficult for a program director, the management of good employees is often ignored. An employee who performs well must be recognized and sufficiently rewarded. When good work goes unrewarded, the results can be equally demoralizing to the program staff. Unfortunately, one cannot always reward with promotions, since a position for promotion must be vacant, and the promotion must be well deserved.

Finally, administrators must examine their own personalities in order to develop management techniques and styles with which they are comfortable and which result in productive and loyal staffs who enjoy their work. Not all program directors have the personality to be effective administrators and be well-liked. Most, however, have the abilities to be good administrators and respected by their staff. The "good guy" image is a trap in which many inexperienced administrators unknowingly place themselves. All administrators must know their own qualities and how they can best perform as an integral part of the overall program.

One method of determining effectiveness as an administrator of a program is to create both informal and formal mechanisms for staff input and performance review. Although not all program directors are capable of doing this on an informal basis, there is no excuse for failure to create a formal review process. Everyone on the staff should have the opportunity to evaluate the performance of the supervisors, as they, in turn, expect to be evaluated by them.

STAFF RECRUITMENT

In recruiting staff for cardiac rehabilitation programs, it is important to realize that coronary artery disease (CAD) is a multifactoral disease and consequently requires collaboration of a variety of health professionals working together.[1-4] Staff selection is based on program objectives and should not be accomplished by the capricious addition of individuals as the program develops and grows.

Staff recruitment should be well conceived, organized, and in accordance with the long-range objectives of the institution.[5,6] This approach ensures that personnel will be well suited for their jobs and that the staff positions will be necessary for the program's overall operation.

The development of in-depth job descriptions is the first step in the recruitment process. Often, general job descriptions are developed for distribution, and detailed descriptions are provided to those who actually apply. Figure 10–1 is an example of a general job description for the position of program director with responsibilities for exercise testing and cardiac rehabilitation in a hospital setting. This description should be widely distributed to appropriate agencies, institutions, and individuals who may provide candidates for the position. Frequently, it is also desirable to place advertisements in appropriate professional journals, as illustrated in Figure 10–2.

The detailed job description explains all aspects of the particular position to the applicant, including the scope of responsibilities, administrative and clinical responsibilities, communications, staff development and interactions, qualifications for the job, and a description of specific tasks to be performed. There should be no question in the applicant's mind regarding the details of the position. An awareness of one's job is not only important for employment but also for future performance reviews. A thorough understanding of the detailed job description will most likely result in the selection of the highest qualified candidate who will, in turn, be the most satisfied and productive employee on the job.

Finally, it is important that all applicants for a position receive a response regardless of the particular merits of the applicants. Failure to respond to a job applicant is discourteous and results in bad public relations.

CERTIFICATION

A number of agencies and organizations currently offer various levels of certification for health professionals working in exercise testing, adult fitness, and cardiac rehabilitation. It is strongly recommended that program administrators urge their staffs to pursue certifications that are most relevant to their job descriptions. The quality of a program is clearly enhanced by personnel who are up to date and well trained. The following sections briefly review the certification programs that are most relevant to personnel working in exercise-related fields.

American Heart Association

The American Heart Association (AHA) offers basic cardiac life support (BCLS) certification to the general public and health professionals.[7] This certification is an absolute requirement for all staff working in exercise and rehabilitation programs. BCLS involves the initial recognition and management of cardiopulmonary arrest and includes closed chest cardiac compression, mouth-to-mouth ventilation, and management of the obstructive airways. In addition the AHA has also developed advanced cardiac life support (ACLS) certification, which includes intubation, defibrillation, intravenous techniques, recognition and treatment of cardiac arrhythmias, and acid–base management.[7] ACLS certification is recommended for personnel working in cardiac rehabilitation programs but may not be necessary for adult fitness personnel.

POSITION AVAILABLE
EXERCISE PHYSIOLOGIST/DIRECTOR OF CARDIAC REHABILITATION
AND EXERCISE TESTING

Position

Faculty appointment at the (university) and Director of Cardiac
Rehabilitation and Exercise Testing at (hospital or clinic)
Medical Center.

Qualifications

Ph.D. or equivalent. Management experience with postoperative and
postmyocardial infarction patients; experience, demonstrated competency in diagnostic and functional exercise testing; thorough knowledge of
preventive, intervention, rehabilitation programs; administrative experience in cardiac rehabilitation; teaching and research productivity as university faculty member.

Salary

Commensurate with qualifications.

Available

July 1, 1987

Apply to

Search and Screen Committee: Exercise Physiologist
(Address)

Deadline

May 15, 1987

Fig. 10–1.   General job description.

American College of Sports Medicine

One of the more prestigious certification programs for personnel working in exercise testing, adult fitness, and cardiac rehabilitation has been developed by the American College of Sports Medicine (ACSM).[8] Various levels of certification are offered including exercise test technologist, exercise leader, fitness instructor, exercise specialist, and program director. Each certification level is developed according to specific behavioral objectives and requires passing a written and practical examination. Over 1,500 health professionals have been certified by the ACSM since 1975. The ACSM has published the *Guidelines for Exercise Testing and Prescription*,[8] which describes the specific learning objectives for each level of certification. This publication, now in its third edition, has become a very important resource for program staff.

American Fitness in Business

Formed in 1975, American Fitness in Business (AFB) now consists of over 3,000 members. Formerly the American Association of Fitness Directors in Business and Industry (AAFDBI), this organization has become one of the most active and influential in the field of adult fitness.[9]

American Physical Therapy Association

Certainly one of the most stringent certifications is the cardiopulmonary specialty

Announcement—Job Description

POSITION OPENING
EXERCISE PHYSIOLOGIST
DIRECTOR OF CARDIAC REHABILITATION
AND EXERCISE TESTING
(Hospital or Clinic) MEDICAL CENTER
and
FACULTY POSITION
at
(Name of University)

1. Effective Date

   June or July 1, 1980 (optional).

2. Rank

   Associate or Professor, depending upon experience.

3. Salary

   $35,000 to $45,000 (annual salary).

4. Position Description

   The position consists of a dual appointment through the (name of
   university) and the (hospital or clinic) of (city). The position is within
   the Department of (department) and the (department or section)
   of (hospital or clinic). The University (description, i.e., size, faculty,
   facilities, curriculum). The (section) of the (hospital or clinic) (description,
   i.e., services provided, subspecialties, number of beds, facilities).

7. Applicant Requirements

   Applicants must have extensive clinical experience in the management of
   postoperative and postmyocardial infarction patients from early inpatient
   rehabilitation through complete recovery. The individual must also have a
   thorough understanding and considerable experience in diagnostic and
   functional exercise testing. The applicant must have administrative experience in the area of cardiac rehabilitation and exercise testing and be
   interested in sportsmedicine. The applicant must be interested in research
   and publishing and possess a Ph.D. or the equivalent degree. A minimum
   of five years of clinical experience is recommended but not required.

8. Applications

   Send application letter, vita, and references to:

   _____

   _____

9. Deadline Date for Receipt of Applications

   May 1, 1987

Fig. 10–2. Sample journal advertisement.

offered by the American Physical Therapy Association (APTA). Formed in 1984, the APTA's minimal criteria for candidacy is 10,400 hours (5 years) of practice in the field, of which 3 years should be full-time patient care in cardiovascular disease of both an acute and rehabilitation nature. Additional requirements for candidacy are 1 year of both educational and administrative responsibilities, plus current ACLS certification.[10]

Young Men's Christian Association

The YMCA offers several levels of certification for exercise program staff. The Physical Fitness Specialist and Specialist Advanced[11] have met the basic needs of the YMCA Physical Director, while the YMCArdiac Therapy Program[12] certification has attempted to meet the needs of personnel involved in cardiac rehabilitation programs. The YMCArdiac Therapy Program is impressive in that it covers all aspects of program operation, as well as other involved staff positions including medical director, program nurse, fitness director, nurse supervisor, fitness leader, and business administrator.

Additional Certifications

There are a number of additional certifications available from other groups involved in adult fitness programs.[13,14] Several dance associations offer certifications.[14,15] It is estimated that there currently are over 50 different certification programs for dance exercise specialist,[15] with the Aerobics and Fitness Association of America alone having certified over 7,000 individuals since 1983.[13]

JOB DESCRIPTIONS

The staff working in cardiac rehabilitation and adult fitness programs includes personnel for hospital phase I and II cardiac rehabilitation, freestanding phase II programs, community-based and freestanding phase III and IV programs, and adult fitness programs. Figures 10–3 and 10–4 illustrate the possible staff relationships and administrative schematics for phase I, II, and III programs. Figure 10–5 describes the responsibilities of the individual positions on the cardiac rehabilitation team.

The following discussion considers the job descriptions of administrative staff, exercise testing personnel, and personnel assigned to cardiac rehabilitation and adult fitness programs.

ADMINISTRATIVE STAFF

Advisory Board

Members of an advisory board serve for the purposes of offering general direction, establishing policies and procedures, and providing overall expertise to program operation. The board should meet regularly and have officers elected by the entire group. The normal time commitment for a board member is 3 to 5 years without remuneration. It is important that the advisory board represent a cross section of the community served by the program. Members of the board both individually and as a group can be instrumental in the program's development and eventual success by virtue of their influence in the community.

Medical Director

The medical director is ultimately responsible for clinical policies and procedures of a cardiac rehabilitation program and may have a similar role in adult fitness programs as well. The medical director should have a background in the specialty of internal medicine and optimally be board certified in the subspecialty of cardiovascular diseases. BCLS and ACLS certification is expected for exercise testing and cardiac rehabilitation responsibilities. The medical director should have practical

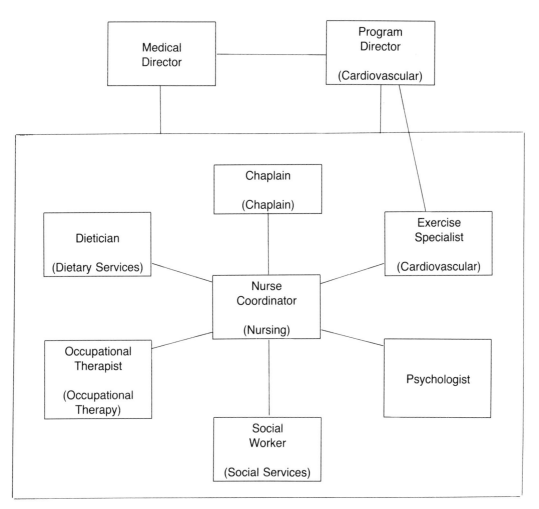

Fig. 10–3.   Staff relationships, phase I: inpatient program. Courtesy of Dr. Sherry Zigon, Director of CR, Research Medical Center, Kansas City (Fort Worth, Texas, ACSM).

experience and expertise in all aspects of the program including exercise testing, exercise prescription, and cardiac rehabilitation. In addition, the medical director should be a liaison to the program's advisory board, the program staff, and the referring and participating physicians.

Program Director

The program director is responsible for the daily operation of the program and usually has a major role in planning and developmental efforts. This individual must have skills in administrative and budgetary matters, personnel manage-ment, and patient care activities. The program director must work closely with the medical director and other administrative personnel in dealing with day-to-day problems. In addition to administrative responsibilities, this person must have a firm grasp of exercise physiology and the applications of prescriptive exercise for cardiac rehabilitation and preventive health mainte-nance. Ideally, the program director should have a master's or doctorate in physical education, health education, exercise physiology, or a related field. Some program directors are physicians with interests in cardiac rehabilitation and pre-

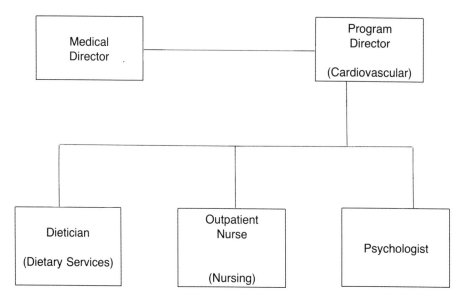

Fig. 10–4. Staff relationships, phase II and III: outpatient programs. Courtesy of Dr. Sherry Zigon, Director of CR, Research Medical Center, Kansas City (Fort Worth, Texas, ACSM).

ventive medicine. Finally, the program director should be certified by the ACSM[8] and, if possible, have ACLS certification by the AHA.[7]

Business Manager

A business manager may be employed on a part-time or full-time basis with specific responsibilities for the business aspects of the program.[12] Programs that function as a service of a hospital, medical clinic, or community-based adult fitness setting may have staff assigned the duties of business manager. The background of the individual should include accounting, budgeting, personnel management, insurance claims, and payroll procedures. Normally, the individual will have a degree in business management or business administration, perhaps with a specialization in hospital administration.

Secretarial/Clerical

Secretarial and clerical duties may be performed by part-time staff for a small program, although this is unusual. Normally a full-time secretary is required for most programs. Receptionist and telephone duties are usually a part of this position. Other responsibilities include filing of insurance claims, processing laboratory and exercise data, correspondence, case reports, and typing research papers. Word-processing experience is strongly recommended as a prerequisite for this job.

Lawyer

As with the business manager, a lawyer is usually part-time or on retainer.[16–18] In the developmental stages of a program, there are often questions for which a legal opinion is helpful. For example liability status of the program and personnel, legal implications of specific policies and practices, formulating legal documents, and questions of copyrights and incorporation are all areas where legal advice is useful. Once the program is operational, legal opinions may be necessary to resolve liability matters, assist in obtaining delinquent fees and preparation of documents for local and state health system agencies, negligence issues, and lawsuits.[17,18]

Medical Director (Cardiologist, M.D.)
Provides medical direction for all phases of the program. Provides informal consultation to team members and relays information to attending physicians.

Program Director (Exercise Physiologist, Ph.D., A.C.L.S.)
Provides direction and guidance for overall quality of all phases of the program. Interacts with the medical staff and administration on behalf of the program. Consults with all members of the team as needed. Assists with coordination of the inpatient and outpatient program. Directs and implements all aspects of outpatient program including prescriptions.

Cardiovascular Clinical Nurse Specialist (R.N., C.C.R.N., A.C.L.S.)
Functions as a coordinator of the inpatient program. Works with medical director, attending physicians and other team members to establish and implement the plan of care. Provides educational programs for inpatients and staff. Accepts responsibility for evaluating the program's effectiveness, and updating it as needed.

Outpatient Nurse (R.N., C.C.R.N., A.C.L.S.)
In conjunction with the program director, implements the outpatient program (Phases II & III), including patient assessment, education and supervision of ECG telemetered and non-telemetered exercise therapy. Directs staff during medical emergency until relieved by physician of Code Blue team.

Exercise Specialist (Physical Therapy or Nursing background, B.C.L.S., A.C.L.S. preferred)
In conjunction with the referring physician and the program director, decides the appropriate exercise level for the patient, both in the hospital and upon discharge. Supervises, monitors and documents the patient's response to exercise. Communicates this response to other team members. Aids in deciding and suggesting the appropriateness of the patient for the outpatient program.

Occupational Therapist (Certified O.T.)
Aids the Phase I patient in adapting to a therapeutic functional activity level through didactic presentations of energy conservation and work simplification principles. Demonstrates the compensatory techniques and discusses the application of the principles and techniques in both home and work settings. Serves as a consultant to the staff and the team.

Dietitian (R.D.)
Provides personalized nutritional counseling to the inpatient and family after assessing dietary habits. Routinely provides basic and intermediate nutritional counseling. Provides indepth counseling as ordered by the physician. Provides scheduled classes for the outpatient. Serves as a consultant for the team, staff, and outpatients.

Social Worker (M.S.W.)
Provides psychosocial assessment, social casework and referral to community resources for identified needs in inpatients. Participates in discharge planning. Serves as a consultant to the staff and the team.

Chaplain (Member of hospital chaplain staff)
Offers support to inpatient and family allowing them an opportunity to express anxiety and concerns. Participates in the team meeting. Serves as resource for staff and team.

Psychologist (M.S.; Ph.D. preferred)
Conducts group and individual sessions on stress management and relaxation techniques.

Fig. 10–5.   Composition and responsibilities of the cardiac rehabilitation team. Courtesy of Dr Sherry Zigon, Director of CR, Research Medical Center, Kansas City (Fort Worth, Texas, ACSM).

EXERCISE TESTING PERSONNEL

Electrocardiogram Technician

Some exercise testing laboratories have both an electrocardiogram (ECG) technician and an exercise test technologist, although in most instances one individual performs both functions. The ECG technician is responsible for all ECG aspects of the exercise test including preparation of recording and monitoring equipment, calibration, skin preparation, operation of the equipment during the test, and processing of ECG data after the test. Many freestanding programs use nurses as ECG technicians during exercise testing.

Exercise Test Technologist

The exercise test technologist requires a level of competency above that of the ECG technician. This individual is responsible for explaining the test to the patient, obtaining the history and informed consent, demonstrating and operating the exercise equipment, taking blood pressures during the test, and processing all the test data for the attending physician. An ACSM certified exercise testing technologist is also familiar with the equipment and procedures for respiratory gas analyses, body composition analyses, strength and flexibility assessments, and other related fitness parameters.[8] ACSM certification, therefore, is strongly recommended for exercise test personnel working in cardiac rehabilitation and adult fitness programs.

Physician

The attending physician in an exercise testing laboratory must have a thorough background in cardiology including ECGs, exercise physiology, and basic and advanced cardiac life support.[19,20] The physician should be familiar with each patient being tested and the purpose of the test. The physician should send reports and appropriate ECG data to the referring physician. During the testing procedures the attending physician is in charge and must supervise the performance of other exercise test personnel.

ADULT FITNESS PERSONNEL

Program Director

The responsibilities of a program director in an adult fitness program will differ greatly from those working in cardiac rehabilitation. Figure 10–6 illustrates the results of a survey of 110 corporate fitness program directors.[21] Fifty-one percent of those surveyed represented a company of 10,000 employees or more, and only 7% worked for companies having less than 500 employees. The length of employment varied from less than 5 years (7% of fitness directors) to more than 30 years (26%). The survey revealed that corporate fitness directors spend most of their time planning, budgeting, and evaluating programs, and they spend the least amount of time attending conventions and conferring with other directors.

Figure 10–7 illustrates the various levels of ACSM certification for personnel working in either cardiac rehabilitation or preventive (adult fitness) programs.[8] In Figure 10–8, the relative competencies of the ACSM preventive tract are charted. The Fitness Leader certification has been refined to include those working in the military, dance instructors, and general adult fitness personnel.

Exercise Specialist

The exercise specialist should have an understanding of all aspects of therapeutic exercise and is generally considered a senior member of the program.[22–24] Responsibilities should include preparing exercise prescriptions, supervision during exercise training, recognition and management of orthopedic injuries, rehabilitation activities, and administration of BCLS.[7] The ex-

S M T W T F S

Activity	Time spent 1 = greatest, 9 = least
Planning programs	1
Budgeting	2
Attending staff conferences	3
Evaluating programs	3
Developing policies	4
Reading and studying	4
Attending employee group conferences	5
Attending program events	5
Consulting	6
Fundraising	7
Attending local, state, and national conventions	8
Conferring with other corporate directors	9

Fig. 10–6. Typical director's month. From Sawyer, T.H.: The employee program director. Parts 1–3. Corporate Fitness and Recreation, Aug./Sept.: 1985, Oct./Nov.: 1985, Dec./Jan.: 1986.

ercise specialist is also expected to keep up-to-date with the exercise literature and clinically apply appropriate advances in exercise therapy resulting from research. ACSM certification is recommended.[7]

Fitness Instructor

The fitness instructor is supervised by the exercise specialist and is responsible for leading the exercise classes. The individual must be knowledgeable in warm-up and stretching techniques, forms of aerobic exercise, strength and flexibility exercises, interpreting exercise prescriptions, motiva-

tional techniques, cool-down exercises, and BCLS. ACSM certification is recommended.[8]

CARDIAC REHABILITATION

The multidisciplinary team approach to cardiac rehabilitation has become widely accepted for both hospital and freestanding, or community-based, facilities. Personnel for phase I generally include the patient's primary care physician, attending physicians, nurses, physical therapists, nutritionists, and social workers and/or psychologists. An even larger team may be uti-

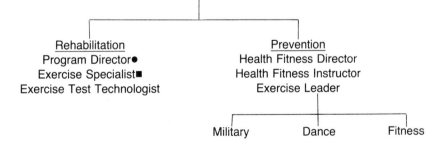

Preventive/Rehabilitation Certification

Rehabilitation
Program Director●
Exercise Specialist■
Exercise Test Technologist

Prevention
Health Fitness Director
Health Fitness Instructor
Exercise Leader

Military   Dance   Fitness

●Also meets behavioral objectives for Health Fitness Director
■Also meets behavioral objectives for Health Fitness Instructor

Fig. 10–7. American College of Sports Medicine (ACSM) preventive/rehabilitation certification, as developed and maintained by the ACSM Preventive/Rehabilitation Exercise Program Committee.

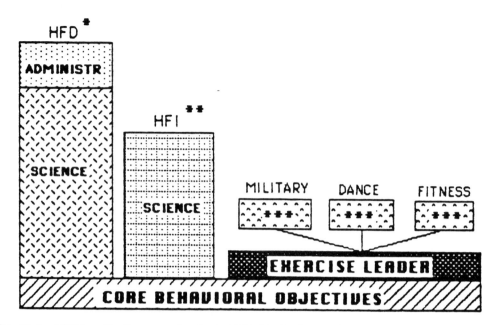

Fig. 10–8. ACSM certification preventive tract, 1987. *Health fitness director, **Health fitness instructor, ***Specialty interest.

lized for phase II programs.[25] The following discussion considers the team approach to each phase of cardiac rehabilitation.

Phase I

In phase I the floor nurse may be actively involved in exercising individual patients in the patient's room or on the hospital corridors. It is important for the nurses to know what particular "step" each patient is on and the appropriate clinical parameters to follow. In addition nurses usually participate in the education process. A great deal of the progress made by the patient during these critical days in the hospital is the result of the support and assistance provided by nursing personnel.

In addition to nursing involvement in phase I exercise programs, the physical therapist is often an integral part of the team. The therapist is particularly valuable for assessing musculoskeletal dysfunction and in designing corrective exercises to be used in conjunction with those normally performed during all phases of cardiac rehabilitation.

The phase I team also includes various patient educators, who may be nurses or other health educators. Patient education is an ongoing process that encompasses all phases of rehabilitation. During phase I the emphasis is on the patient's particular health problems in the hospital and on introducing the concept of healthy life-styles.

The primary physician is important in providing the necessary continuity of care for the patient while in the hospital and will most likely be responsible for the patient after hospital discharge. Active participation by the primary physician in the rehabilitation program can be very beneficial in achieving the long-term goals of the total program.

A cardiologist or internist is recommended as the clinical supervisor of the phase I program to assist the rehabilitation staff with medical questions or other problems that may arise.[19,20] This individual should be familiar with the patients participating in the program and be able to assist the primary physicians in advancing their patients through the progressive "steps" of the program. Finally, the clinical supervisor should follow patient progress in the exercise and educational components of the program and make recommendations whenever appropriate.

Phase II

The staff of a phase II program usually consists of an exercise specialist, a rehabilitation nurse, and a supervising physician. In addition, an education specialist may be involved in providing the educational activities of the program, although other members of the staff can also carry out these responsibilities. The patient's primary physician is also considered to be a member of the rehabilitation team, although not necessarily present during the exercise sessions.

The exercise specialist in phase II is responsible for the exercise activities and must be very familiar with each patient's exercise prescription and clinical status.[8,22-25] The exercise specialist usually has a background in nursing, physical therapy, physical education, or health education and should be ACSM certified.[8] In addition to being responsible for the exercise prescription, this individual provides patient support in efforts to modify risk factors and promote healthy life-styles.

The primary task of the rehabilitation nurse in phase II is to monitor both the patient's ECG response to exercise and symptoms.[12] This individual should be ACLS certified and well trained in recognition of cardiac arrhythmias and in managing cardiac emergencies.[9]

An education specialist provides educational information to patients and teaches behavioral skills necessary to modify risk factors and other unhealthy life-styles. These activities often take place in small groups rather than the one-on-one setting of phase I. This individual is usually part-time, although a large phase II program may require a full-time person. The same

person may also participate in phase I teaching activities.

The supervising physician for phase II is generally not involved with the daily operation of the program but is needed to evaluate clinical problems and manage any medical emergencies that may arise. This individual must be in the vicinity of the exercise area and immediately available to respond to emergencies. ACLS certification is also required.[9] The physician's presence during the exercise sessions often provides motivational and emotional support to the patients.

The patient's personal physician must be kept informed about patient progress throughout the duration of the program. The physician's enthusiastic support of the program is often well received by the patient and may become a strong motivating factor for continued participation. Frequent progress reports detailing symptoms and response to exercise should be sent to the primary physician in order to provide continuity of care, readjustment of medications, and assist in other clinical decisions.

Phases III and IV

The personnel for phase III and IV programs usually consist of fitness instructors, exercise specialists, nurses, education specialists, supervising physicians, and the primary care physicians.

The fitness instructor has specific responsibilities for the safe and effective conduct of the exercise class. Attention to the exercise prescription, warm-up, aerobic activities, cool-down, and prevention and care of exercise-related injuries are the responsibilities of this individual. ACSM certification is strongly recommended.[8]

As in phase II, the exercise specialist is primarily responsible for the exercise program and reports to the program director. Supervision of the fitness instructor, preparation of exercise prescriptions, providing support to patients, managing records and forms, and providing BCLS are among the responsibilities of the exercise specialist. Certification by the ACSM is also expected for this position.[8]

Nurses, patient educators, supervising and primary physicians all have roles comparable to phase II cardiac rehabilitation programs, and their specific responsibilities are described in the previous section.

SUPPORT PERSONNEL

Many support personnel may be needed to provide important services to adult fitness and cardiac rehabilitation programs. These include, but are not limited to, nutritionists, mental health workers, occupational therapists, volunteers, students, and AHA workers.

Nutritionists

Nutrition specialists or dieticians are important members of the health-care team.[26–30] These individuals may work on a one-on-one basis with patients, or they may teach classes involving patients, family members, and others. Dietary management of hyperlipidemia, low-salt diets, and weight management are the primary responsibilities of the nutritionists, although the behavioral management of these problems may be provided by patient education and mental health workers.

Mental Health Workers

Many cardiac rehabilitation programs utilize the services of mental health workers (psychologists and social workers) to assist in managing the psychological, behavioral, and social problems of the patients. Services include patient assessments, counseling, and behavioral interventions when appropriate to favorably affect the patients' long-term outcomes.[31,32]

Occupational Therapists

A return to gainful employment is a concern for many cardiac patients. Unfortu-nately, for a variety of reasons, many patients do not return to their previous employment after myocardial infarction (MI) or heart surgery, and they often do not return to employment at all.[33] The role of the occupational therapist is to provide the necessary assistance to determine new avenues of employment along with the appropriate reeducation. The cardiac rehabilitation program should be concerned with identifying patients in need of vocational counseling and providing the necessary expertise and motivation to return them to productive life-styles.

Volunteers

Volunteers can also play a significant role in adult fitness and cardiac rehabilitation programs. The volunteer forces may consist of former patients and family members, interested citizens in the community, students from various colleges and universities, and AHA personnel.

Lay personnel, including former patients, family members, and others, can contribute by participating in coronary clubs, "mended heart" clubs, and related organizations. Counseling and advice to spouses, family members, and friends can often be provided by these individuals. Often, the patients themselves eventually become volunteers and provide similar services to new patients.

Students in various curricula can also be of assistance to a program. Graduate and undergraduate students in health education, physical education, recreation, social work, physical therapy, occupational therapy, nursing, exercise physiology, and medicine are often interested in clinical hours, student teaching, clinical assignments, and internships. These students may have valuable skills in areas of patient education, exercise testing, and exercise therapy. A program should strive to develop strong cooperative relationships with local educational institutions for placement of students.

The local affiliates of the AHA can often assist in providing personnel and expertise to cardiac rehabilitation and adult fitness programs. Areas of participation include fund raising, patient education, public relations, and research. The AHA has a major commitment to cardiac rehabilitation and prevention, and it is therefore important to keep local affiliates informed of program developments.

CONCLUSIONS

Successful organization and administration of adult fitness and cardiac rehabilitation programs revolve around the staff of those programs. There is no single factor of more importance to the overall success or failure of a program as its staff. Appropriate staffing with well-defined responsibilities, recruited through the best methods possible, helps to ensure a successful program.

REFERENCES

1. Brock, L.L.: Administrative consideration. *In* Coronary Heart Disease: Prevention, Detection, Rehabilitation with Emphasis on Exercise Testing. Edited by S.M. Fox, III. Denver, Department of Professional Education, International Medical Corp., 1974.
2. Haskell, W.L.: The allied health professional. *In* Exercise Testing and Exercise Training in Coronary Heart Disease. Edited by J.P. Naughton, H.K. Hellerstein, and I.C. Mohler. Orlando, Fla., Academic Press, 1973.
3. Morse, R.L.: Personnel for exercise programs. *In* Exercise and the Heart: Guidelines for Exercise Programs. Edited by R.L. Morse. Springfield, Ill., Charles C Thomas, 1972.
4. Stoedefalke, K.G.: The physical educator's role in exercise programs. *In* Exercise Testing and Exercise Training in Coronary Heart Disease. Edited by J.P. Naughton, H.K. Hellerstein, and I.C. Mohler. Orlando, Fla., Academic Press, 1973.
5. Johnson, M.P.: Staffing sources: Where to find good people. IRSA Club Business, Sept.:25, 1985.
6. Stevens, J.: How to hire the employees you want. IRSA Club Business, Sept.:27, 1985.
7. Standard and Guidelines for Cardiopulmonary Resuscitation (CPR) and Emergency Cardiac Care (ECC). JAMA, 255:2905, 1986.
8. American College of Sports Medicine: Guidelines for Exercise Testing and Prescription. 3rd Ed. Philadelphia, Lea & Febiger, 1986.
9. Patton, R.W.: Implementing Health Fitness Programs, Champaign, Ill., Human Kinetics, 1986.
10. Cardiopulmonary Speciality Council, Board for Certification of Advanced Clinical Competence. Alexandria, Virginia, American Physical Therapy Association, 1984.
11. National Council of YMCAs: Leadership training and development. *In* The Y's Way to Physical Fitness. Edited by C.R. Myers, L.A. Golding, and W.E. Sinning. Emmaus, Pa., Rodale Press, 1973.
12. Fry, G., and Berra, K.: YMCArdiac Therapy. National Council of YMCAs. Chicago, Ill., 1981.
13. Gorney-Cooper, P. (ed.): Aerobics: Theory and Practice. Sherman Oaks, Calif., Aerobics and Fitness Association of America, 1985.
14. I.D.E.A., Industry and certification examination. Bulletin of Information, San Diego, International Dance Exercise Association, 1986.
15. Basic facts on forty seven training organizations. Dance Exercise Today, Jan./Feb.:42, 1985.
16. Morgan, S.: A crusade for quality. Corporate Fitness and Recreation, Oct./Nov.: 21, 1985.
17. Abbott, R.A.: Medicolegal considerations in professional service. *In* Cardiac Rehabilitation: Exercise Testing and Prescription. Edited by L.K. Hall, G.C. Meyer, and H.K. Hellerstein. Jamaica, N.Y., SP Medical & Scientific Books, 1984.
18. Herbert, D.L., and Herbert, W.G.: Legal Aspects of Preventative and Rehabilitation Exercise Programs. Canton, Ohio, Professional and Executive Reports and Publications, 1985.
19. Obma, R.: Physician Supervision. *In* Adult Fitness and Cardiac Rehabilitation. Edited by P.K. Wilson. Baltimore, University Park Press, 1975.
20. Wenger, N.K.: The role of the physician in exercise testing and exercise training. *In* Exercise Testing and Exercise Training in Coronary Heart Disease. Edited by J.P. Naughton, H.K. Hellerstein, and I.C. Mohler. Orlando, Fla., Academic Press, 1973.
21. Sawyer, T.H.: The employee program director. Parts 1–3. Corporate Fitness and Recreation, Aug./Sept.: 1985, Oct./Nov.: 1985, Dec./Jan.: 1986.
22. Christina, J.: The fitness professional: What to look for in a qualified director. Athletic Purchasing and Facilities, July:38, 1982.
23. Collingwood, T.R.: Fitness leadership: Ingredients for a Winner. Athletic Purchasing and Facilities, Aug.: 18, 1982.
24. Oldridge, N.B.: What to look for in an exercise class leader. Physician Sportsmed., 5:85, 1977.
25. Wilson, P.K., and Hall, L.K.: Personnel of adult fitness and cardiac rehabilitation programs. JOHPER, 1984.
26. Flipse, B.G.: Diet and nutritional concerns of the cardiac patient. *In* Cardiac Rehabilitation: Exercise Testing and Prescription. Edited by L.K. Hall, G.C. Meyer, and H.K. Hellerstein. Jamaica, N.Y., SP Medical & Scientific Books, 1984.
27. Storlie, J., and Jordan, H.A. (eds.): Behavioral Management of Obesity. Jamaica, N.Y., SP Medical & Scientific Books, 1984.
28. Storlie, J., and Jordan, H.A. (eds.): Evaluation

and Treatment of Obesity. Jamaica, N.Y., SP Medical & Scientific Books, 1984.

29. Storlie, J., and Jordan, H.A. (eds.): Nutrition and Exercise in Obesity Management. Jamaica, N.Y., SP Medical & Scientific Books, 1984.

30. Wagstaff, M., and Beman-Mattfeldt, M.: The fitness opportunity for dietetic educators and practitioners. J. Am. Dietetic Assoc. *84*:1464, 1984.

31. Hall, L.K.: Psychological concerns of the cardiac patient. *In* Cardiac Rehabilitation: Exercise Testing and Prescription. Edited by L.K. Hall, G.C. Meyer, and H.K. Hellerstein. Jamaica, N.Y., SP Medical & Scientific Books, 1984.

32. Reith, C.A.: Avoiding post hospital adjustment problems. *In* Cardiac Rehabilitation: Exercise Testing and Prescription. Edited by L.K. Hall, G.C. Meyer, and H.K. Hellerstein. Jamaica, N.Y., SP Medical & Scientific Books, 1984.

33. Streater, S.E., and Erlandson, R.J.: Social and vocational considerations in cardiac rehabilitation. *In* Cardiac Rehabilitation: Exercise Testing and Prescription. Edited by L.K. Hall, G.C. Meyer, and H.K. Hellerstein. Jamaica, N.Y., SP Medical & Scientific Books, 1984.

11

FACILITIES AND EQUIPMENT

Considerable information is available to assist the program director with facility planning and development, and equipment selection.[1-6] Standards have been developed by the American College of Sports Medicine (ACSM)[3] and the American Heart Association (AHA)[4] that are recommended for cardiac rehabilitation and exercise testing equipment and facilities. The purpose of this chapter is to discuss specific facility and equipment requirements for cardiac rehabilitation, exercise testing, and adult fitness programs.

FACILITIES

The most important elements of any successful program are good personnel and the adequacy of the facility. Personnel requirements are discussed in Chapter 10. Facility planning and development for different types of programs are discussed in this chapter.

Phase I

Most of the cardiac rehabilitation services provided in phase I are done at the patient's bedside and in adjacent corridors and stairwells.

Some hospital programs, particularly those with active cardiovascular surgery, have separate exercise facilities for low-level, monitored physical activity. Coronary artery bypass surgery patients and other cardiac patients with less severe disease might benefit from a more vigorous inpatient program than that which is normally conducted at bedside (Chapter 12). Figures 11-1 to 11-4 are examples of phase I exercise areas. Although not required, shower rooms can be provided for patients who are able to exercise more vigorously. A separate room should also be planned for individual and group counseling and teaching. Sufficient space should be provided to accommodate at least 5 to 10 persons. The teaching/counseling room should be quiet, well lighted, pleasantly decorated, and easily accessible.

Phase II—Hospital

The requirements of a phase II program facility are substantially greater than phase I. Adequate space is needed for stress testing, patient education and counseling, supervised–monitored exercise classes, offices for the staff, business office, patient reception, waiting area for guests, dressing rooms, and shower facilities.

If phase II is conducted in a hospital setting, the primary considerations are adequate space for the program, patient accessibility, and appearance. These considerations are discussed later in the chapter in the section on freestanding facilities.

The facility is planned with consideration of the objectives established by the administration and the allocated financial resources. In a small hospital with limited cardiology services, a phase II program might occupy 1,000 square feet including

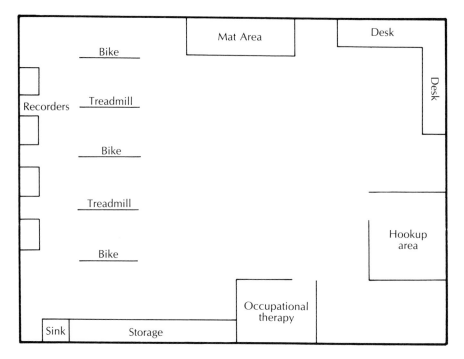

Fig. 11–1.   Phase I, facility A.

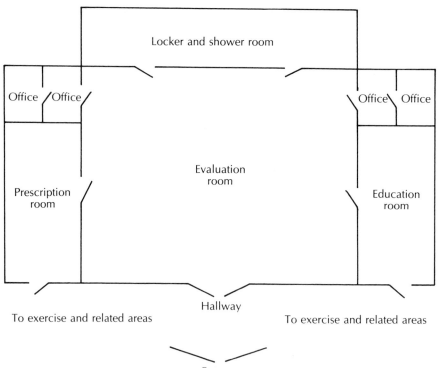

Fig. 11–2.   Phase I, facility B.

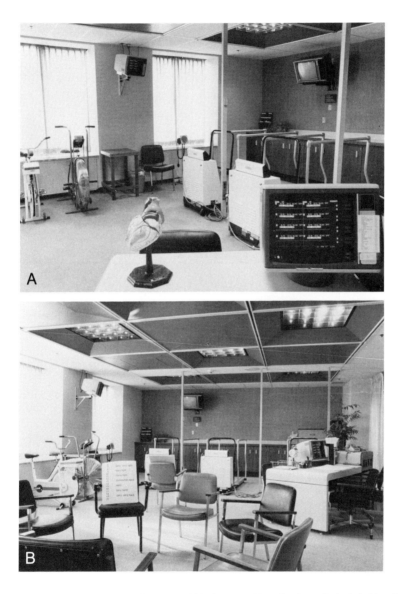

Fig. 11–3.   *A, B,* Phase I exercise area. (Courtesy of MidAmerica Heart Institute; St. Luke's Hospital of Kansas City; Patricia Caldwell, Coordinator, David Venner, photographer.)

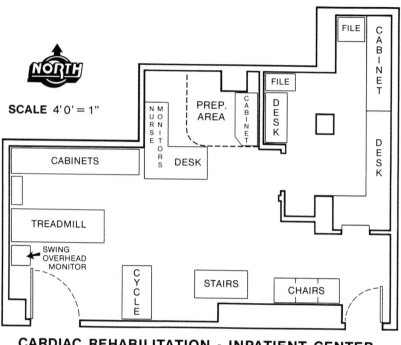

CARDIAC REHABILITATION - INPATIENT CENTER
MOUNT SINAI MEDICAL CENTER, MILWAUKEE, WI.

Fig. 11–4. Phase I cardiac rehabilitation facility. (Courtesy of Mount Sinai Medical Center, Milwaukee, Wisconsin; Neil Oldridge, Ph.D., Director.)

a room to exercise two to four patients at one time, dressing and shower facilities, and a small office. A large hospital with active cardiology and cardiovascular surgery programs is likely to have a program considerably larger in scope and occupy several thousand square feet. The total space could accommodate stress testing, human performance research, teaching and patient counseling, exercising 8 to 12 patients at one time, office space, reception and waiting areas, and dressing and shower facilities. In some hospital programs an exercise room might also be used for phase III as well as phase II. Examples of various-sized phase II facilities are presented in Figures 11–5 to 11–10.

Phase II—Freestanding

Freestanding phase II programs are becoming increasingly prevalent and necessitate special consideration to meet their unique needs. For example the location of the center should receive careful attention. A feasibility study should identify the approximate geographic center of the prospective patient population. Exact location is determined by accessibility, appearance of the surrounding area, internal environment, and financial resources.

A good location is one that is easily accessible by automobile and public transportation. Since compliance decreases beyond a 20- to 30-minute drive,[7,8] it is important to choose a site that includes a large population base within that driving distance. If the center is located away from the main highway and necessitates a lot of back-street driving, then the population base is reduced. Accessibility should also take into account parking availability, ease of entrance and exit, and finding the facility once inside the building.

The internal and external environment are also important. Is the surrounding area

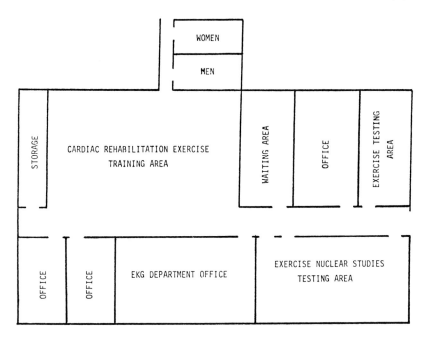

EXERCISE CENTER, DIVISION OF CARDIOLOGY, CREIGHTON UNIVERSITY - ST. JOSEPH HOSPITAL
    *scale: 1 inch = 8 feet

Fig. 11–5.   Exercise center. (Courtesy of Creighton University—St. Joseph Hospital, Omaha, Nebraska; Mark A. Williams, Ph.D., Director.)

safe, pleasing to the eye, and conducive to an exercise program? Is the internal environment aesthetically pleasing? Should the center be located on the ground floor with easy walk-in, or is a higher floor better because of the view? Is basement space, which has fewer distractions and is generally less expensive, a good choice? All of these questions are important and influence the patient's decision whether or not to participate.

Financial resources have a significant effect on the environmental questions. How much money can be budgeted for rent, renovations, or the purchase of property? Large buildings with open areas may have considerable aesthetic appeal, but can be very costly to maintain and have a lot of unusable space. Basement space usually requires renovations to make it more appealing. The best advice in considering these questions is to thoroughly research alternatives and choose carefully. Look at

a variety of locations, taking each of these questions into consideration. The final selection should offer the best chance that the program will succeed, even though it might not be the first choice for some reasons.

After the site has been chosen and the amount of space determined, specific plans for the facility need to be prepared. One of the initial steps suggested to simplify this process is to employ the services of an architect,[9] preferably one with experience in planning exercise facilities. An architect may not be necessary for all projects, especially if the facility requires only simple construction, or is identical to a previous center. In general, however, an architect saves money for the project and better ensures a finished product that is functional and pleasant.

The architect must balance several elements: (1) aesthetics—the appearance of the facility; (2) technology—construction

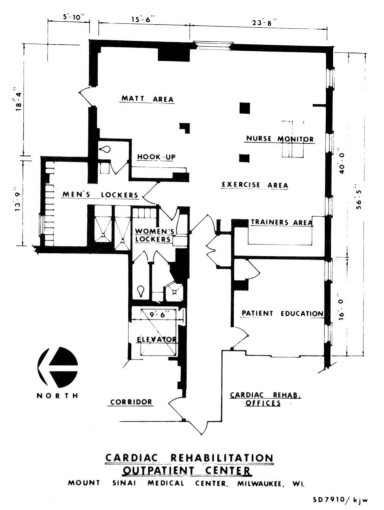

Fig. 11–6.   Phase II cardiac rehabilitation facility. (Courtesy of Mount Sinai Medical Center, Milwaukee, Wisconsin.)

and control of the facility's internal environment; (3) economics—the project budget; and (4) function—the purpose of the facility. Once these elements are clear in the mind of the architect, it is possible to advance to the next stage.[9]

There are four distinct phases in the development of the project.[9]

1. Conceptual design: taking ideas and putting them into a general layout
2. Developmental design: developing specific plans for each room
3. Construction documents and bidding: the final plans and taking bids for construction

4. Construction: The job of supervising construction is the responsibility of the general contractor. The architect, however, can do on-site inspections and serve in the role of liaison to the contractor. Remember that the architect is working for the project managers, and they must set the financial limitations of the construction.

SPACE REQUIREMENTS FOR PHASE II

The most important factor in allocating space in a center is a realistic estimate of the program's size. What is the number of

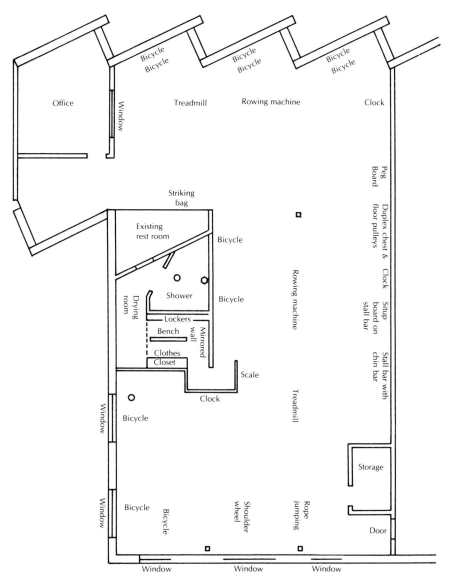

Fig. 11–7. Phase II, facility A.

patients likely to use each part of the facility at a given time? A spacious facility may look nice, but it may not be functional if the space is not well utilized.

The following suggestions of room size are offered for specific areas within a traditional center. These guidelines may have to be adjusted in order to correspond with the services that are scheduled and the priority attached to these services.

Exercise Room

In the exercise room 100 square feet of space should be allocated for each patient. For example if individual classes are planned for six to eight patients, then 600 to 800 square feet of space should be planned. The actual space that is usable for exercise is going to be less when equipment, cabinets, drinking fountain, sink, counter top, and decorative items are

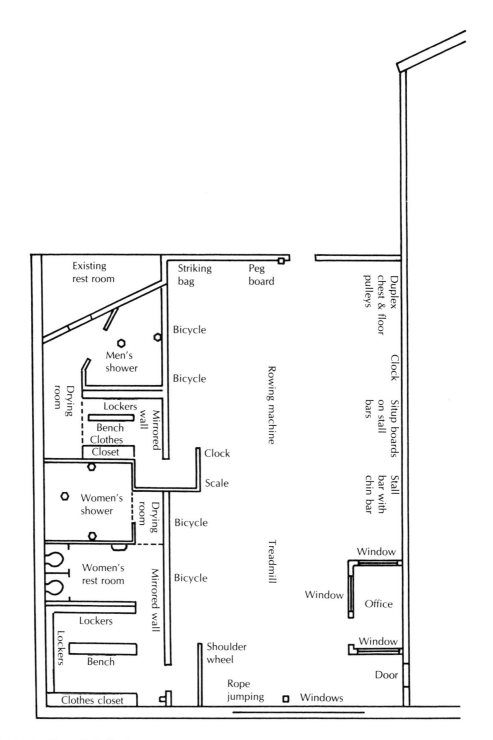

Fig. 11–8.   Phase II, facility B.

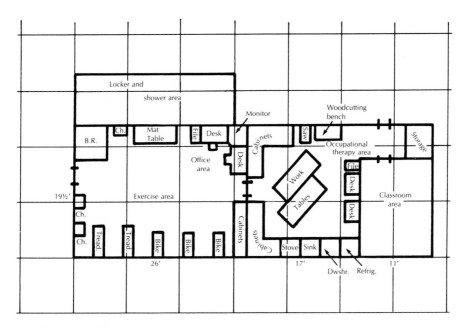

Fig. 11–9. Phase II, facility C.

added. If the minimal amount of space is all that is available, the use of mirrors helps to give the room a larger appearance.

Exercise Testing

The exercise testing room requires about 100 square feet to test one patient at a time. If more than one test is performed at the same time, an additional 75 to 100 square feet per station is recommended. If back-to-back tests are planned, an adjacent area is required for patient preparation. Otherwise, an additional 50 square feet should be set aside in the stress test room. The area must comfortably accommodate test personnel, equipment, and supplies. Sufficient room is also needed to manage any emergency that might occur in the test area. Finally, a small amount of space, a desk, and telephone should be designated for the physician to dictate reports, make and receive telephone calls, and utilize time effectively between tests.

Conference Room

The conference room should be large enough to accommodate 10 to 20 persons comfortably. Sessions that are conducted in a classroom seating arrangement might be slightly larger. If the classes are to be informally conducted and emphasize class interaction and comfort, the amount of space increases. A minimum of 300 square feet is suggested for a conference room. The room should be quiet, well lighted, and provide an atmosphere that is pleasant and encourages learning. The conference room should have a built-in chalk board, screen, dimmer lights, and be well equipped with audiovisual equipment.

Locker and Shower Area

The dressing area must be large enough for the number of patients who are finishing an exercise class plus those reporting for the subsequent class. Since the ratio of males/females is at least 2:1 in the prevalence of coronary heart disease (CHD), then a larger area is required for men. Two shower stalls are usually adequate for men and one for women for class sizes of eight or less. It is suggested that 150 to 200 square feet be reserved for each dressing and shower area.

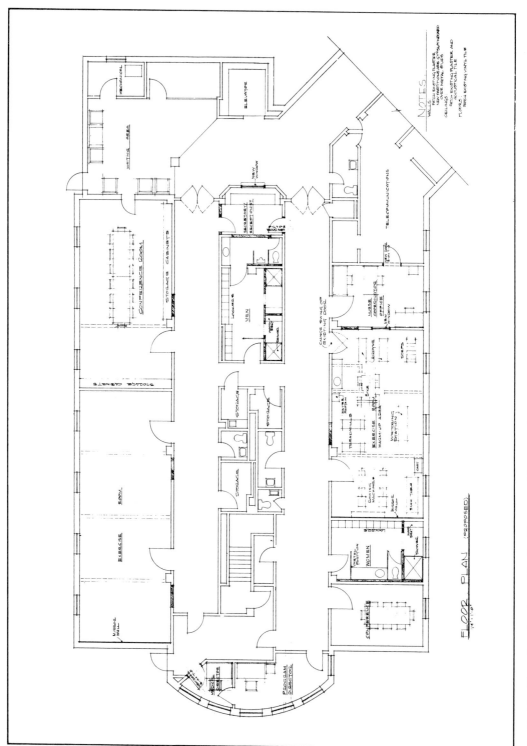

Fig. 11–10. Floor plan of a phase II facility. (Courtesy of Peninsula General Hospital and Medical Center, Salisbury, Maryland; Jeanne Ruff, Director.)

Office Space

There should be sufficient office space for three or more professional staff to allow for a minimum of 40 to 50 square feet per person. The program director requires a private office that is large enough to meet with several visitors at one time.

The business office must be large enough to accommodate secretarial space, office equipment and supplies, and adequate room for file cabinets. Enough file space should be planned to house patient records for at least 3 years. In general the business office should be at least 100 to 150 square feet. If the business office is also used for patient reception, then the area will have to be larger. Keep in mind that a growing program eventually needs additional business staff and filing space. Filing space can be reduced with efficient utilization of computers (Chapter 9).

Waiting Area

If a general waiting area is not available within the building, or is not convenient, then a room must be planned to accommodate awaiting patients and their guests. Enough room should be planned for one visitor per patient, since a spouse, relative, or friend often accompanies the patient. Usually, 100 square feet is sufficient for a waiting area.

Additional Facilities

If the facility is to be a showcase, then additional space might be required for such things as a research laboratory, staff lounge, library, or increased conference and teaching space.

In summary the amount of space required for a phase II program of 200 to 300 patients a year is approximately 2,000 to 3,000 square feet.

Layout

After space requirements have been defined, the layout of the floor plan should be developed, taking into consideration traffic patterns, patient privacy, business operations, light, noise, and environmental factors.

TRAFFIC PATTERNS. The layout of the facility should be designed so that there is minimal interference among the different aspects of the program. This helps to ensure patient privacy. In general, patients do not want to be frequently interrupted or observed. They often resent outside visitors, especially nonprofessionals. Therefore, it is best to restrict the number of visitors, and when they are present, to be sure to introduce these persons so that the patients know who they are and the purpose of the visit. The traffic pattern must also plan for patient safety. In the case of an emergency, the patient must be reached easily for treatment. There should also be ample room for emergency equipment and personnel and patient evacuation.

BUSINESS OPERATIONS. The business office should be located to minimize interference from classes. Patient registration should also be organized so that it does not interfere with patient activities. Because conversation in the business office is often personal, this area should be quiet and private.

LIGHT AND NOISE. There should be minimal noise from one room to another. For example it is undesirable to locate the conference room contiguous to a noisy exercise area. Areas of increased noise should be located away from areas where quiet is important. All rooms should be adequately lighted and use natural light sources whenever possible.

Environmental Factors

The location of facility rooms with regard to the surrounding outside environment is important. If the area around the center is picturesque, then every effort should be made to take advantage of this. The rooms that would benefit from a nice view should be designed with expanses of windows and positioned so that the view can be enjoyed. Outside noise and light should also be considered in order to minimize distractions. If outdoor facilities are used, the weather should be taken into account. Temperature and humidity should be within acceptable ranges, 20° to 24° C (68° to 75° F) and less than 60%, respectively.[10,11] Other factors to consider are noise and air pollution, sunlight, wind, and safety. Outdoor facilities are encouraged when feasible, especially for long-term programs. The patient needs to be confident that vigorous physical activity can be engaged in safely outside of the environmentally controlled exercise laboratory. During phase II, however, the principal objectives are to maximize physical and psychological benefits and minimize outside distractions.

Phases III and IV and Adult Fitness

Current thinking for many programs is to combine cardiac rehabilitation and fitness facilities into large multipurpose complexes. The logic of this approach is to offer all aspects of the program under one roof. There is a distinct logistic advantage to this approach, assuming that adequate space is available. The major disadvantage is financial. Large, complex, and multipurpose facilities are expensive to design, construct, and maintain. Extreme care must be given to completing a thorough market survey in order to demonstrate the financial and usage feasibility of a large center. If it is determined that the multipurpose complex is the desirable approach to take, then professional planning and design assistance should be solicited.

Facilities vary considerably in size, shape and layout for phases III and IV and adult fitness programs. Phases III and IV can be conducted in a facility similar to phase II and can accommodate small groups at a time. Or, a similar layout can be used but of increased size to accommodate larger numbers of patients. Another option is the large, multipurpose exercise facility that is used both for cardiac rehabilitation and adult fitness.

Figures 11–10 to 11–20 provide a series of floor plans and other illustrations of facilities that include exercise areas of various types, conference rooms, dressing and shower areas, exercise test laboratories, physical therapy, massage, whirlpools, sauna and steam rooms, pro shops, restaurant and lounge facilities, and open space for planters, decorations, and other designer items to make the environment attractive. Additional facility information is found elsewhere.[1,2,9,12,13]

Exercise Testing Laboratory

The laboratory areas needed to service cardiac rehabilitation and adult fitness programs must be developed with special attention to purpose and available space. Figure 11–21 illustrates a laboratory floor plan of approximately 1,800 square feet, which provides a variety of services. This design is compact enough to be contained in a large truck as a mobile laboratory or in a hospital or clinic where available space is limited. Figure 11–22 is a floor plan of a laboratory providing similar services in 4,000 square feet of space. When space is at a premium, ceiling electrocardiogram (ECG) scopes and treadmills sunk into the floor should be considered.

In most laboratories and exercise rooms, electrical requirements can be met by the standard 115 voltage. However, if there might be a need for 220 voltage in the future, it is better and less expensive to put in a line at the beginning rather than having to rewire later. A sufficient number of electrical outlets including floor and ceiling strip outlets every 6 to 12 feet should be planned. The electrical system should also be designed with isolated transformers and outlets on different circuits to avoid overloading the system, voltage surges, and circuit breaker problems. This is particularly important in the installation of any computer equipment, which can be sensitive to

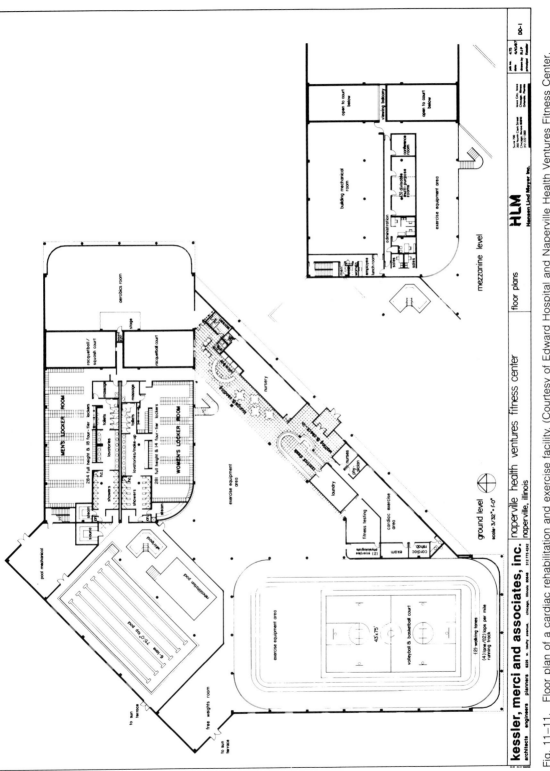

Fig. 11–11.   Floor plan of a cardiac rehabilitation and exercise facility. (Courtesy of Edward Hospital and Naperville Health Ventures Fitness Center, Naperville, Illinois.)

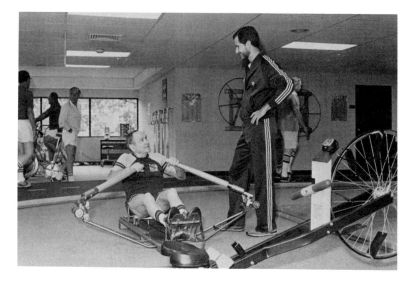

Fig. 11–12. Exercise area for cardiac rehabilitation and adult fitness. (Courtesy of The Health Institute, St. Luke's Hospital, Kansas City, Missouri, David Venner, photographer.)

voltage changes. Two- and three-phase electrical circuits are important and often require special lines. Plans should be made in advance for the possibility of dual testing if that is a likelihood.

Since water supply is needed in the testing and exercise areas, careful plans must be made. Because plumbing is very expensive, plans for locating sinks, drinking fountains, and showers should keep cost in mind. Adequate space, water supply, and drainage need to be considered if underwater weighing is going to be included.

Finally, the aesthetic needs of cardiac re-

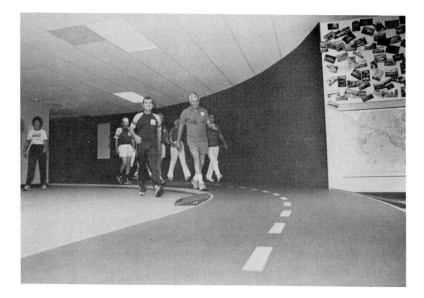

Fig. 11–13. Exercise track for cardiac rehabilitation and adult fitness. (Courtesy of The Health Institute, St. Luke's Hospital, Kansas City, Missouri, David Venner, photographer.)

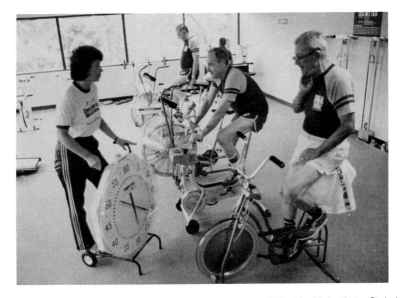

Fig. 11–14. Supervised exercise on stationary bicycles. (Courtesy of The Health Institute, St. Luke's Hospital, Kansas City, Missouri, David Venner, photographer.)

habilitation and adult fitness centers should be given careful attention. Unless someone on the staff is experienced in interior design, a professional should be consulted. If the center is to be a showcase facility, the services of an interior designer are even more important. The facility should be pleasant in appearance, with colored walls, murals, pictures, hanging plants, mirrors, stereo music, and carpeting. Areas designated for phases I and II should avoid looking like a hospital and should be brightly colored, well decorated, and comfortable.

EQUIPMENT

Selecting the best equipment to meet the needs of a program has become increasingly complex. This is especially true for expensive electronic equipment such as stress testing and ECG monitoring systems. Electronics have changed substantially in versatility and computer utilization. At the same time competition for sales of these products has become intense. To make the best choice of equipment requires an unbiased expert opinion or taking the time

necessary to become thoroughly familiar with the various systems. If you take the latter approach, you should become sufficiently well educated to ask the appropriate questions and to comprehend technical answers. If the salesperson cannot answer these questions adequately, then you need to seek out the person who can. Comparative prices, technology, service availability, agreements, future needs, and possible compatibility with other systems/components must be investigated.

In the following sections equipment requirements are discussed for each phase of cardiac rehabilitation and adult fitness.

Phase I

The equipment used in most phase I programs is relatively minimal. The exercise program is usually conducted at bedside and requires light weights (1 or 2 lbs.), blood pressure apparatus, a watch with a sweep hand, and perhaps some small game balls. In a few phase I programs, exercise bikes are used in the patient's room for more vigorous activity. A few centers also have a separate room to exercise phase I patients. The equipment needs of a dedi-

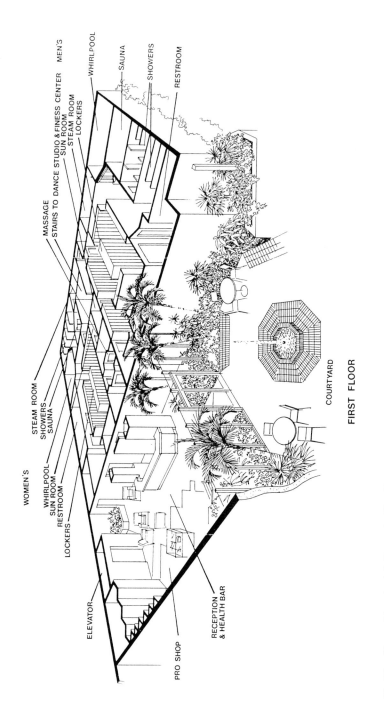

FIRST FLOOR

Fig. 11–15. Phase IV and adult fitness facility. (Courtesy of The Health Institute and Spa of Indigo Lakes, Daytona Beach, Florida; Michael McCaffrey, Designer and Manager.)

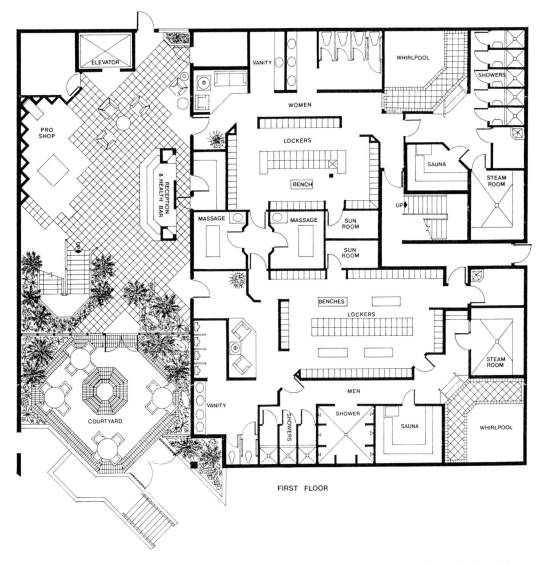

Fig. 11–16.   Phase IV and adult fitness facility. (Courtesy of The Health Institute and Spa of Indigo Lakes, Daytona Beach, Florida; Michael McCaffrey, Designer and Manager.)

cated phase I exercise room are discussed later in this chapter.

Audiovisual equipment and supplies are usually extensive in phase I because of the emphasis on patient education and lifestyle modification. A typical list of items includes several types of projectors, tape recorders and players, films, slides, flip charts, manuals, books, filmstrips, and a variety of handout materials. If ECG monitoring is done in phase I, then a decision must be made concerning the best choice

of equipment. If a central monitoring station is used in the patient unit, it can also be used to observe patient responses to exercise. If a central station is not available or is insufficient to monitor the number of patients who are exercising, then a portable system should be considered. Portable units are moderately priced and can easily be transported. Since ECG monitoring is often required for reimbursement and its use enhances patient safety, some type of a system is necessary. In phase I programs

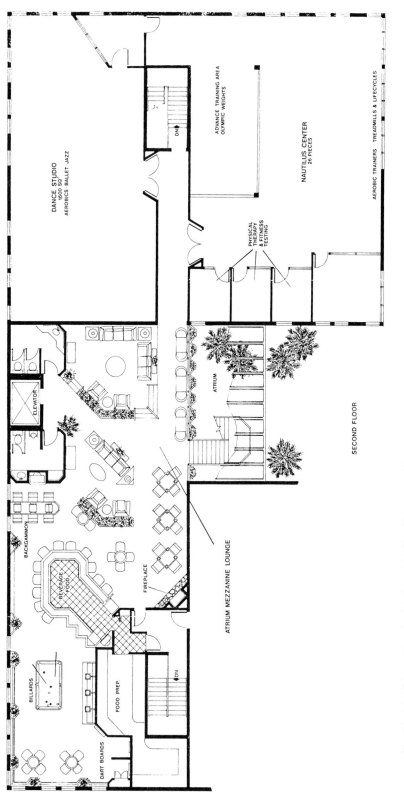

Fig. 11–17. Phase IV and adult fitness facility. (Courtesy of The Health Institute and Spa of Indigo Lakes, Daytona Beach, Florida; Michael McCaffrey, Designer and Manager.)

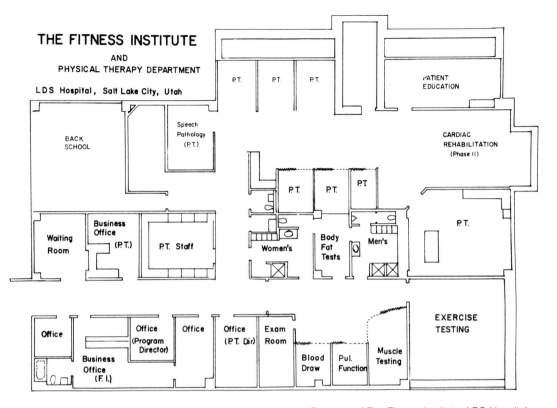

THE FITNESS INSTITUTE
AND
PHYSICAL THERAPY DEPARTMENT

LDS Hospital, Salt Lake City, Utah

Fig. 11–18. Cardiac rehabilitation and adult fitness facility. (Courtesy of The Fitness Institute, LDS Hospital, Salt Lake City, Utah.)

that have a separate room for exercise, the equipment needs are similar to those in phase II. The most notable difference between phases I and II exercise is the emphasis on lower body activity for postsurgical patients in phase I due to their inability to do much upper body work following surgery.

Phase II

Phase II exercise programs are generally equipped with exercise devices for both upper and lower body. These include arm and leg ergometers, rowing machines, treadmills, wall pulleys, shoulder wheels, and step devices. At least one heavy-duty treadmill is recommended to handle the markedly obese patient.

Electrocardiographic monitoring devices consist of telemetry or hard wire systems. Although telemetry is more common than hard wire, the latter can be just as good when used properly and is much less expensive.

With the availability of so many excellent monitoring systems, selecting the best one can be difficult. Questions that are important to consider include cost, reliability, availability of service, simplicity of maintenance, ease of use, and equipment features. It is very important that those who use the equipment have input into the selection.

The principal use of monitoring equipment is for the detection and documentation of arrhythmias and significant ischemic changes. Ischemic changes may be more difficult to assess as a result of reduced frequency response of most telemetry systems, lead placement errors, or poor patient preparation. Careful patient preparation should be emphasized at all times. Monitoring system, electrode place-

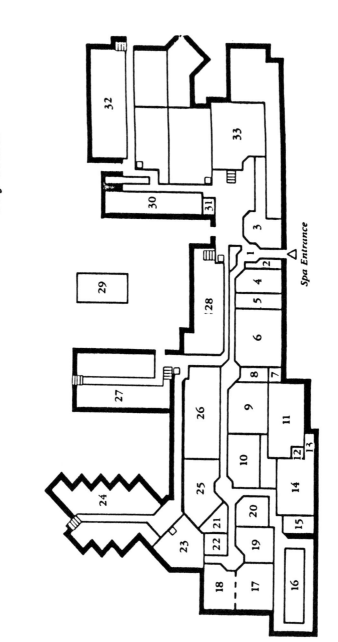

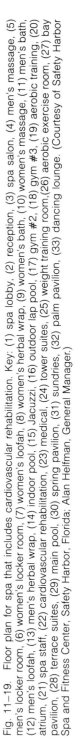

Fig. 11–19.   Floor plan for spa that includes cardiovascular rehabilitation. Key: (1) spa lobby, (2) reception, (3) spa salon, (4) men's massage, (5) men's locker room, (6) women's locker room, (7) women's loofah, (8) women's herbal wrap, (9) women's bath, (10) women's massage, (11) men's bath, (12) men's loofah, (13) men's herbal wrap, (14) indoor pool, (15) Jacuzzi, (16) outdoor lap pool, (17) gym #2, (18) gym #3, (19) aerobic training, (20) atrium, (21) spa staff, (22) cardiovascular rehabilitation, (23) medical, (24) tower suites, (25) sundries, (26) aerobic exercise room, (27) bay pavilion, (28) terrace suites, (29) main pool, (30) spring pavilion, (31) sundries, (32) palm pavilion, (33) dancing lounge. (Courtesy of Safety Harbor Spa and Fitness Center, Safety Harbor, Florida; Alan Helfman, General Manager.)

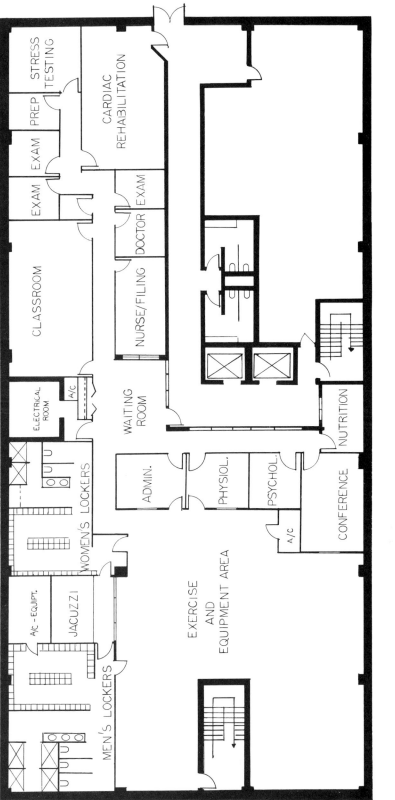

Fig. 11–20. Floor plan of cardiac rehabilitation and adult fitness facility. (Courtesy of North Arundel Cardiac Rehabilitation/Fitness Center, Glen Burnie, Maryland; Linda Carlson, Designer.)

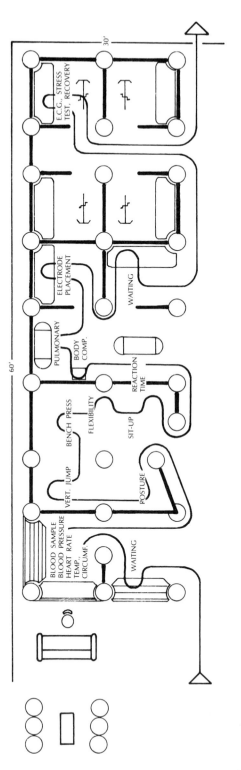

Fig. 11–21.   Laboratory design, restricted space. Used with permission of La Von Johnson, Ph.D., Fitness Monitoring, Fontana, Wisconsin.

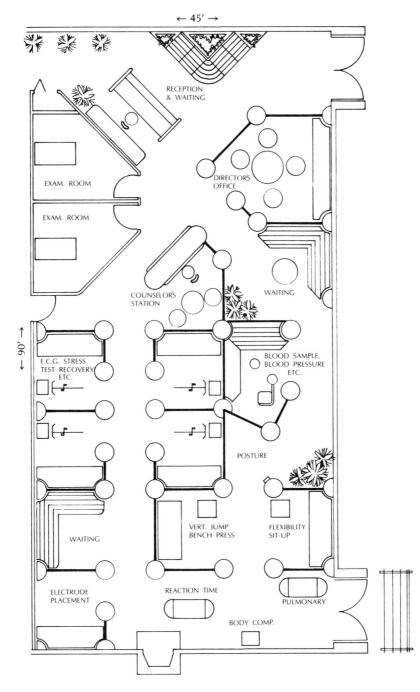

Fig. 11–22. Laboratory design, expanded space. Used with permission of La Von Johnson, Ph.D., Fitness Monitoring, Fontana, Wisconsin.

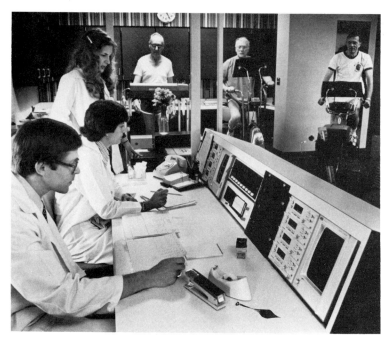

Fig. 11–23.   Phase II, ECG monitoring systems, Mt. Sinai Medical Center, Milwaukee, Wisconsin. Photo courtesy of Michael Pollock, Ph.D.

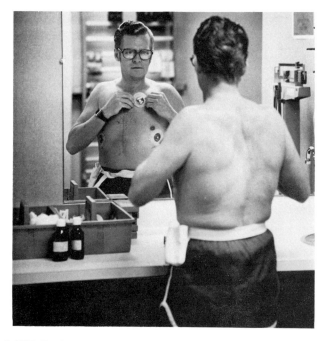

Fig. 11–24.   Phase II, ECG "hookup area," Mt. Sinai Medical Center, Milwaukee, Wisconsin. Photo courtesy of Michael Pollock, Ph.D.

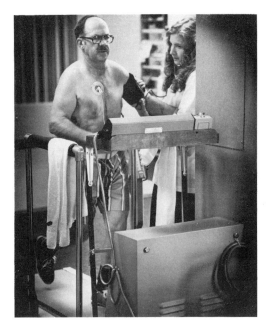

Fig. 11–25. Phase II, exercise, Mt. Sinai Medical Center, Milwaukee, Wisconsin. Photo courtesy of Michael Pollock, Ph.D.

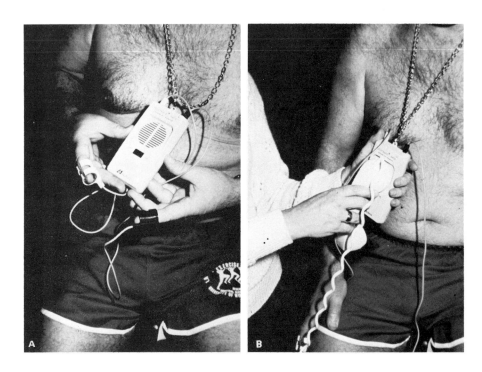

Fig. 11–26.   Telephone ECG. *A*, Finger cups. *B*, Telephone (Lead I).

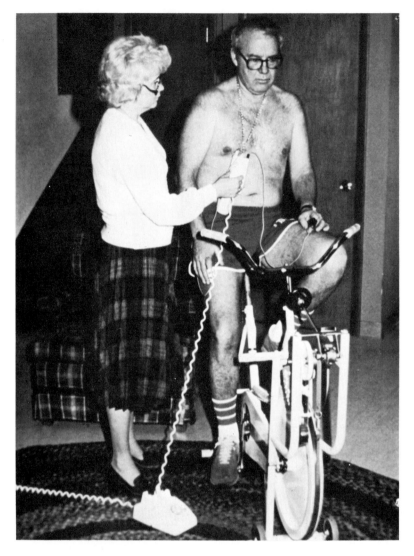

Fig. 11–27.   Patient telephoning in ECG.

ment, and transmitter attachment are shown in Figures 11–23 to 11–25.

Some features of newer monitoring equipment are storage of arrhythmias, miniature transmitters, transmitters that can be used underwater, and "trending" devices, which can display and later print average heart rates and frequency of arrhythmias. Each of these features has some benefit, but they can also create additional work for the staff. Because the primary function of monitoring equipment is to detect and document arrhythmias, some of these features might seldom be used.

Choosing the best stress test equipment can also be difficult and time-consuming. A plethora of stress test systems are available today. Some systems are quite expensive and sophisticated in their electronics, information retrieval, and patient information printouts. There are also excellent low-cost systems that provide only the basic needs, that is, a multichannel recorder, scope with nonfade capability, and a treadmill. Since cardiac rehabilitation patients have already had their disease diagnosed, many of the sophisticated features are not necessary. Ultimately, the choice of equip-

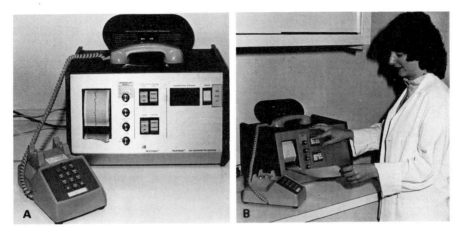

Fig. 11–28. Telephone ECG being received at medical facility (*A* and *B*).

ment depends on its intended use and available financial resources. The AHA manual on standards for equipment provides an excellent guideline for equipment needs.[4]

Transtelephonic ECG systems are becoming increasingly utilized for home monitoring of exercise training. The equipment is particularly useful in assessing patients between discharge from the hospital and entrance into the phase II program, or at the conclusion of the monitored program for patients with significant ar-

rhythmias. In addition, since phase II is not feasible for some patients due to distance from the center, having returned to work, and lack of transportation, telephonic electrocardiography may be a reasonable alternative. Before selecting telephonic equipment, the system's capabilities must be understood. Although several systems are available, some are not sufficiently sensitive to assess ischemic changes. Figures 11–26 to 11–28 illustrate the transmitter and receiving units. Figures 11–29 and 11–30 illustrate a new transtelephonic te-

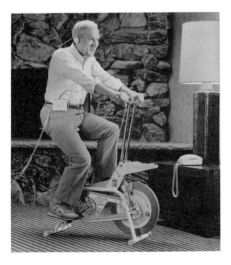

Fig. 11–29. Transtelephonic telemetry system: patient monitoring. (Courtesy of FutureCare Systems, Minneapolis, Minnesota.)

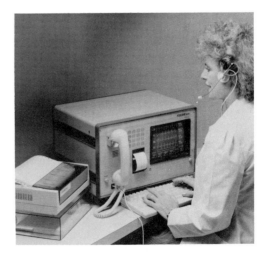

Fig. 11–30. Transtelephonic telemetry system: receiving monitor and print-out. (Courtesy of FutureCare Systems, Minneapolis, Minnesota.)

Table 11–1. A Summary of Resistance Equipment

Four Classifications of Weight Equipment
1. Isotonic
2. Isokinetic
3. Variable resistance
4. Accommodating resistance

Available Equipment and Product Names
  Isotonic equipment
    Free weight equipment
      Benches, racks
        Chrome-plated finish (Paramount, Universal)
        Painted finish (Badger, Polaris, Eagle, Muscle Dynamics)
      Plates, bars
        Standard bore (1 to $1\frac{1}{16}$ inch diameter) or Olympic bore ($2\frac{1}{4}$ inch diameter) (Ivanko, Sonata, York)
      Dumbbells (Ivanko, Sonata, York)
        Fixed weight
         i. Cast-iron plates
         ii. Chrome-plated plates
         iii. Rubber-coated plates
        Solid
         i. Cast-iron
         ii. Chrome-plated
      Direct-resistance pulley systems
        Chrome-plated finish (Paramount, Universal)
        Painted finish (Badger, Muscle Dynamics, Polaris)
  Variable resistance equipment
    Selectorized weight stack machines
      Elliptical cam-style varied resistance
        Chain drive
         Chrome-plated finish machines (Nautilus)
         Painted finish machine (Badger, Muscle Dynamics)
        Cable drive
         Chrome-plated finish machine (Paramount, Universal)
         Painted finish machines (Eagle)
        Belt drive
         Painted finish machines (David)
      Lever-style varied resistance
        Chrome-plated finish machines (Nautilus, Paramount, Universal)
        Painted-finish machines (Nautilus, Badger, Polaris, Muscle Dynamics)
      Indirect pulley system-style varied resistance
        Chrome-plated finish machines (Paramount, Universal)
        Painted finish machines (Eagle, Badger, Polaris)
    Computerized electromagnetic resistance (resistance set and controlled electronically)
      Double positive resistance (no negative resistance)
        Painted finish machines (Paramount, Muscle Dynamics, Toro)
  Accommodating resistance equipment
    Pneumatic resistance
      Chrome-plated finish machines (Keiser)
    Hydraulic resistance
      Double positive resistance (no negative resistance)
        Chrome-plated finish machines (Hydra, Zone)
        Painted finish machines (Hydra)
  Isokinetic equipment (includes only variable resistance equipment with controlled speed of movement)
    (Cybex, Biodex, Kim Com)

Table 11–1. Continued

Manufacturers' Addresses and Phone Numbers

Badger Fitness Equipment
1010 Davis Avenue
S. Milwaukee, WI 53172
(414) 764-4068

Eagle Fitness Systems by Cybex
2100 Smithtown Avenue
Ronkonkoma, NY 11779

Ivanko Barbell Company
P.O. Box 1470
San Pedro, CA 90733
(213) 514-1155

Keiser Sports Health Equipment
411 S. West Avenue
Fresno, CA 93706
1-800-228-7800

Muscle Dynamics Corp.
17022 Montanero Street, #5
Carson, CA 90746
(213) 637-9500

Nautilus Sports Medical Industries
P.O. Box 1783
Deland, FL 32721-1783
1-800-874-8941

Paramount Fitness Equipment Corp.
6450 E. Bandini Blvd.
Los Angeles, CA 90040-3185
1-800-421-6242

Polaris
3515 Sweetwater Springs Blvd.
Spring Valley, CA 92077
1-800-858-0300

Universal Gym Equipment
930 27th Avenue S.W.
Cedar Rapids, IA 52406
(319) 365-7561

Zone Industries, Inc.
7114 W. Jefferson Ave.
Suite 100
Lakewood, CO 80235
(303) 969-8910

(Courtesy of ACT Equipment Incorporated, Ft. Lauderdale, Florida; Dean Bauer, President.)

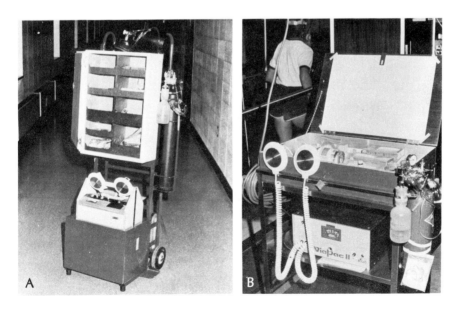

Fig. 11–31. CPR crash carts. *A*, Mobile exercise areas. *B*, Exercise testing facility. LaCrosse Exercise Program, University of Wisconsin, LaCrosse, Wisconsin.

Table 11–2.   Emergency Cart Contents

TOP OF CART
Defibrillator
Tube of electrode paste
3 Suction catheters (2 adult, 1 child)
6 Disposable electrodes (3 No. 2255T, 3 No. 2259T)
1 Roll ECG paper
1 Disposable T & A suction tip (Yankauer suction)
1 N66 connecting tubing
1 Angle needle valve with suction bottle, 1-K66, 1-N52
   connecting tubing and suction container ring/or
   suction machine with connecting tubing

BACK OF CART
Massage Board

SIDE OF CART
Clipboard with medic forms
PMR-2 resuscitation bag with O_2 demand valve and
   medium respiration mask (assemble all parts together)

FIRST DRAWER—MEDICATIONS
2 Aminophylline 500 mg/20 ml ampules
2 Metaraminol bitartrate (Aramine) 10 mg/ml to 10
   ml (1% vial)
3 Atropine 1 mg/10 ml (Bristoject)
6 Bretylium tosylate 50 mg/ml 10 ml ampules
2 Calcium chloride 10% 1 gm (Bristoject)
3 Digoxin (Lanoxin) 0.5 mg/2 ml ampules
2 Dopamine 200 mg/5 ml ampules
4 Epinephrine injection (adrenalin) 1 mg/10 ml
   (1:10,000 Bristoject)
1 Glucagon 1 mg/1 ml ampules
1 Glucose 25 g/50 ml 50% ampules
2 Isoproterenol (Isuprel) 0.2 mg/ml 5 ml ampules
2 Furosemide injection 100 mg/10 ml
3 Lidocaine 2% (Xylocaine) 100 mg/5 ml (Bristoject)
1 Lidocaine 2 g 50 ml vial
2 Naloxone (Narcan) 0.4 mg/ml ampules
2 Norepinephrine bitartrate (Levophed) 1 mg/ml 4
   ml ampules
2 Procainamide (Pronestyl) 500 mg/ml 2 ml ampules
3 Propanolol (Inderal) 1 mg/ml ampules
4 7.5% Sodium bicarbonate 44.6 mEq 50 ml (Bristoject)
2 Solu-Cortef 100 mg/2 ml vial *or* hydrocortisone sodium succinate injection
2 Solu-Cortef 500 mg/4 ml vial *or* hydrocortisone sodium succinate injection
2 Diazepam (Valium) 10 mg/2 ml ampules
2 Verapamil hydrochloride 5 ml (2.5 mg/ml)

(MEDICATION—ADDED LABELS)
(Place under appropriate medication)
5 Lidocaine 2 g/500 D5W
2 Dopamine 400 mg/250 D5W
2 Isoproterenol (Isuprel) 1 mg/250 D5W
2 Procainamide (Pronestyl) 2 g/500 D5W
2 Norepinephrine (Levophed) 4 mg/250 D5W
6 Bretylium 2 g/500 D5W

SECOND DRAWER
1 Laryngoscope handle
2 Curved blades No. 2 and No. 3
2 Straight blades No. 2 and No. 3
1 Extra bulb for laryngoscope blade
2 C or D batteries (depends on what size laryngoscope
   handle requires)
1 9-volt battery
1 Curved Kelly
1 Lidocaine ointment
1 Tube Lubrafax
2 Adaptors No. MAR 2750
1 Nasal airway I.D. 8.0 mm No. 340080

1 Oxymetazoline hydrochloride (Neo-Synephrine)
   1/4%
1 Benzoin 3 oz.
2 30 ml syringe (disposable)
2 4 × 4 packages of gauze
1 Roll 1-inch white adhesive tape
Assortment of airways (sm, med, lg)
1 Sterile scissors
1 Sterile endotracheal stylet
1 Adult magill forceps (sterile)
Endotracheal tubes: 2 No. 7; 2 No. 7.5; 2 No. 8; 2
   No. 8.5; 2 No. 9

Table 11–2.   Continued

THIRD DRAWER

Syringes with needles:
  4 3 ml with 20-1½ needle
  4 6 ml with 22-1½ needle
  4 12 ml with 20-1½ needle
Needles:
  3 No. 18 Jelco 1¼ inch
  3 No. 20 Jelco 1¼ inch
  4 No. 19 minicath
  2 No. 21 minicath
  2 No. 23 minicath
  4 No. 25 g ⅝ inch
  3 No. 19 g 1½ inch
  2 No. 16 g 1½ inch
  3 No. 23 g 1 inch
  4 No. 18 spinal 3½ inch

Syringes:
  3 60 ml syringes
  3 35 ml syringes

Miscellaneous Supplies:
  1 Roll medication labels
  3 Tourniquets
  1 Roll 1-inch adhesive tape
  18 Medium alcohol preps
  3 Tegaderm dressings

FOURTH DRAWER

1 Pac tray (Argon) 8.5 fr.
1 Deseret catheter No. 3172
1 Deseret catheter No. 3174
1 Subclavian jugular catheter No. 755
3 Packages 3-0 silk (684H)
1 50 ml 1% lidocaine (Xylocaine)
1 2-inch Adhesive tape
1 No. 11 Knife blade

1 No. 3 Knife handle
1 Iodine prep solution (2 oz)
4 4 × 4 gauze sponges
Gloves:
  1 pr. size 7
  1 pr. size 7½
  1 pr. size 8

FIFTH DRAWER

4 500 ml D5W
3 500 ml Ringers Lactate
2 250 ml D5W
2 Minibags 50 ml, D5W
8 Nonvented I.V. sets (No. 86-01-0)
2 Nonvented secondary I.V. sets (No. 86-21-0)

1 Travenol I.V. set (No. 2C0001)
2 Extension sets (2C0065)
2 3-way stopcocks
1 Salem sump tube 18 Fr.
1 Disposable Asepto syringe
1 Volume infusion set 52-02-0

BOTTOM OF CART—RESPIRATORY EQUIPMENT

1 Large respiratory mask
1 Nebulizer set-up (Purified Water 500)
1 Nebulizer adaptor cap
1 Prefilled disposable humidifier
1 Adult aerosol mask
1 Nasal cannula

1 Oxygen connecting tubing
1 Blood sampling kit
1 T-piece
1 Instant ice transporter
1 Large-bore tubing
Assortment of airways

  Note: On 3 to 11 or 11 to 7 shift, if any respiratory equipment cannot be replaced, notify Respiratory Therapy
    Supervisor.

OTHER

Break-type lock is installed on each Medic Cart. The purpose of the bend and break lock is to ensure to
  everyone that the contents of the cart are intact without difficulty in gaining entrance to the cart. If for
  any reason the lock is not intact, the Pharmacy or Central Processing should be called for a new lock.

(Courtesy of Peninsula General Hospital and Medical Center, Salisbury, Maryland.)

lemetry system that can monitor real-time ECG responses to exercise.

Other large items of electronic equipment that should be considered during planning are computers and word processors. These can be used for the preparation of forms, data collection, storage and analysis of data, physician reports, accounting, and billing purposes. Computer equipment is covered more thoroughly in Chapter 9.

Phases III and IV and Adult Fitness

Much of the same exercise equipment used in phase II can also be utilized in the phase III program. In addition exercise equipment that can be used in low-level organized games and provides a variety of activities should be selected. Phase IV and adult fitness might also include resistance equipment. These systems are summarized in Table 11–1.

Since patient compliance is one of the most important indicators of success, it is important to include activities that are easily available to the patient and fun to continue. In most cases phase III and IV are nonmonitored or intermittently monitored. In the latter situation portable monitoring or using a defibrillator-monitor with see-through paddles is most appropriate. This system is illustrated in Chapter 14.

Emergency equipment including defibrillator, monitor, drug supplies, oxygen, crash cart and resuscitation equipment must be available in all phases of the program (Figure 11–31). Table 11–2 specifies those items that should be included on an emergency crash cart. A standard procedure should be devised for regularly checking the equipment. Expiration dates of drugs are checked routinely, and the defibrillator should be test fired at least once a day.

Equipment and supplies similar to that recommended for phase I should be available for the other phases of the program.

Since patient education and life-style modification are an on-going process, these programs should become a routine part of rehabilitation.

The plethora of equipment and innovations in modern facilities for multipurpose, clinically oriented, or adult fitness facilities necessitates keeping current with such items as design, technology, and pricing. The following list of resource information is recommended for those who desire to keep abreast of equipment and facility developments:

1. Corporate Fitness and Recreation: The Journal for Employee Health and Services Programs. Brentwood Publishing Corporation, 825 S. Barrington, Los Angeles, CA 90049. (The Buyer's Guide Issue is particularly useful.) Published bimonthly.
2. Athletic Business. Athletic Business Publications, Inc., 1842 Hoffman St., Suite 201, Madison, WI 53704.
3. Athletic Purchasing and Facilities. P.O. Box 7006, 1842 Hoffman St., Suite 201, Madison, WI 53704. Published monthly.
4. Fitness Management. Leisure Publications, Inc., 3923 West 6th Street, Los Angeles, CA 90020. Published bimonthly.
5. Fitness in Business: Comprehensive Programming for Employee Health and Fitness. AFB: The Association for Employee Health and Fitness, 428 East Preston Street, Baltimore, MD 21202. Published bimonthly.
6. Club Business, The Magazine of the International Racquet Sports Association. 112 Cypress Street, Brookline, MA 02146. Published monthly.
7. Patton, R.W., Corry, J.M., Gettman, L.R., and Graf, J.S.: Implementing Health/Fitness Programs. Champaign, Ill., Human Kinetics Publishers, 1986.

CONCLUSIONS

Information for planning and developing facilities were discussed in this chapter.

In addition suggestions were made concerning the different aspects of a facility. Equipment required for a program and suggestions to aid in the selection process also were presented. Final decisions are influenced by financial resources and the objectives of the program.

REFERENCES

1. Wilson, P.K., Fardy, P.S., and Froelicher, V.F.: Cardiac Rehabilitation, Adult Fitness, and Exercise Testing. Philadelphia, Lea & Febiger, 1981.
2. Pollock, M.L., Wilmore, J.H., and Fox, S.M.: Exercise in Health and Disease. 2nd Ed. Philadelphia, W.B. Saunders, 1984.
3. American College of Sports Medicine: Guidelines for Exercise Testing and Prescription. 3rd Ed. Philadelphia, Lea & Febiger, 1986.
4. Exercise Standards Book. Dallas, American Heart Association, 1979.
5. Guidelines for Cardiac Rehabilitation Centers. Los Angeles, American Heart Association, Greater Los Angeles Affiliate, 1982.
6. Theurnissen, W.: Planning facilities, the role of the exercise specialist. J. Phys. Ed. Rec., 49:27, 1978.
7. Oldridge, N.B.: Compliance and exercise in primary and secondary prevention of coronary heart disease: A review. Prev. Med., 11:56, 1982.
8. Franklin, B.A.: Exercise program compliance: Improvement strategies. In Behavioral Intervention in Obesity. Edited by J. Storlie and H.A. Jordan. Jamaica, N.Y., Spectrum Publications, 1984.
9. Ferreri, J.P.: Successful strategies for facility planning. Atlantic Business, Jan.:46, 1985.
10. Yaglou, C.P.: Temperature, humidity and air movement in industries. The effective temperature index. Am. J. Physiol., 58:439, 1927.
11. Karpovich, P., and Sinning, W.E.: Physiology of Muscular Activity. Philadelphia, W.B. Saunders, 1971.
12. Patton, R.W.: Trends in Facility Design. Fitness in Business, 1:73, 1986.
13. Patton, R.W., Corry, J.M., Gettman, L.R., and Graf, J.S.: Implementing Health/Fitness Programs. Champaign, Ill., Human Kinetics, 1986.

INPATIENT, OUTPATIENT, ADULT FITNESS EXERCISE AND LIFE-STYLE MANAGEMENT PROGRAMS

INPATIENT CARDIAC REHABILITATION

Cardiac rehabilitation is traditionally divided into several different phases. The major objectives of phase I include patient and family education, ambulation and low-level exercises designed to prevent problems associated with prolonged bedrest, and preparation for a return to a more active life-style after hospital discharge. Phase II is an early posthospitalization program that consists of physician-supervised and -monitored exercise classes, patient and family education, and behavioral self-management training. These classes are usually held in a hospital or freestanding facility. Phase II goals include increased physical work capacity, enhanced psychosocial well-being, and improved clinical status. Phase III programs are usually home-based or community-based programs where the main objective is to achieve a level of function compatible with each patient's occupational and recreational interests. Finally, phase IV programs are a continuation of phase III and represent the long-term maintenance phase after recovery. Phase IV programs for cardiac patients are comparable to most adult fitness programs designed for healthy individuals. This chapter discusses phase I exercise programs and inpatient education.

THE PHASE I PROGRAM: INPATIENT EXERCISE

The initial phase of cardiac rehabilitation should be started as soon as the pa-
tient's condition has stabilized.[1,2] Low-level exercise during the hospital stay has been shown to be safe,[3] feasible,[4] and beneficial,[5] although there may be no improvement in cardiovascular fitness from such low-level activities.[6]

The attending physician is responsible for determining the appropriate time to start phase I. The coronary care nurse and cardiac rehabilitation personnel should also play an active role in assessing eligibility and recommending suitable candidates to the program. These include patients with diagnosed MI or other cardiovascular diseases; patients recovering from coronary artery bypass surgery, angioplasty, or other cardiovascular procedures; and patients with significantly elevated risk factors for coronary heart disease (CHD) who are hospitalized for other reasons. Cardiac exercise programs may be contraindicated if any of the conditions listed in Table 12–1 are present.

Entrance to phase I begins with a written referral from the patient's attending physician (Fig. 12–1). The inpatient program is usually the responsibility of a cardiac rehabilitation nurse; other cardiac rehabilitation personnel, cardiac nurses or physical therapists may also contribute to the program. Close communication is required among the program staff and between the staff and attending physician.

Starting the Program

Prior to initiating the exercise program, information should be obtained regarding

Table 12–1. Contraindications for Phase I Exercise

Intractable and/or recurrent chest pain
Heart failure
Uncontrolled arrhythmias
Shock
Resting systolic blood pressure over 200 mm Hg
Resting diastolic blood pressure over 100 mm Hg
Moderate to severe aortic stenosis
Acute systemic illness or fever
Third-degree heart block
Active pericarditis or myocarditis
Recent embolism
Thrombophlebitis
Resting ST displacement greater than 3 mm
Uncontrolled diabetes
Orthopedic problems that would prohibit exercise

the patient's medical history and current clinical status. This provides an excellent opportunity for interaction with the staff nurse regarding rehabilitation activities. Pertinent information is recorded on the patient information form (Fig. 12–2). A meeting is then arranged with the patient and family in order to carefully explain the program's objectives and procedures.

Cardiac exercises begin at a low level of exertion and continue in a stepwise fashion throughout hospitalization. The patient is advanced through a series of passive, active, and resistance exercises in the supine, sitting, and upright positions (Figs. 12–3 to 12–18). Most patients are able to begin with active exercise, although passive exercises are occasionally warranted for those with extensve myocardial damage or other complications. The patients are also encouraged to move their legs and feet on their own in order to minimize venous stasis (Figs. 12–5 to 12–9). Each step of the program is outlined on an exercise program sheet and separate exercise cards (Fig. 12–19). Supervised exercise sessions are recommended at least two times per day and usually last 10 to 15 minutes, including time for informal education and conversation.

Exercise sessions may be led by a cardiac rehabilitation nurse, physical therapist, exercise specialist, or cardiac nurse. Most sessions are conducted at the bedside and

adjacent corridors or stairwells. Electrocardiogram monitoring is generally recommended during exercise and may be required for reimbursement. A central monitoring station is most common, although portable monitors are available to use when a central station is not in place.

In some hospitals patients are advanced to a monitored exercise program that is conducted in a separate facility specifically established for that purpose. These more advanced activities are especially appropriate for surgical patients or others who may be more aggressively treated. These programs appear to be safe and beneficial,[7] although data to compare these programs with traditional phase I programs are unavailable. Phase I group facilities are discussed in Chapter 11.

Organizational Procedures

Separate exercise programs are presented in Figure 12–19 for post-MI and postsurgical patients. Postsurgical patients usually can be exercised more aggressively, since there is little or no permanent damage to the myocardium. Generally, patients are progressed one or two steps each day. The amount of exertion increases from 1.0 to 4.0 metabolic equivalents (METs), or between 1.0 and 5.0 kcal/min per session.[8–11] For those individuals who are in monitored phase I exercise programs, the sessions last from 5 to 20 minutes for postinfarct patients and for 5 to 30 minutes for postsurgical patients, several times a day.[7,12] Exercise usually consists of treadmill walking or bicycle ergometry in the monitored program.

The progress of the patient is reviewed daily by the rehabilitation staff. Prior to exercise or advancing to a higher level, the patient is evaluated for pulse, blood pressure, electrocardiogram (ECG) waveform and rhythm, muscular and joint limitations, dizziness, appearance, and symptoms. Activity cards, detailing objectives and procedures for the day, are left at the

REFERRAL FORM
(to be completed by physician)

Patient's Name_____ Date_____
          Last   First   Middle Initial

Address_____ _____
          Street   City   State   Home Telephone

Birth Date_____ Age_____ Spouse's Name_____

Insurance Company_____ Policy No._____

Diagnosis: _____Bypass Surgery   _____Myocardial Infarct
               _____Cardiac Patient   _____Angioplasty
               _____Symptomatic Coronary Artery Disease (Angina)
Other:_____ Explain_____

Specific Cardiac Information_____

Other Limitations_____

Date of Most Recent Hospital Admission_____

| | | | Date | Physician |
Medications	Dosage	Frequency	Prescribed	Prescribing

Please fill in information below if possible:
Date of Examination_____
1. Urine: sp. gr._____ Alb._____ Glucose_____ Micro._____
2. Complete blood count: Hbg_____ Hct_____ WBC_____ Diff._____
3. ECG, 12 lead (enclose copy)_____
4. Blood pressure: Systolic R_____ L_____ Diastolic R_____ L_____
5. Cholesterol _____mg%; HDL _____mg%; LDL _____mg%; Triglycerides _____
mg%
6. Exercise Stress Test Results (enclose, if available)_____

Impression of above information_____

Signed _____, M.D.

Type or Print:

Name of Physician_____
Address_____
Phone_____

Fig. 12–1. Referral form.

Scheduled for Stress_____   Program Adm._____
_____   Hospital Adm._____
                                            Discharge_____
NAME_____   Birth Date _____/_____/_____
ADDRESS_____   Age_____
_____   Phone #_____
Spouse's Name_____
Place of Employment_____
Phone #_____
Referring Physician_____
Attending Physician_____

DIAGNOSIS:_____
_____

RISK FACTORS:_____
_____

CHOLESTEROL:_____
ARTERIOGRAM RESULTS:_____
_____

ACTIVITY:_____   _____
MEDICATIONS:_____   _____
              _____   _____
              _____   _____
              _____   _____
DIET:_____

Fig. 12–2.   Patient information form.

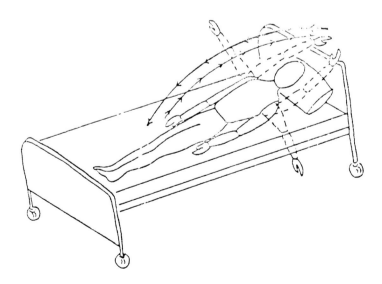

Fig. 12–3.   Phase I shoulder exercises: abduction, adduction, flexion, and extension. Adapted from Phase I, Peninsula General Hospital and Medical Center, Salisbury, Maryland.

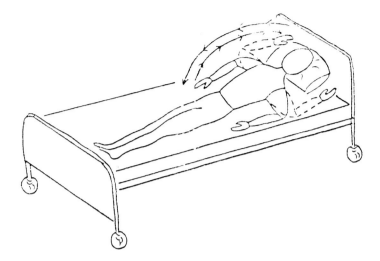

Fig. 12–4.   Phase I shoulder exercises: internal and external rotation. Adapted from Phase I, Peninsula General Hospital and Medical Center, Salisbury, Maryland.

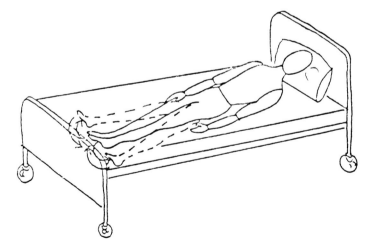

Fig. 12–5.   Phase I hip exercises: abduction and adduction. Adapted from Phase I, Peninsula General Hospital and Medical Center, Salisbury, Maryland.

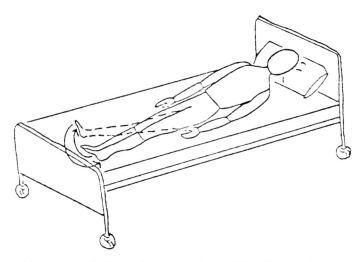

Fig. 12–6. Phase I hip exercises: flexion and extension. Adapted from Phase I, Peninsula General Hospital and Medical Center, Salisbury, Maryland.

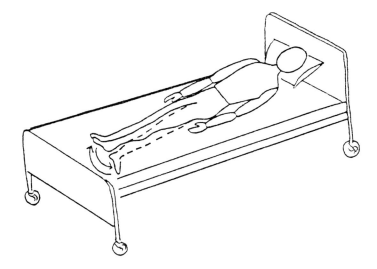

Fig. 12–7. Phase I hip exercises: internal and external rotation. Adapted from Phase I, Peninsula General Hospital and Medical Center, Salisbury, Maryland.

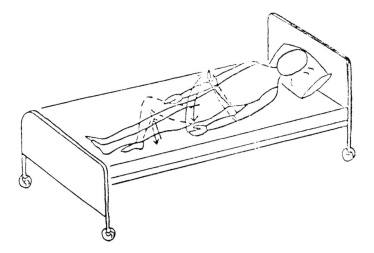

Fig. 12–8.   Phase I knee and elbow exercises: flexion and extension. Adapted from Phase I, Peninsula General Hospital and Medical Center, Salisbury, Maryland.

bedside to be reviewed with the patient. Heart rate and blood pressure are recorded immediately preceding and following each exercise session. Physiologic and clinical responses to exercise are reported to the staff nurse in charge and are documented in the physician's progress notes.

Objectives of Exercise

The objectives of phase I exercises are:
1. To decrease deconditioning problems that are associated with prolonged bedrest, that is, muscle atrophy, pulmonary emboli and infection, postural hypotension, and general circulatory deterioration.
2. To reassure patients that they are not permanently incapacitated.
3. To provide a setting for patient interaction with the exercise leader.
4. To reduce the length of the hospital stay.

Program Personnel

CARDIAC REHABILITATION NURSE. The cardiac rehabilitation nurse usually as-

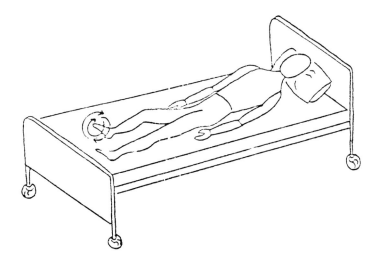

Fig. 12–9.   Phase I exercise: foot circles. Adapted from Phase I, Peninsula General Hospital and Medical Center, Salisbury, Maryland.

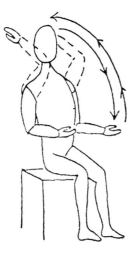

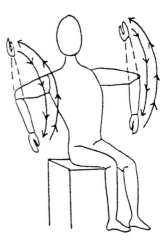

Fig. 12–12. Phase I shoulder exercises: internal and external rotation. Adapted from Phase I, Peninsula General Hospital and Medical Center, Salisbury, Maryland.

Fig. 12–10. Phase I shoulder exercises: flexion and extension. Adapted from Phase I, Peninsula General Hospital and Medical Center, Salisbury, Maryland.

sumes the leadership role of a phase I program. The nurse is responsible for coordinating the efforts of the rehabilitation team, leading exercises, and directing patient education. The role of the cardiac rehabilitation nurse is elaborated throughout the chapter.

PHYSICAL THERAPIST. The physical therapist may be involved in all aspects of the exercise program. In addition the therapist

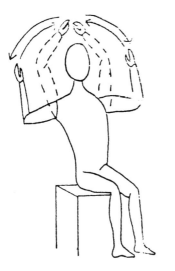

Fig. 12–11. Phase I shoulder exercises: abduction and adduction. Adapted from Phase I, Peninsula General Hospital and Medical Center, Salisbury, Maryland.

is particularly valuable in assessing musculoskeletal dysfunction associated with joint immobility.

When joint mobility has been impaired, a physical therapist may prescribe additional exercises to those already being done in order to meet the specific needs of the patient. Sometimes it is necessary to continue with physical therapy following discharge from the hospital. Although the order to continue therapy is given by the attending physician, the recommendation of the cardiac rehabilitation staff is valuable. Physical therapists who work with cardiac patients should be trained to recognize adverse cardiovascular signs and symptoms.

EXERCISE SPECIALIST. The exercise specialist may lead phase I exercises and teach patients about the value of long-term physical activity. The exercise specialist does not have the clinical expertise of the nurse, but should become familiar with all aspects of the program that affect patient safety.

CARDIAC NURSE. Staff nurses should also be actively involved in cardiac rehabilitation. They can lead exercises and participate in patient education. Their activities should be closely coordinated with those of the cardiac rehabilitation staff. In some in-

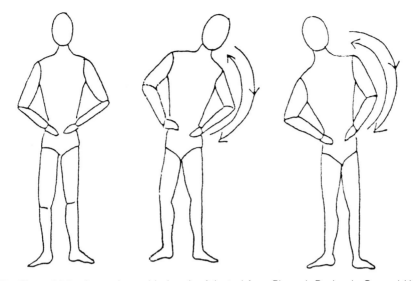

Fig. 12–13. Phase I lateral exercises: side bends. Adapted from Phase I, Peninsula General Hospital and Medical Center, Salisbury, Maryland.

stances the staff nurses will assume the major role in the conduct of the program, particularly in small hospitals where full-time rehabilitation programs do not exist. Participation and cooperation of the nursing staff are very important to the success of the program.

It is suggested that in-service presentations be provided to the nursing staff so that they better understand the goals of cardiac rehabilitation. In-service education is important to train nurses in the correct procedures for exercise, what to look for in the patient's condition, and the proper documentation of activities and responses to exercise. The nursing staff should play a role in assessing the patient's readiness for advancement in the program. Nurses

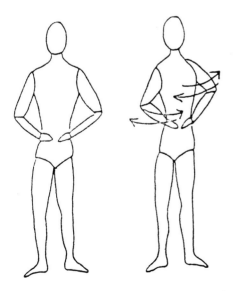

Fig. 12–14. Phase I exercises: trunk twisting. Adapted from Phase I, Peninsula General Hospital and Medical Center, Salisbury, Maryland.

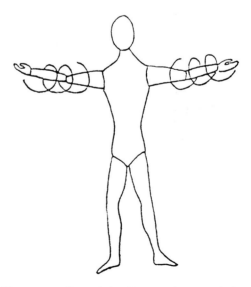

Fig. 12–15. Phase I shoulder exercise: arm circles. Adapted from Phase I, Peninsula General Hospital and Medical Center, Salisbury, Maryland.

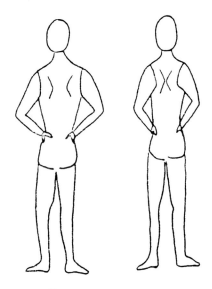

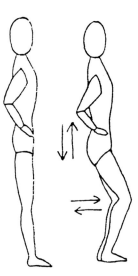

Fig. 12–16. Phase I shoulder exercise: scapular adduction. Adapted from Phase I, Peninsula General Hospital and Medical Center, Salisbury, Maryland.

Fig. 12–17. Phase I exercise: slight knee bends. Adapted from Phase I, Peninsula General Hospital and Medical Center, Salisbury, Maryland.

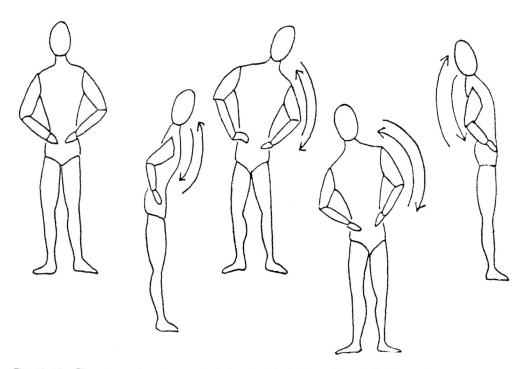

Fig. 12–18. Phase I exercise: four-way body bends. Adapted from Phase I, Peninsula General Hospital and Medical Center, Salisbury, Maryland.

Five to ten repetitions of each exercise will be performed.

STEP 1

Active Range of Motion to all extremities while lying in bed using proper breathing. <u>Shoulder:</u> abduction, adduction, flexion, extension (Fig. 12–3), internal and external rotation (Fig. 12–4). <u>Hip:</u> abduction, adduction (Fig. 12–5), flexion, extension (Fig. 12–6), internal and external rotation (Fig. 12–7). <u>Knee and elbow:</u> flexion and extension (Fig. 12–8). <u>Active foot:</u> circling at least one time per hour (Fig. 12–9). <u>Surgical patients:</u> up in chair two times daily, ambulation with assistance in room.

MET level: 1.0 to 1.5

STEP 2

Repeat all exercises as in Step 1. <u>Surgical patients:</u> with bed at 45° angle. Up in chair ad lib, at least two times daily. Short walks with assistance in room and corridor.

MET level: 1.0 to 1.5

STEP 3

Repeat all exercises as in Step 2 with mild resistance. <u>Surgical patients:</u> exercises done while sitting on bed. Increase walking, chair sitting as in Step 2.

MET level: 1.0 to 2.0

STEP 4

Active Range of Motion to all extremities while sitting using mild resistance and proper breathing. <u>Shoulder:</u> exercise done with flexed elbow (Figs. 12–10 to 12–12). <u>Surgical patients:</u> up ad lib in room without assistance. Longer walks in hall with assistance at least two times daily.

MET level: 1.5 to 2.0

STEP 5

Repeat exercises of Step 4 with moderate resistance and proper breathing. Walk to tolerance, not more than 50 feet. <u>Surgical patients:</u> exercises in standing position with 1- to 2-pound weights, lateral side bends, trunk twists (Figs. 12–13 and 12–14). Continued walking.

MET level: 1.5 to 2.0

Fig. 12–19.   Cardiac rehabilitation phase I exercise program, Peninsula General Hospital and Medical Center, Salisbury, Maryland. *Phase I exercise description.* (Documentation of the patient's heart rate/blood pressure responses to the exercises and comments are found on the cardiac rehabilitation progress record). (MET, metabolic equivalent.)

STEP 6

Active Range of Motion activities to all extremities with 1- to 2-pound weights while standing. Shoulder: add arm circles (Fig. 12–15, scapular adduction (Fig. 12–16). Walk to tolerance, not more than 100 feet. Surgical patients: walking ad lib without assistance.

MET level: 1.5 to 2.0

STEP 7

Repeat exercises in Step 6. Walk to tolerance, not more than 200 feet. Surgical patients: repeat Step 6. Add slight knee bends (Fig. 12–17); continue walking, walk down one flight of stairs with assistance (up on elevator).

MET level: 1.5 to 2.5

STEP 8

Repeat exercises in Step 7. Walk to tolerance, not more than 300 feet. Surgical patients: repeat Step 7. Continue walking, walk down two flights of stairs with assistance (up on elevator).

MET level: 1.5 to 2.5

STEP 9

Repeat exercises in Step 8. Add slight knee bends, fourway body bends (Fig. 12–18). Walk to tolerance, walk down one flight of stairs with assistance (up the elevator). Surgical patients: up one flight of stairs, down one.

MET level: 2.0 to 2.5

STEP 10

Repeat exercises in Step 9. Down two flights of stairs with assistance. Surgical patients: Repeat Step 9.

MET level: 2.0 to 2.5

STEP 11

Repeat exercises in Step 10. Down one flight of stairs and up with assistance.

MET level: 2.5 to 3.0

Fig. 12–19 (Continued).

should also be familiar with other features of the program, even though they may not be actively involved. To do so fosters a greater feeling of participation and motivates the staff nurse to play an active role in the program. If the nurses have an active role, they are more likely to be enthusiastic. The result is better patient care and more highly motivated patients.

PHYSICIAN. A physician is responsible for referring the patient into the program. In this capacity the referring physician paves the way for cardiac rehabilitation personnel and therefore needs to be aware of patient progress. A few words of encouragement by the physician is extremely important in motivating the patient.

Figure 12–20 outlines phase I personnel and responsibilities.

When To Start Exercise

The decision to start cardiac rehabilitation is made by the referring physician, who may be a cardiologist or primary care doctor. The exercise program should be initiated as soon as the patient's condition has stabilized and takes several factors into consideration: ECG waveform and rhythm, symptoms, enzymes, and examination. The physician maintains the prerogative to alter the program at any time in accordance with the patient's clinical status. The rate of advancement is dependent on the patient's daily progress.

Under certain circumstances some patients may be instructed to exercise on their own. Although unsupervised exercise is generally not recommended, it may occa-

Patient/Physician

Cardiovascular Clinical Specialist

1. Identify appropriate referrals—follow up with M.D.
2. Direct patient "rounds" twice weekly.
3. Caseload of "problem patients" identified.
4. Discharge planning consultation as necessary.
5. Follow-up document to referring MD.
6. Chair cardiac rehabilitation committee.
   Members: nursing, medicine, physical therapy,
   fitness institute, dietary, social services.
7. Coordination of class schedule.
8. Maintenance/revisions of instructional materials.
   Written
   Audio

Physical Therapy

1. Patient visit daily
2. Identification of appropriate progression of levels
3. Home program
4. Teaching classes as identified

Nursing

1. Primarily coordination of patient care
2. Exercises with patients following level instructions
3. Teaching classes as identified and arranged

Fitness Institute

1. Predischarge visit with those patients not entering phase II
2. Teaching classes as identified
3. Home program/phase II
4. Outpatient program/phase II

Fig. 12–20. Cardiovascular center at LDS hospital. Cardiac rehabilitation program: organizational structure and responsibilities. Phase I, inpatient program.

CONTENT OF GROUP SESSIONS	TEACHING DATES	INSTRUCTOR	COMMENTS
Risk factors			
Sexuality			
Physical activity			
Diet			
Initial assessment			
Follow-up			
Psychosocial adjustment			
Family adjustments			
Content of individual sessions			
Orientation to phase I			
Orientation to phase II			
Home walking program			
Home stationary bike program			
Discharge planning			

INDIVIDUAL
TEACHING NEEDS

Fig. 12–21.   Education flow sheet. Cardiac rehabilitation for the inpatient.

Table 12–2.   Topics for Individual Patient Classes

Preoperative teaching for coronary artery bypass surgery
Orientation to cardiac rehabilitation—phase I
Orientation to cardiac rehabilitation—phase II
Orientation to critical care environment
Anatomy of the heart; disease and the healing process
Home walking and home stationary bicycle program and pulse taking
Angina pectoris
Medications

Table 12–3.   Topics for Group Classes

Family adjustment
Psychosocial adjustment to coronary artery disease
Inpatient rehabilitation program—nutrition intervention
Coronary disease risk factors
Physical activity and coronary artery disease
Sexual activity and coronary artery disease

sionally be appropriate and necessary. If the patient can be monitored from a central station, unsupervised exercise might be a better alternative than canceling the exercise session. Physician approval is required.

The cardiac rehabilitation staff regularly reviews the patient's progress. Positive feedback can be very encouraging for the patient and reinforces the goal of an active and healthier life-style.

Exercise Testing

At the conclusion of the inpatient program, a low-level exercise test is often performed. This test may be carried out before or shortly after discharge, depending on clinical circumstances. The safety of such tests has been well documented.[13–16] The purpose of the low-level test is to determine more precisely the functional capabilities of the patient and to provide specific rec-

CLASS SCHEDULE

Group classes available:

Monday	2:00–2:30 P.M.		Hypertension
	2:30–3:00 P.M.		Smoking and Heart Disease
Tuesday	2:00 P.M.		Physical Activity and Heart Disease
Wednesday	2:00 P.M.		Adjustment of Life-style—The Beat Goes On
Thursday	11:00 A.M.		Diet and Coronary Heart Disease
Friday	10:15 A.M.		You Don't Have to Be Crazy To Be Scared

Fig. 12–22. Sample class schedule. St. Catherine Hospital. Department of Cardiac Rehabilitation.

ommendations for posthospitalization activities. Pre- and postdischarge exercise testing are discussed thoroughly in Chapter 5.

PHASE I EDUCATION

Purpose

Education and behavior modification are integral parts of phase I. They are ongoing and include sessions for individuals and groups that cover a wide variety of subjects. The purpose is to enable the patient and family to better cope with the hospitalization, render physical and emotional support to enhance recovery, and assist in identifying appropriate life-style modifications. The topics selected should be

taught carefully and cogently. It is best to identify the most important objectives of each session in advance, concentrate on them, and not try to do too much. Periodic reinforcement of the material is suggested.

Personnel

Although patient education and behavior modification are usually the responsibility of the cardiac rehabilitation staff, a multidisciplinary approach is recommended. The professional staff might conceivably consist of physicians, nurses, social workers, dieticians, psychologists, exercise specialists, occupational and physical therapists, and other professionals (chaplain, health educator) who can provide a meaningful contribution.

	Monday	Tuesday	Wednesday	Thursday	Friday	Saturday	Sunday
A.M.	Exercise—PT Visit	Exercise—PT Visit	Exercise—PT Visit	Exercise—PT Visit	Exercise—PT Visit	Exercise—PT Visit	Exercise—PT Visit
10:00 to 10:45	Class—Risk Factors	Class—Diet	Class—Discharge	Class—Activity	Class—Emotional Reactions	—	—
P.M.	Exercise—With Nurse	Exercise—With Nurse	Exercise—With Nurse	Exercise—With Nurse	Exercise—With Nurse	Exercise—With Nurse	Exercise—With Nurse
3:45 to 4:30	Class—Activity	Class—Emotional Reactions	Class—Risk Factors	Class—Diet	—	Class—Activity	—
6:30 to 7:15	—	—	—	—	Class—Discharge	—	Class—Discharge

PT, physical therapist

Fig. 12–23. Cardiovascular center at LDS hospital. Cardiac rehabilitation program. Phase I: classes and exercise schedule.

During your hospital stay your activity will gradually increase with the supervision of the medical staff. This is to facilitate your recovery and subsequent discharge from this hospital. Self-care and activity levels, along with suggested exercises, are listed here so you know exactly what you may do. Help us with your progress by doing only what your physician and nurses feel is allowable for your individual condition. It would be helpful to have a wristwatch during your stay, after you leave the ICU, to monitor the exercise period.

	SELF-CARE	BEDSIDE ACTIVITIES	SUPERVISED EXERCISE	SPECIFIC LEARNING OBJECTIVES
LEVEL 1	Feed self Use bedside commode Wash hands/face Brush teeth	Sit up in bed with firm back support	Passive ROM all extremities Active plantar/dorsiflexion Ankle circles Diaphragmatic breathing	Patient will understand purpose of cardiac rehabilitation and importance of adhering to limits and levels of advancement
LEVEL 2	Bathe self at bedside Wash hands/face/upper body/personal area Nurse assist with back and legs Comb hair Shave self	Dangle legs on side of bed Sit up in chair/20 min *not* at same time as meals or immediately before or after another activity such as bathing Light reading	Active assisted ROM all extremities Ankle exercises Shoulder shrugs Diaphragmatic breathing	
LEVEL 3	Bathe self at bedside or in front of sink sitting in chair Nurse assist with back and legs	Walk to bathroom in room with assistance Sit up in chair as tolerated Bedside chair for meals	Active ROM all extremities Ankle exercises Shoulder shrugs Diaphragmatic breathing Supine: flex knees to 75° NOTE: LEVEL 1 to 3 exercises are to be done 3 times per day; once with PT, twice with nursing	Teach pulse monitoring Reinforce cardiac class concepts
LEVEL 4	Take warm shower if appropriate	Bedside chair as tolerated Bedside chair for meals Bathroom first time and assist if needed	1 min each, 3 times per day: Supine flex knees to 75° Sitting flex knees to 75° Sitting knee extender Sitting push and pull 3-min walk 3 times per day or 150-ft walk 3 times per day	Teach importance/purpose of warm-up exercises Reinforce cardiac class concepts
	Take warm shower if appropriate	Bedside chair as tolerated Bedside chair for meals Bathroom first time and assist if needed	3-min walk or 150-ft walk at *least* 3 times per day, but may walk as many times as desired	

LEVEL 5	Take warm shower, if desired	Increase bedside chair sitting time as tolerated Bathroom privileges	1.25 min each, 3 times per day: Supine flex knees to 75° Sitting with lateral trunk bender Standing push and pull Walk down one flight of stairs (ride elevator up) once per day 4-min walk 3 times per day or 200-ft walk 3 times per day at least, and may walk as many times as desired	Review home activity class Review appropriate exercise equipment for home
LEVEL 6	Continue as above standing self-care	Continue with bedside chair and bathroom privileges	1.5 min each, 3 times per day: Sitting hip flexion Standing arm extender Standing lateral trunk bender Ride elevator down and walk up one flight of stairs once per day 5-min walk 3 times per day or 350 feet walk 3 times per day at least, and may walk as many times as desired	Patient demonstration pulse monitoring Patient demonstrate warm-up activities
LEVEL 7	Up ad lib	Up ad lib	1.5 min each, 3 times per day: Standing knee flexion Standing arms overhead Standing lateral bend Walk up and down one flight of stairs once per day 6-min walk 3 times per day or 400-ft walk 3 times per day at least, and may walk as many times as desired	

Additional notes on supervised exercise:
Heart rate and blood pressure are recorded before and after each exercise session.
Beginning with LEVEL 4, heart rate is monitored before each timed exercise, patient is given 1-min rest, and then heart rate is monitored again.
Supervised exercise will be done one time by physical therapist and twice by nursing staff.
ROM = range of motion.

Fig. 12–24.   Cardiovascular center at LDS hospital. Daily levels for patients.

When To Start Education

Patient education should be initiated early during hospitalization[17,18] and should involve members of the patient's family and/or friends when possible and appropriate. In some instances education may precede the start of exercise. For most patients education can start almost immediately, e.g., "Introduction to the CCU." In the case of surgery patients, presurgical teaching is valuable and appropriate to prepare the patient and family for the upcoming procedure and aftermath. Individual and group sessions for patients usually last from 15 to 45 minutes. The classes are shorter at the beginning. Longer sessions can be planned for family members and friends.

Curriculum

The subject matter of each session should be documented on the exercise card, in the physician's progress notes, and on the cardiovascular education flow sheet (Fig. 12–21). The nurses should utilize assessment skills to ascertain patient readiness. The nurses must also be able to identify "teachable moments" and the appropriateness of the material to be covered. Topics that are generally covered in individual patient sessions are listed in Table 12–2.

Education classes also are planned for the family. Long-term adherence can be enhanced greatly when the attitude of the spouse is positive, as opposed to either neutral or negative.[19] It has also been shown that risk factors are often similar among members of a household.[20,21] Education sessions for the family are scheduled regularly and are usually led by the cardiac rehabilitation staff. Sessions should last approximately 45 to 60 minutes and are informally structured to allow for any questions.

As the patient's condition improves, regularly scheduled group classes are encouraged. These classes should be conducted in a pleasant environment to facilitate learning. The patients can ambulate or be transported to a classroom with other patients and family members. Appropriate classes are recommended by the cardiac rehabilitation staff according to individual needs. Regularly scheduled group classes might include those listed in Table 12–3. Sample class schedules are presented in Figures 12–22 and 12–23. Figure 12–24 summarizes phase I exercise, bedside activities, self-care, and individual education sessions.

CONCLUSIONS

Phase I programs have been shown to be safe and beneficial. Since these programs are initiated within a few days of hospital admission, the cardiac rehabilitation nurse and referring physician need to carefully monitor the patient's progress. Although the cardiac rehabilitation nurse is usually responsible for progressing the patient through exercise and education, the physician can alter the program at any time. In this sense the most important goals of phase I are probably patient safety and developing a positive attitude in the patient about life-style modification following discharge from the hospital.

REFERENCES

1. Noble, B.J.: Cardiac rehabilitation: Psychological implications. In Research and Practice in Physical Education. Edited by R.E. Stadulis, C.O. Dotson, V.L. Katch, and J. Schick. Champaign, Ill., Human Kinetics, 1977.
2. Hackett, T.P., and Cassem, N.H.: Psychological adaptation in convalescence in myocardial infarction patients. In Exercise Testing and Exercise Training in Coronary Heart Disease. Edited by J.P. Naughton, H.K. Hellerstein, and I.C. Mohler. Orlando, Fla., Academic Press, 1973.
3. Wenger, N.K.: Critical evaluation of cardiac rehabilitation. Chest, 71:317, 1977.
4. Graber, A.L.: Cardiovascular disease prevention programs in a community hospital. J. Tenn. Med. Assoc., 70:95, 1977.
5. Gilliland, M.M., and Jones, W.L.: A quest for earlier and more organized rehabilitation of the coronary patient. South Dakota J. Med.,29:7, 1976.
6. Sivarajan, E.S., et al.: Treadmill test responses to

an early exercise program after myocardial infarction: A randomized study. Circulation, 65:1420, 1982.

7. Pollock, M.L., et al.: Exercise prescription for rehabilitation of the cardiac patient. *In* Heart Disease and Rehabilitation. Edited by M.L. Pollock and D.H. Schmidt. New York, John Wiley & Sons, 1986.

8. The Committee on Exercise: Exercise Testing and Training of Individuals With Heart Disease or at High Risk for Its Development. Dallas, The American Heart Association, 1975.

9. Carpenter, T.M.: Tables, factors, and formulas for computing respiratory exchange and biological transformations of energy. Washington, D.C., Carnegie Institution of Washington Publication 303C, 1964.

10. Zohman, L.R., and Tobis, J.S.: Cardiac Rehabilitation. Orlando, Fla., Grune & Stratton, 1970.

11. German, M.A.: Energy expenditure in passive and active range of motion exercises. Unpublished master's thesis. Cleveland, Ohio, School of Nursing, Case Western Reserve University, 1975.

12. Pollock, M.L., Ward, A., and Foster, C.: Prescription of exercise in a cardiac rehabilitation program. *In* Cardiac Rehabilitation: Implications for the Nurse and Other Health Professionals. Edited by P.S. Fardy, J.L. Bennett, N.L. Reitz, and M.A. Williams. St. Louis, C.V. Mosby, 1980.

13. Ibsen, H., et al.: Routine exercise ECG three weeks after acute myocardial infarction. Acta Med. Scand., 198:463, 1975.

14. Ericsson, M., et al.: Arrhythmias and symptoms during treadmill testing three weeks after myocardial infarctions in 100 patients. Br. Heart J. 35:787, 1973.

15. DeBusk, R., Houston, N., and Markiewicz, W.: Prognosis of early postinfarction exercise testing. Circulation, 54(suppl. 2): 9, 1976.

16. Wohl, A.J., et al.: Cardiovascular function during recovery from acute myocardial infarction. Circulation, 64(suppl. 2): 147, 1976.

17. Cassem, N.K., and Hackett, T.P.: Psychological rehabilitation of myocardial infarction patients in the acute phase. Paper supported by NIH grants PHS 43-67-1443 + 5-KO 1 HL 13781-02, Boston, Massachusetts General Hospital, 1974.

18. Cassem, N.H., and Hackett, T.P.: Psychiatric consultation in a coronary care unit. Ann. Intern. Med., 75:9, 1971.

19. Heinzelmann, F.: Social and psychological factors that influence the effectiveness of exercise programs. *In* Exercise Testing and Exercise Training in Coronary Heart Disease. Edited by J.P. Naughton, H.K. Hellerstein, and I.C. Mohler. Orlando, Fla., Academic Press, 1973.

20. Mjos, O.D., et al.: Family study of high density lipoprotein cholesterol and the relation to age and sex. Acta Med. Scand., 201:323, 1977.

21. Sackett, D.L., et al.: Concordance for coronary risk factors among spouses. Circulation, 52:589, 1975.

13

PHASE II CARDIAC REHABILITATION

Phase II of cardiac rehabilitation is a supervised outpatient program of individually prescribed exercise that is usually accompanied by continual electrocardiogram (ECG) monitoring and life-style modification classes. The exercise program is based on an individualized prescription that specifies intensity, duration, frequency, and mode of activity.[1–5] The details of formulating an exercise prescription have been described in Chapter 6. Life-style modification and management, which must accompany physical activity, is an ongoing process described in Chapter 15.

OBJECTIVES OF PHASE II

The objectives of phase II follow:

1. Enhance cardiovascular function, physical work capacity, strength, endurance and flexibility
2. Detect arrhythmias and other ECG changes during exercise that are contraindicated for physical activity
3. Educate patients on the proper mechanics of exercise
4. Work with patients and family members on an appropriate program of life-style modification and management
5. Enhance the psychological outlook of the patients
6. Prepare the patients physically, mentally and emotionally for a return to work and for resumption of normal familial and social roles
7. Provide the patients with guidelines for long-term home-based exercise or supervised exercise, that is, phases III and IV

The objectives are best attained through a well-planned program that might be hospital based or in a physician-directed free-standing clinic. The purpose of this chapter is to outline and discuss the main points that need to be considered in planning a phase II program. These include patient eligibility, equipment and facility, personnel, entering the program, the exercise routine, patient monitoring, adaptation to training, untoward events, emergency procedures, advancement to long-term exercise, nonhospital-based programs, motivation and adherence, education, and life-style modification.

PATIENT ELIGIBILITY

Entrance into phase II requires a written physician referral. Patients are generally eligible if they have any of the following diagnoses:

1. documented myocardial infarction (MI)
2. coronary artery bypass surgery or angioplasty
3. stable angina pectoris

Patients with elevated risk factors can also

benefit from a structured program that is supervised and monitored. Although occasionally approved for reimbursement, preventive programs are generally paid out of pocket.

EQUIPMENT AND FACILITY

Equipment and facilities are discussed in detail in Chapters 7 and 11. Specific equipment that is recommended for phase II includes the following:

1. exercise devices that utilize upper and lower extremities
2. electrocardiogram monitoring equipment, either telemetry or hard wire
3. stress testing equipment for patient evaluation
4. emergency apparatus such as defibrillator, medications, oxygen, suction, and other items required for resuscitation

The exercise facility must provide sufficient space for patients to exercise comfortably and be closely supervised. Approximately 100 square feet of space is recommended for each patient in the class. If the program is designed to accommodate eight patients in an exercise class, then approximately 800 square feet of floor space is needed. Although a larger room may appear impressive to the casual observer, the ability of the staff to supervise closely could be impaired. The facility should be pleasing to the eye and environmentally controlled. Additional space should be allocated for offices, dressing and shower rooms, and education and life-style management classes.

PERSONNEL

The number of staff and their professional expertise is determined by the size and scope of the program. The most important member of the staff is the coronary-trained nurse, who is responsible for reading and interpreting ECGs and responding to any emergency. Usually, this is an RN with appropriate training, although other professionals who have undergone proper training can be used. This person should also be capable of communicating effectively with physicians, taking the lead in emergencies, and leading patient education and life-style management classes. As a general rule, one nurse handles up to four patients per exercise class.

An exercise specialist is a valuable addition to the nurse in order to ensure that the patient is exercising correctly and to answer questions that arise concerning home exercise. The exercise specialist is usually involved in exercise testing, exercise prescription, and life-style classes. In some programs a physical therapist assumes the role of exercise specialist.

The medical director or other physician assigned to the program can make a significant contribution just by being present. Although generally not in direct supervision of the exercise class, the physician must be immediately available to assist with emergencies. All nonphysician personnel are under the direct supervision of the physician who should have a reasonable understanding of exercise physiology and be well trained in cardiology.

Additional staff for phase II include professionals for education and behavior modification (e.g., nutritionists, psychologists, social workers, etc.). Student interns, volunteers familiar with leading exercise, and the patients themselves can also be utilized. Patients who serve as exercise leaders help to enhance self-confidence in new patients, who can thus visualize the amount of progress that they can make. Other support staff are discussed in Chapters 7 and 10. It is suggested that all members of the staff be certified in basic cardiopulmonary resuscitation (CPR) and have regular practice sessions for emergency procedures. Those responsible for patient monitoring should be certified in advanced cardiac life support (ACLS).

ENTERING THE PROGRAM

Entrance into phase II necessitates a comprehensive evaluation that consists of medical and life-style history, physical examination, laboratory blood tests, physical fitness assessment, and an exercise stress test. These are discussed in detail in Chapters 3 to 5.

Orientation

Once referred, eligible patients and their family members or friends are invited to attend a patient orientation. The purpose of the orientation is to introduce the staff, show the facility, demonstrate the use of equipment, explain the procedures of exercise, discuss the financial requirements, and provide an opportunity for questions and answers. Orientation sessions may be conducted individually or in small groups. If possible it is desirable to show an exercise class in progress. The orientation should make the patient more comfortable with the program.

THE EXERCISE ROUTINE

A typical exercise routine consists of patient preparation, warm-up, exercise training, cool-down, and relaxation.

Patient Preparation

Before coming to class the patient is given a list of preexercise instructions (Table 13–1). At the beginning of the session, the patient is taught to properly cleanse the appropriate area of the skin for electrodes (Fig. 13–1). After the electrodes are self-applied, the patient usually weighs in and responds to a series of questions from the nurse. A resting heart rate, blood pressure, and ECG rhythm strip are obtained. The patient is now ready to begin the warm-up.

Warm-up

A thorough warm-up is necessary at the beginning of each exercise training session.

Table 13–1. Patient Instructions Before Exercise

1. Do not eat a large meal at least 2 hours prior to the exercise session. A small snack is fine.
2. Alcohol should not be consumed before exercise.
3. Do not drink beverages with caffeine, i.e., coffee, tea, coke, etc., at least 2 hours prior to exercise.
4. Do not smoke at least 1 hour prior to exercise.
5. Wear comfortable clothing to exercise, i.e., gym shorts, loose-fitting slacks, sneakers, socks, loose-fitting blouse or shirt, etc.
6. Please be prompt! Try to arrive 10 to 15 minutes prior to the scheduled time of the exercise class in order to get ready.
7. If you experience any unaccustomed symptoms of pain, discomfort, or soreness, let the nurse know before starting to exercise.
8. Inform the nurse of any changes in medications before exercising.
9. Bring a lock to the class to secure your valuables.

The benefits of the warm-up have been well studied and reviewed.[4,6,7] Physiologically, the purpose is to increase circulation, thereby augmenting oxygen delivery to needed muscle tissue; improve flexibility; and elevate body temperature. As muscle

Electrode Attachments

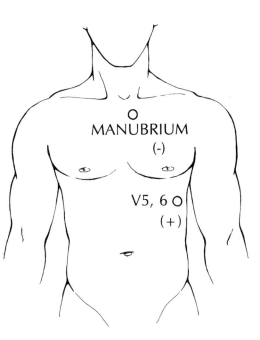

Fig. 13–1. Electrode attachments.

temperature rises, its viscosity is decreased and efficiency of contraction is increased.[8,9] Warm-up also reduces the potential for muscle pulls and musculoskeletal injury.

The warm-up should also concentrate on muscle groups with specific weaknesses; for example hip flexibility and abdominal-strengthening exercises are helpful to prevent injuries of the lower back, the most common disabling orthopedic problem in adults.[8,10] In addition proceeding with strenuous exertion without adequate warm-up increases the incidence of myocardial ischemias.[11,12] This might be attributable to myocardial demands increasing more rapidly than oxygen is supplied[13] and could precipitate angina pectoris or an MI. Increasing coronary circulation through a gradual progression of effort reduces this possibility.[7,11,12] Therefore, the value of warm-up has implications for preventing myocardial damage as well as musculoskeletal injury. A sample of warm-up activities is provided in Figure 13–2.

Exercise Training

The goal is to exercise at a sufficient target heart rate to attain a training threshold. The target heart rate and workout schedule are provided on an exercise prescription card (Fig. 13–3), which is given to the patient at each session. The intensity of effort should be increased gradually until this level is attained. The heart rate should be maintained for the duration of the session (continuous training), or interspersed with brief periods of rest (intermittent training). With intermittent training more work is possible at a higher heart rate and the same amount of work can be performed with less exertion, because the rest period between bouts of exercise allows time for metabolic waste products to be eliminated.[8,10] Table 13–2 lists heart rate, oxygen uptake, pulmonary ventilation, and blood lactate responses during continuous and intermittent training.

Dynamic–rhythmic and aerobic activities are emphasized. Exercises are designed to incorporate upper and lower extremity muscle groups, using, for example, the bicycle ergometer, arm ergometer, treadmill, wall-pulley, steps, arm crank, and rowing machine. The patient usually exercises 5 to 10 minutes on these different modalities, with 1 minute between devices.

Cool-Down

It is important to taper off gradually following exercise. The supply of energy reserves must be replenished and waste by-products of metabolism need to be removed.

Sufficient cardiac output following exercise needs to be maintained. This is accomplished by enhanced venous return due to the massaging action of contracting and relaxing muscles on the veins, thereby increasing stroke volume in accordance with the Frank-Starling Principle.[9,14] When vigorous exercise is suddenly terminated, particularly if the person remains upright, there is a tendency for blood to pool in the lower extremities, which results in reduced return to the heart. The concomitant effect is elevated heart rate and increased myocardial oxygen demand ($M\dot{V}O_2$). Hypotension, decreased blood flow to the brain and accompanying light-headedness, dizziness, or fainting are other possible results. Maintaining adequate circulation also enhances removal of metabolic wastes, especially lactic acid, and reduces the possibility of muscle soreness subsequent to exercise.[9,15]

During cool-down, physical activity is continued at a low level of effort. In particular it is advisable to continue to exercise those muscles that were utilized during training in order to pump the lactic acid from these areas. Movement of large muscle groups is particularly beneficial to maximize the massaging action and to maintain adequate systemic circulation.

PROGRESSION OF THE PATIENT

The patient is advanced throughout phase II as adaptation to exercise occurs.

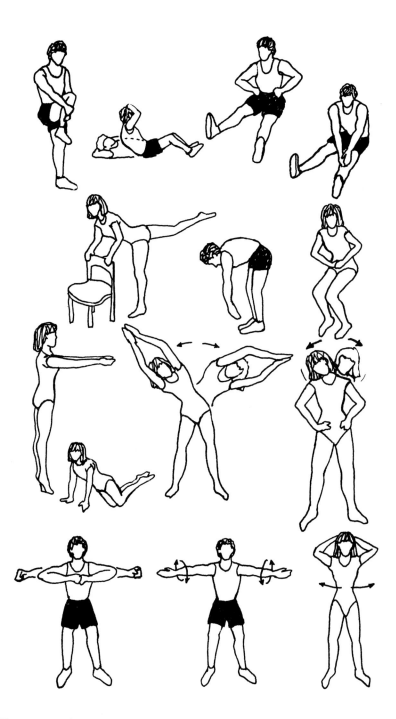

Fig. 13–2.   Warm-up exercises.

Name_____
                Last   First

Target Heart Rate_____

Device and Order	Work Load	Adjusted Work Load

Fig. 13–3. Exercise Prescription Card.

The rate of progression is tied to the rate of improvement. Although evaluated on an individual basis, the average patient is reviewed for an increase in the target heart rate at the end of each 4 weeks. Typically, the heart rate prescription is increased by 5%. Therefore, if the patient starts the exercise program at 75% of maximal heart rate, it would be increased to 80% at the fifth week and to 85% at the ninth week. Increases in work loads occur whenever it is necessary to elevate the heart rate to attain the desired target.

RELAXATION TECHNIQUES

Relaxation exercises can be effective at the end of cool-down[16] and have been observed to reduce heart rate, blood pressure, and cardiac arrhythmias.[17–20] Relaxation should be initiated after sufficient cool-down because lying down postexercise may increase $M\dot{V}O_2$ via the LaPlace relationship.

Relaxation techniques are particularly valuable for individuals who find it difficult to slow down. Too often the hectic pace of

Table 13–2. Physiologic Responses to Intermittent Training and Continuous Training[a]

Type of Exercise		Oxygen Uptake (liters/min)	Pulmonary Ventilation (liters/min)	Heart Rate (beats/min)	Blood Lactic Acid (mg/100 ml)
Continuous 2160 kpm/min		4.60	124	190	150
Intermittent 2160 kpm/min					
Work	Rest				
½ min	½ min	2.90	63	150	20
1 min	1 min	2.93	65	167	45
2 min	2 min	4.40	95	178	95
3 min	3 min	4.60	107	188	120

[a]Adapted from Åstrand, P.O., and Rodahl, K.: Textbook of Work Physiology. New York, McGraw-Hill, 1970.

the day is carried over into the training session. Typically, such individuals rush into the exercise session, often late, try to hurry through the class, rush to the shower and on to the next appointment without ever taking a moment to slow down. One questions whether any benefit is being derived for those who approach exercise in this manner. Relaxation exercises ensure at least a brief respite from such frantic activity. These exercises should be encouraged at other times of the day and might also be helpful to improve sleep habits. Instructions for relaxation exercises are provided in Table 13–3. The basic technique is to concentrate on breathing while alternating contraction and relaxation of muscle groups.

PATIENT MONITORING

Electrocardiogram monitoring is considered an important adjunct to patient safety in most cardiac rehabilitation centers. However, not all programs believe that continual monitoring is necessary for all patients. Consequently, several questions need to be addressed: Is ECG monitoring necessary in phase II of cardiac rehabilitation? Do all patients need to be moni-

Table 13–3. Instructions for Relaxation Exercises

1. Close eyes and relax (in a supine position)
2. Take a deep breath . . . . and relax. Concentrate on your breathing. Allow 10 to 15 sec between commands.
3. Again, a deep breath . . . . and relax.
4. Now, contract the muscles in one arm (either one) . . . . and relax.
5. Repeat with opposite arm.
6. Contract the muscle in one leg . . . . and relax.
7. Repeat with opposite leg.
8. Now contract the muscles of an arm and the leg of the opposite side . . . . and relax.
9. Repeat with other arm and leg.[a]

[a]Initially, an assistant might check that the muscles are being completely relaxed. If they are, one should be able to lift the designated limb with no muscular resistance.

tored? For how long should monitoring be continued? Is ECG monitoring more necessary with certain modes of exercise than others?

The current clinical opinion favors continual ECG monitoring for all cardiac patients who enter into vigorous exercise programs soon after discharge from the hospital. The rationale for this is that patients adhere better to the heart rate prescription, they are less anxious and apprehensive about exercising, and program safety is better ensured through the increased likelihood of detecting arrhythmias.[21–23] Table 13–4 illustrates the frequency of significant arrhythmias that occurred during a 12-week phase II program.[24] In this instance significant arrhythmias were defined as ventricular tachycardia, ventricular bigeminy or trigeminy, ventricular coupling, and more than five ventricular contractions per minute.[24]

These data are similar to findings reported elsewhere.[22] In this study[24] significant arrhythmias were detected in 50% of the patient population during the 12-week program compared to 12% during stress testing. Although the frequency of significant arrhythmias decreased in weeks 8 to 12, 13% of the total population experienced new events during this time. Clearly, most patients with significant arrhythmias were detected during the initial 7 weeks of the program, although a sufficiently large number were observed after week 7 to warrant monitoring for the entire 12 weeks. It is interesting to note that at least one new patient each week exhibited a new, significant arrhythmia. On the basis of these results, ECG monitoring is recommended for at least 7 weeks and can be justified for as long as 12 weeks.

Electrocardiogram monitoring is also recommended whenever the exercise prescription is increased. Having the patient exercise while being monitored, even if only for two to four sessions, enhances program safety. Short-term monitoring is also recommended for patients who are unable

Table 13–4. Frequency of Significant Arrhythmias During 12-Week, Phase II, Monitored Exercise

Week of Program	Total Patients With Significant Arrhythmias	New Patients With Significant Arrhythmias
1	14	14
2	15	8
3	15	5
4	14	8
5	18	6
6	18	2
7	18	5
8	13	1
9	10	1
10	18	3
11	12	1
12	13	1

Data from Fardy, P.S., Doll, N., and Williams, M.: Monitoring cardiac patients: How much is enough? Physician Sportsmed., *10*:146, 1982.

to participate in phase II exercise due to logistical problems. These patients can then be provided with safer guidelines to continue exercise in a home-based program. Careful self-monitoring is taught, although this approach is limited by the fact that contraindicating signs may appear at levels of exercise that are asymptomatic and thereby go undetected.[22,25]

Electrocardiogram monitoring is also useful for patients with a history of frequent, complex multiform ventricular arrhythmias. Monitoring of these patients during phase II exercise is an effective and relatively inexpensive procedure for assessing medication effectiveness as compared to serial exercise testing or Holter monitoring.[22,26,27] Monitoring can also help to determine if arrhythmias occur at a heart rate threshold and if they occur more frequently with certain types of activities.

Although there are phase II exercise programs that are unmonitored or have reduced monitoring in the latter stages of the program, the data from Table 13–4 indicate that all patients should be monitored for at least some period of time. Probably, 7 weeks is a minimal recommendation. In further support of patient monitoring is evidence that no fatal events have occurred in continually monitored programs of 352,000 and 888,460 patient hours of experience.[28,29] Perhaps unmonitored programs are less aggressive, have patients with lower risk, or do not enroll patients into the program as quickly.

ADAPTATION TO TRAINING

Some of the most important information used to assess patient progress is available from records of the exercise sessions. For this reason equipment with quantifiable work loads is strongly urged in order that progress can be documented (Fig. 13–4) and explained objectively to the patient. Periodic updates of the exercise prescription and patient feedback are valuable to provide information and motivation.

In noncardiacs training adaptation may begin to be evident in as few as 4 to 6 weeks, although some changes may take considerably longer to occur.[30] The rate and magnitude of change can vary considerably among individuals, with some persons exhibiting improvement quickly, while in others the process may be much slower. The amount of damage to the myocardium also affects the rate of improvement. Patients with normally functioning ventricles have a significantly better chance to improve

Name_____ Date _____Target Heart Rate_____
           Last   First

Have you had any health problems since your last exercise session? _____

Have you taken your medication today? Yes_____ No_____

Have there been any medication changes? Yes_____ No_____

Resting Heart Rate_____   DEVICES: A = Arm Ergometer
Resting Blood Pressure_____/_____   B = Bicycle
Recovery Blood Pressure_____/_____   R = Rowing Machine
                                                                 S = Step
                                                                 T = Treadmill

EXERCISE DATA

Order	Exercise Device	Work Load	ECG Changes	Signs and Symptoms	Exercise Heart Rate	Recovery Heart Rate
0.	Warm-Up					
1.						
2.						
3.						
4.						
5.						
6.						
7.	Relax					

Average Exercise Heart Rate_____

Comments:_____
_____
_____

Fig. 13–4. Exercise Training Session.

compared with those with ventricular dysfunction.[31] Finally, infarct and bypass surgical patients seem to adapt to exercise similarly.[32]

UNTOWARD EVENTS

The chance of life-threatening untoward events occurring in phase II is small.[23,28,29] Proper medical supervision, continual patient monitoring, individualized exercise prescription, adhering to correct guidelines for exercise, and having the necessary equipment and supplies to deal with untoward events all help to promote a safe program. Untoward events may be further reduced by teaching patients to monitor themselves. Since physical exertion can be perceived accurately, it is possible to gauge the correct intensity of exercise.[33–35] However, subjective feelings alone may not accurately reflect hemodynamic events. Asymptomatic abnormalities might occur even though the level of exertion is perceived as light.[22,25] Relying solely on subjective criteria could unnecessarily expose one to increased risk if exercise were continued when there was reason to stop. Potential untoward signs and symptoms are presented in Table 13–5.

Emergency Procedures

A plan for dealing with emergencies should be developed that describes procedures and routines for cardiorespiratory care, personnel assignments and responsibilities, plans for patient transfer and hospitalization, and other procedures that pertain to handling emergencies.

The entire staff should be certified in basic CPR, and in the case of the freestanding facility, at least one staff person should be available at all times who is certified in ACLS.

Unless a physician is present for all exercise sessions, the cardiac rehabilitation nurse is designated as team leader during emergencies. The nurse's responsibility is to assist in the emergency and determine a plan of action. Standing physician orders should be available (Fig. 13–5).

In the case of an emergency, someone is designated responsible to monitor and record continuous ECG tracings, notify the medical director, and call a medical code. The patients are instructed to leave the training room to a station where they are supervised by other members of the cardiac rehabilitation staff. The team leader is responsible to see that the following steps are performed: CPR, possible defibrillation, setting up an intravenous infusion, inserting an airway if needed, providing oxygen, and preparing medications until the arrival of the physician. Immediately after the initial care, the personal physician should be contacted if possible. The patient is transferred to the emergency room at the discretion of the physician responding to the emergency call. The medical director or cardiac rehabilitation nurse is responsible for scheduling periodic reviews of emergency procedures including mock calls. Emergency procedures are outlined by the American College of Sports Medicine (ACSM).[36]

ADVANCEMENT TO LONG-TERM EXERCISE

Exit from phase II should signal the beginning of a long-term commitment to exercise for the patient. At this time the uncomplicated MI or coronary artery bypass surgery patient needs to be reassured that return to a normal life-style is within reach. The patient must be made to understand that regular exercise and life-style management are necessary in order to sustain the improvements that have been started. Before the patient advances to more strenuous exercise, a clinical decision must be made that the patient is ready. Most pro-

Table 13–5. Common Untoward Signs and Symptoms During and Following Exercise[a]

During Exercise	Following Exercise
Angina pectoris	Insomnia
Chest discomfort	Excessive excitement
Skipped beats	Exhilaration
Excessive dyspnea	Weakness
Uncoordination	Fatigue
Lightheadedness	Muscular cramping
Faintness	Skeletal muscular pain
Syncope	Gastrointestinal disturbances
Cold sweat	Nausea
Undue muscle soreness	Vomiting
Fatigue	

[a]Based on Hellerstein, H.K., et al.: Principles of exercise prescription: For normals and cardiac subjects. *In* Exercise Testing and Exercise Training in Coronary Heart Disease. Edited by J.P. Naughton, H.K. Hellerstein, and I.C. Mohler. Orlando, Fla., Academic Press, 1973.

8/84 R9/84
9/86 2/87

1. FIRST NURSE (The role of the "First Nurse" is crucial in achieving ultimate patient survival.)
   a. Open airway
   b. Insert Oral Airway
   c. Begin bag-to-mouth breathing (4 breaths), using STAT Blue Resuscitation Bag.
   d. Feel for Carotid Pulse—If Absent:
      (1) Immediately, begin Cardiac Massage—15 Compressions—2 Breaths (at the rate of 80 Compressions/Minute).
   e. Call for Help
   f. If return of pulse, breathing, and consciousness:
      (1) Notify Physician
      (2) Medic Cart to Room
      (3) Continue Assessment
   g. If no pulse, no breathing, and unconscious, continue CPR. . . .

2. SECOND NURSE
   a. Dial 11 and announce "MEDIC"—area, room number and attending physician. Speak slowly and distinctly.
   b. Take area medic cart to room
   c. Assist first nurse with breathing or massage. With 2 rescuers, the compression rate is maintained at 80/minute giving 1 breath between 5th and 6th compression (approximately 10–12 breaths/minute).
   d. Assist therapist with airway, suction oxygen 100%.
   e. Roll patient onto compression board (from area's Medic Cart).

3. AREA NURSE
   a. Stay in room to describe events leading to arrest.

4.   SUPERVISOR

   | 1. Verify "MEDIC" announced |
   | 2. Chart to room |
   | 3. Page attending M.D. STAT |
   | 4. Isolate other patients |
   | 5. Direct and control traffic |
   | 6. Obtain extra supplies/equipment |
   | 7. Maintain records |

ALS NURSE: Nurses with advanced life support training as required in their work area (i.e., 2W, 2E, ICU, CCU, ED, PACU, CARDIAC REHAB). Upon physician arrival, assists with intubation, drug administration, emergency pacing, etc.

Fig. 13–5. Physician's Order Sheet.

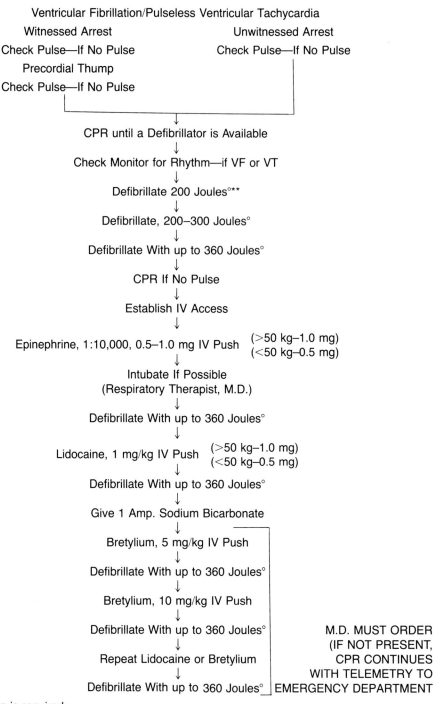

Ventricular Fibrillation/Pulseless Ventricular Tachycardia

Witnessed Arrest	Unwitnessed Arrest
Check Pulse—If No Pulse	Check Pulse—If No Pulse
Precordial Thump	
Check Pulse—If No Pulse	

CPR until a Defibrillator is Available
↓
Check Monitor for Rhythm—if VF or VT
↓
Defibrillate 200 Joules°**
↓
Defibrillate, 200–300 Joules°
↓
Defibrillate With up to 360 Joules°
↓
CPR If No Pulse
↓
Establish IV Access
↓
Epinephrine, 1:10,000, 0.5–1.0 mg IV Push   (>50 kg–1.0 mg) (<50 kg–0.5 mg)
↓
Intubate If Possible
(Respiratory Therapist, M.D.)
↓
Defibrillate With up to 360 Joules°
↓
Lidocaine, 1 mg/kg IV Push   (>50 kg–1.0 mg) (<50 kg–0.5 mg)
↓
Defibrillate With up to 360 Joules°
↓
Give 1 Amp. Sodium Bicarbonate
↓
Bretylium, 5 mg/kg IV Push
↓
Defibrillate With up to 360 Joules°
↓
Bretylium, 10 mg/kg IV Push
↓
Defibrillate With up to 360 Joules°
↓
Repeat Lidocaine or Bretylium
↓
Defibrillate With up to 360 Joules°

M.D. MUST ORDER
(IF NOT PRESENT,
CPR CONTINUES
WITH TELEMETRY TO
EMERGENCY DEPARTMENT

**If defibrillation is required:
  (1) Apply paste to paddles, set at 200.
  (2) WHILE THE DEFIBRILLATOR IS BEING CHARTED, the person to execute defibrillation announces: "Ready to Defibrillate."
  (3) Just prior to defibrillation, this person announces, "Everybody back" or "Everybody off" while visually checking to see no one is in danger of receiving a shock.
  (4) A 5 second wait should be made between the two calls to assure everyone has had time to get back. Remember, the person who holds the paddles is responsible for the safety of others at the bedside.
  CAUTION: Oxygen running to the patient to be defibrillated must be removed from patient immediately prior to administering the shock. After the shock is given, oxygen may be resumed.

Fig. 13–5. Physician's Order Sheet (Continued).

Ventricular Fibrillation
Ventricular Tachycardia

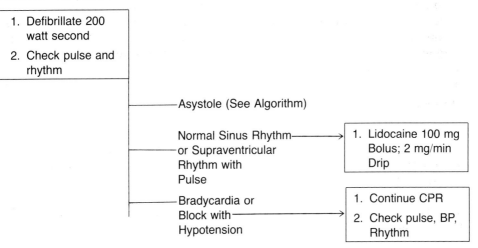

ASYSTOLE (Cardiac Standstill)

ASYSTOLE (CARDIAC STANDSTILL)

If Rhythm is Unclear and Possibly Ventricular

Fibrillation, Defibrillate as for VF. If Asystole is Present

Continue CPR

Establish IV Access

Epinephrine, 1:10,000 0.5–1.0 mg IV Push   (>50 kg–1.0 mg)
(<50 kg–0.5 mg)

Intubate When Possible
(Respiratory Therapist/MD)
Give 1 Amp. Sodium Bicarbonate
Atropine, 1.0 mg IV Push (Repeated in 5 min.)   MD. MUST ORDER,
IF PRESENT, CPR
Consider Pacing   CONTINUES WITH
TELEMETRY TO
EMERGENCY
DEPARTMENT

NSR or Supraventricular
Rhythm with Pulse

1. Check Pulse,
   BP, Rhythm

Bradycardia or Block with
Hypotention (Rate <50, BP
<90 Systolic)

1. Continue CPR
2. Check pulse, BP,
   rhythm

Fig. 13–5. Physician's Order Sheet (Continued).

grams have an exit criterion for allowing patients to advance to phase III and phase IV.[2] The medical director must also assess other clinical parameters before making decisions on the patient's capacity for outside activities, returning to work, driving, sexual activity, and so on.

The long-term program usually is conducted at a community site suitable for large numbers, for example, a YMCA, Jewish Community Center (JCC), university, or public school gymnasium. The alternative is for the patient to continue exercising in an unsupervised setting. This may be less desirable than a supervised program but is sometimes necessary because of logistic problems and other considerations. Telephonic electrocardiography can be used to make home programs more safe and effective.[37] Patients in unsupervised programs should be reevaluated periodically to assess their progress and update the exercise prescription. Long-term programs are discussed in detail in Chapter 14.

NONHOSPITAL-BASED PROGRAMS

Physician-directed, freestanding facilities have become a viable alternative to hospital-based phase II programs. These programs are generally similar to hospital-based centers in facility design, equipment, and personnel. The advantages of the freestanding facility are more economical management and that it provides a financial incentive to physician-owners, making them more likely to refer patients. Conduct of the program is similar whether hospital based or freestanding.

An option to both the hospital-based and freestanding facility is to exercise at home. In the case of a home exercise program, the patient needs careful instructions and guidelines. The patient must be taught how to exercise, accurately monitor the heart rate, recognize untoward signs and symptoms, and understand the benefits of exercise. A schedule should be developed so that the patient periodically returns to the exercise center to be evaluated and progressed appropriately.

The home program can be made simpler and safer if telephone ECG is utilized when applicable. With this equipment real-time ECGs or 1 or 2 minutes of taped ECGs are obtained and transmitted by a standard telephone to the cardiac rehabilitation center. Some of the real-time ECG transmission systems place restrictions on activity, time of transmission, and possibly clarity of the ECG. These systems are illustrated in Chapter 11.

In deciding on the advisability of a home-based program, the benefits of group dynamics in the supervised and monitored setting must be weighed against those factors that make a supervised program less feasible. It is also important that the patient's physician render a clinical judgment as to whether a home-based program would be safe. A miniprogram that is hospital based and up to 2 weeks in duration is suggested as a way to obtain information about the patient prior to deciding on the safety of a home program. This also provides the staff with an opportunity to become more familiar with the patient, give the patient the best exercise prescription, increase the patient's confidence and to allay anxieties toward nonsupervised exercise.

MOTIVATION AND ADHERENCE

One measure of the success of a program is adherence. Therefore, attendance should be carefully documented (Fig. 13–6). For adherence to be good, the patients must enjoy the activities and be shown that their efforts are deriving benefit. The exercise leader needs to be enthusiastic, innovative, provide diversification of activity and show that the program is effective. The cardiac rehabilitation nurse must be attentive to patients, provide them with advice and encouragement, and respond to their questions when possible. The nurse must encourage the patient to

Name_____
　　　　　Last　　　　　　　　First

SECTION I Month_____   Month_____

1	2	3	4	5	6	7
8	9	10	11	12	13	14
15	16	17	18	19	20	21
22	23	24	25	26	27	28
29	30	31				

1	2	3	4	5	6	7
8	9	10	11	12	13	14
15	16	17	18	19	20	21
22	23	24	25	26	27	28
29	30	31				

Reasons for absence:_____

Evaluation Date_____

SECTION II Month_____   Month_____

1	2	3	4	5	6	7
8	9	10	11	12	13	14
15	16	17	18	19	20	21
22	23	24	25	26	27	28
29	30	31				

1	2	3	4	5	6	7
8	9	10	11	12	13	14
15	16	17	18	19	20	21
22	23	24	25	26	27	28
29	30	31				

Evaluation Date_____

SECTION III Month_____   Month_____

1	2	3	4	5	6	7
8	9	10	11	12	13	14
15	16	17	18	19	20	21
22	23	24	25	26	27	28
29	30	31				

1	2	3	4	5	6	7
8	9	10	11	12	13	14
15	16	17	18	19	20	21
22	23	24	25	26	27	28
29	30	31				

Evaluation Date_____

Fig. 13–6.　Phase II Attendance Record.

make a lifetime commitment to a healthier life-style.

Motivation plays a key role in adherence. One of the most powerful motivators for persons with a recent cardiac event is likely to be fear of death or of being a "cardiac cripple." As the patient recuperates, the quality of the rehabilitation program assumes a greater importance, that is, the quality of leadership, the social aspects of group participation, and the recognition of improvement.[38,39] Therefore, it is necessary to provide adequate feedback to the patients and encourage group interaction. The latter can be enhanced by planning occasional social events.

Keep in mind that exercise is not easy for most persons. A few are disciplined well enough to exercise by themselves, although most persons find it easier to be in a group[39,40] where they can share the joy and hard work of becoming fit. Motivation and adherence are discussed in greater detail in Chapter 14.

EDUCATION AND LIFE-STYLE MODIFICATION

Although the emphasis of phase II is physical activity, education and life-style management are also important. These need to be part of an ongoing process that includes classes for individuals and groups. Particular attention is given to involve significant family members and friends. Education and life-style programs are generally coordinated by the cardiac rehabilitation nurse, although other professionals should be actively involved, for example, the nutritionist, psychologist, social worker, exercise specialist, occupational therapist, physical therapist, and so on. Education and life-style modification- are covered in depth in Chapter 15.

CONCLUSIONS

Phase II should be the beginning of a program of vigorous physical activity and life-style modification. Good planning, equipment, and facilities are important, although the quality of the staff is the most important factor. It is essential for staff to emphasize from the beginning of phase II that this exercise program is only the start of a life-time commitment. If cardiac rehabilitation is considered "over" at the conclusion of phase II, then it will have been largely a waste of time.

REFERENCES

1. Pollock, M.L.: The quantification of endurance training programs. *In* Exercise and Sport Science Reviews. Vol. 1. Edited by J.H. Wilmore. Orlando, Fla., Academic Press, 1973.
2. Pollock, M.L., Pels, A.E., III, Foster, C., and Ward, A.: Exercise prescription for rehabilitation of the cardiac patient. *In* Heart Disease and Rehabilitation. 2nd Ed. Edited by M.L. Pollock and D.H. Schmidt. New York, John Wiley & Sons, 1986.
3. Pollock, M.L., Wilmore, J.H., and Fox, S.M.: Exercise in Health and Disease: Evaluation and Prescription for Prevention and Rehabilitation. Philadelphia, W.B. Saunders, 1984.
4. Franklin, B.A., Hellerstein, H.K., Gordon, S., and Timmis, G.: Exercise prescription for the myo-
cardial infarction patient. J. Cardiopul. Rehabil., 6:62, 1986.
5. Metier, C.P., Pollock, M.L., and Graves, J.E.: Exercise prescription for the coronary artery bypass graft surgery patient. J. Cardiopul. Rehabil., 6:85, 1986.
6. Franks, B.D.: Physical warm-up. *In* An Analysis and Evaluation of Modern Trends Related to the Physiological Factors for Optimal Sports Performance. Claremont, California, National Coaches Conference, 1976.
7. Foster, C., Dymond, D.S., Carpenter, J., and Schmidt, D.H.: Effect of warm-up on left ventricular response to sudden strenuous exercise. J. Appl. Physiol., 53:380, 1982.
8. Åstrand, P.O., and Rodahl, K.: Textbook of Work Physiology. 2nd Ed. New York, McGraw-Hill, 1977.
9. McArdle, W.D., Katch, F.I., and Katch, V.L.: Exercise Physiology: Energy, Nutrition, and Human Performance. Philadelphia, Lea & Febiger, 1986.
10. Kraus, H., and Raab, W.: Hypokinetic Disease. Springfield, Ill., Charles C Thomas, 1961.
11. Barnard, R.J., et al.: Cardiovascular response to sudden strenuous exercise-heart rate, blood pressure and ECG. J. Appl. Physiol., 34:833, 1973.
12. Barnard, R.J., et al.: Ischemic response to sudden strenuous exercise in healthy man. Circulation, 5:936, 1973.
13. Fardy, P.S., and Hellerstein, H.K.: A comparison of continuous and intermittent multi-stage exercise tests. Med. Sci. Sports, 10:7, 1978.
14. Morehouse, L.E., and Miller, A.T.: Physiology of Exercise. St. Louis, C.V. Mosby, 1971.
15. de Vries, H.: Physiology of Exercise for Physical Education and Athletics. Dubuque, Iowa, William C. Brown, 1966.
16. Fardy, P.S., et al.: Objectives and Procedures for Developing a Cardiac Rehabilitation Program. East Chicago, Ind., St. Catherine Hospital, 1978.
17. Benson, H., Alexander, S., and Feldman, C.L.: Decreased premature ventricular contractions through the use of relaxation response in patients with stable ischemic heart disease. Lancet, 2:380, 1975.
18. Benson, H., et al.: Decreased blood pressure in borderline hypertensive subjects who practice meditation. J. Chron. Dis., 27:163,1974.
19. Benson, H., et al.: Decreased blood pressure in pharmacologically tested hypertensive patients who regularly elicited the relaxation response. Lancet, 1:289, 1974.
20. Patel, C.: Twelve month follow-up of yoga and biofeedback in the management of hypertension. Lancet, 1:62, 1975.
21. Report of the Coronary Drug Project Research Group: The prognostic importance of ventricular premature beats following myocardial infarction. Experience in the Coronary Drug Project. JAMA, 223:1116, 1973.
22. Franklin, B.A.: The role of electrocardiographic monitoring in cardiac exercise programs. J. Cardiac Rehabil., 3:806, 1983.
23. Meyer, G.C.: Telemetry Electrocardiographic Monitoring in Cardiac Rehabilitation: How long?

How often? *In* Cardiac Rehabilitation: Exercise Testing and Prescription. Edited by L.K. Hall. Jamaica, N.Y., Spectrum, 1984.

24. Fardy, P.S., Doll, N., and Williams, M.: Monitoring cardiac patients: How much is enough? Physician Sportsmed., *10*:146, 1982.

25. Williams, M.A., and Fardy, P.S.: Limitations in prescribing exercise. Cardiovasc. Pulmon. Technique, *8*:33, 1980.

26. Ryan, M., Lown, B., and Horn, H.: Comparison of ventricular ectopic activity during 24 hour monitoring and exercise testing in patients with coronary heart disease. N. Engl. J. Med, *292*:224, 1975.

27. Simoons, M., Lap, C., and Pool, J.: Heart rate levels and ventricular ectopic activity during cardiac rehabilitation. Am. Heart J., *100*:9, 1980.

28. Haskell, W.L.: Cardiovascular complications during exercise training of cardiac patients. Circulation, *57*:920, 1978.

29. Van Camp, S.P., and Peterson, R.A.: Cardiovascular complications of outpatient cardiac rehabilitation programs. JAMA, *256*:1160, 1986.

30. Pollock, M.L.: The quantification of endurance training programs. *In* Exercise and Sport Sciences Reviews. Vol 1. Edited by J.H. Wilmore. Orlando, Fla., Academic Press, 1973.

31. Timmons, D.R.: Patients at increased risk of reinfarction and death after myocardial infarction. *In* Cardiac Rehabilitation: Exercise Testing and Prescription. Edited by I.K. Hall, Jamaica, N.Y., Spectrum, 1984.

32. Fardy, P.S., et al.: A comparison of changes between post myocardial infarct and post bypass surgical patients following three months exercise training. Med. Sci. Sports, *11*:101, 1979.

33. Borg, G.: The perception of physical performance. *In* Frontiers of Fitness. Edited by R.J. Shephard. Springfield, Ill., Charles C Thomas, 1971.

34. Noble, B.J., et al.: Perceived exertion during walking and running II. Med. Sci. Sports, *5*:116, 1973.

35. Borg, G.A.: Perceived exertion: A note on "history" and methods. Med. Sci. Sports, *5*:90, 1973.

36. American College of Sports Medicine: Guidelines for Exercise Testing and Prescription. 3rd Ed. Philadelphia, Lea & Febiger, 1986.

37. Pratt, C.M., et al.: Clinical benefits of transtelephonic ECG transmission to monitor home exercise programs in coronary heart disease patients. Med. Sci. Sports Exerc., *15*:120, 1983.

38. Heinzelmann, F.: Social and psychological factors that influence the effectiveness of exercise programs. *In* Exercise Testing and Exercise Training in Coronary Heart Disease. Edited by J.P. Naughton, H.K. Hellerstein, and I.C. Mohler. Orlando, Fla., Academic Press, 1973.

39. Franklin, B.A.: Motivating and educating adults to exercise. JOPER, June:13, 1978.

40. Golding, L.A.: Programs of exercise-program organization. *In* Exercise and the Heart. Edited by R.L. Morse. Springfield, Ill., Charles C Thomas, 1972.

.

14

PHASE III AND IV
AND ADULT FITNESS

Chapter 13 discusses the monitored exercise program that is recommended for cardiac patients following discharge from the hospital (phase II). Although phase II is essential to restore the patient physiologically and psychologically, it is only a prelude to a lifetime commitment to regular exercise and life-style management. This chapter focuses on long-term programs, either cardiac rehabilitation or adult fitness. Table 14–1 outlines the topics discussed.

TYPES OF PROGRAMS

The long-term programs in cardiac rehabilitation are called phases III and IV. Phase III is usually a supervised and intermittently monitored program that immediately follows phase II and lasts 6 months to 2 years. The goal of phase III is continued improvement in physical fitness. Phase IV is an ongoing program of

Table 14–1. Outline of the Chapter

Types of programs
Objectives of long-term programs
Equipment and facility needs
Professional personnel
Exercise training session
Motivation and compliance
Home-based programs
Factors that influence exercise
Potential risks of exercise
Individual progress

physical activity and fitness maintenance that follows phase III.

At the beginning of phase III, intermittent monitoring is suggested to maintain a close vigilance over complicated or at-risk patients. Since long-term exercise programs will also include individuals with no history of coronary disease (i.e., adult fitness), it is necessary to be familiar with each person's medical history. Intermittent monitoring is appropriate for phase III and can be accomplished either with telemetry, a standard electrocardiogram (ECG) recorder with monitor-scope, or defibrillator paddle monitoring.

With defibrillator paddle monitoring, the paddles serve as electrodes (Fig. 14–1) and enable recordings to be obtained quickly. Rapid determination of ECG tracings is extremely important, since even a 30-second delay can result in a significantly decreased heart rate, reduced myocardial oxygen demand, and less probability of significant ECG changes compared to the ECG at a higher heart rate. It is recommended that the equipment selected for patient monitoring have the capability for a 1 cm/mV calibration signal and 12-lead ECG to document abnormalities observed in paddle-obtained records. A 12-lead ECG is necessary to compare with standard hospital records. A single system possessing these capabilities is suggested. The disadvantage of the one-unit "see-through pad-

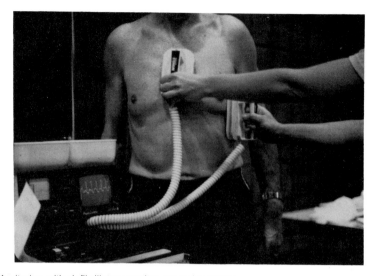

Fig. 14–1. Monitoring with defibrillator–monitor–recorder system.

dles" is that the defibrillator can cause burns if the surface of the paddles gets scratched, and the wires are more likely to break because of frequent use. However, if the equipment is used and stored properly, it is very unlikely that this would occur. Phases III and IV are staffed by professionals capable of recognizing and responding to emergency situations. These are discussed later.

Phase IV maintenance and adult fitness programs are generally nonmonitored and have fewer precautionary considerations than phases II and III, since those who exercise regularly at this level are usually at lower risk. Phase IV is usually supervised by persons trained in physical education. Exercise programs might also be conducted individually at home or at a convenient community location.

Although supervised exercise classes are recommended when possible, it is unrealistic to expect that they will always be available or convenient. Knowing how to exercise correctly is especially important when one is not in a supervised program. If possible, professional guidance should be sought at the beginning so that a safe and beneficial exercise prescription is followed. Guidelines for unsupervised exercise have been described elsewhere,[1–4] and are summarized in Table 14–2.

OBJECTIVES OF LONG-TERM EXERCISE

The objectives of long-term exercise programs are summarized in Table 14–3. After the successful completion of phase II, the patient advances to phase III, which can be conducted at home or in a supervised setting. At this time activities that reflect personal preference are emphasized as well as exercises that do not require special equipment. During phase III the ex-

Table 14–2. Guidelines for Unsupervised Exercise

1. A physical examination including an exercise test should precede vigorous physical activity. This is advisable for everyone and is essential for inactive persons over 40 years of age, those with diagnosed heart disease or risk factors, persons with a family history of premature heart disease, or those who have been sedentary for a long time.
2. Realistic training objectives should be formulated.
3. An exercise prescription should be developed to meet the individual's needs.
4. Exercise sessions should adhere to accepted principles of physical conditioning.
5. Periodic reassessment including upgrading the exercise prescription should follow.

Table 14–3. Objectives of Long-Term Exercise

★ Improved physical condition followed by maintenance
★ Reduction of coronary disease risk factors
★ Increased self-esteem and confidence as new activities are introduced and as the patient is weaned from a supervised–monitored environment
★ Introducing safe and enjoyable activities that may be performed in the usual fitness and recreational facilities
★ Improved awareness of self-monitoring skills
★ Development of life-time exercise habits

ercise prescription is updated periodically to improve on the gains made previously.

In contrast to phase III, phase IV is generally considered a maintenance program when most physical and physiologic measures plateau. Phase IV is also appropriate for the sedentary individual without coronary heart disease (CHD) whose goal is to improve physical fitness and prevent health problems associated with physical inactivity. For these individuals, phase IV emphasizes conditioning at the start and maintenance afterward. Consequently, the objectives and duration of phases III and IV can vary according to individual needs. In general, however, phase IV is a lifetime commitment to regular physical activity and life-style management.

EQUIPMENT AND FACILITIES

Equipment and facilities are discussed in greater detail in Chapters 7 and 11. Equipment and facilities for phases III and IV vary considerably. An imaginative and creative staff is the most important prerequisite for a high-quality and safe program, although certain minimal requirements must be met. Equipment and facility needs are directly influenced by the program's clientele. For example, if exercise sessions are designed primarily for normal individuals or for persons with coronary risk factors but no history of CHD, the needs differ from those programs in which high-risk, postmyocardial infarction (post-MI),

or postcardiac surgical patients predominate. A wider variety of activities is possible and less supervision is necessary for the lower risk population. Under these circumstances a large gymnasium or aquatics facility is safe and desirable. In contrast exercise activities need to be more carefully controlled and the area for exercise should be more carefully selected for individuals who are at increased risk. When a greater number of high-risk patients are exercising, a more confined facility and monitoring is necessary. As physical condition improves, a greater variety of activities is permissible and a better-equipped facility is suggested.

Consideration must also be given to whether the program consists of supervised or unsupervised exercise. The decision as to which is most appropriate depends on the clinical history of the participants. Individuals with coronary disease or who have elevated risk need to be in a more controlled environment than noncardiacs and those at lower risk. At the conclusion of phase II, when continual monitoring is necessary, advancement is made to phase III, where intermittent monitoring is recommended for at least several months and probably on an ongoing basis since the procedures are relatively simple, inexpensive, and unobtrusive.

In most instances phases III and IV are conducted in community exercise facilities rather than in a hospital setting. Since a hospital is mainly associated with treating acute illness, there are advantages to having long-term programs located elsewhere. However, the hospital does provide a greater sense of security and validity to some persons than a nonhospital location.

The amount of available space is important in the design of the activity program. The minimal size recommended would enclose a full-size basketball court, providing sufficient room for a jogging program that is approximately 20 laps to the mile. If the exercise room is much smaller, jogging is more difficult, and the possibility of musculoskeletal injury from frequent turns is increased. When weather permits, outside facilities should be considered for the program. This offers a pleasant environment and helps the patient to realize that exercise is not limited to supervised and envionmentally controlled situations. However, outdoor areas should be clearly outlined so that the program can be reasonably controlled. Traffic patterns, patient visibility, and running surfaces need to be carefully planned. Outdoor cross-country jogging, as an example, should always be under the direction of a staff person and should incorporate the concept of a "buddy system" so that the patient never runs alone.

PROFESSIONAL PERSONNEL

The American College of Sports Medcine has taken a leading role in providing a standard for personnel in cardiac rehabilitation and preventive programs.[5] Other references[6–10] as well as Chapter 10 of this book discuss personnel in detail.

The phase III, community-based program should be supervised by a nurse or physician and one or more exercise professionals. The background for the nurse should be similar to that required for phase II. The nurse should have coronary care training, be able to interpret an ECG, be certified in cardiopulmonary resuscitation, and be able to handle cardiac emergencies. Advanced cardiac life support certification is suggested.

Exercise personnel need to know how to conduct classes as well as to have a basic understanding of the physiology of exercise and kinesiology. Academic training in physical education, recreation, or appropriate allied health science is advisable. The program's participants can also provide assistance in conducting sessions. These persons are excellent as group leaders, once they have learned the appropriate exercises, understand some basic principles of exercise, and have improved their level of fitness sufficiently so as to assume a leadership role. Utilizing program participants is desirable because it demonstrates the level of condition that the cardiac patient can achieve. This is also an excellent means of motivating other participants that a long-term commitment to increased physical activity can be beneficial.

Collaborating with nearby colleges and universities that offer allied health professional preparation programs (i.e., health, physical education, recreation, physical therapy, and nursing) can also be helpful. College administrators and department heads recognize the value of the practical experience and often have programs to accommodate student interns. Usually, arrangements can be made so that students receive credit for an internship, practicum, or independent project. The responsibilities of the student intern might include leading and assisting at exercise sessions, supervising recreational activities, helping with exercise testing, record keeping, patient monitoring, and aspects of program management.

Although there is less clinical need to oversee healthy individuals, supervised classes are still recommended when possible. The presence of qualified personnel can better ensure safe and beneficial activities. This reduces the possibility for injury and enhances the potential for long-term benefit and good adherence. In addition there is a greater chance that exercises are done correctly when the classes are supervised. Other personnel needed to complement exercise include nutritionists, psychologists, and behavior modification specialists. Because CHD disease is a multifactorial problem, it must be dealt with in a multidisciplinary manner.

EXERCISE TRAINING SESSION

Phases III and IV are generally conducted in a community facility such as a school, college or university, YMCA, Jewish Community Center (JCC), or in an unsupervised setting such as a fitness center, health club, or at home. The guidelines for exercise are similar to phase II; that is, the program includes dynamic, aerobic activities for a minimum of 30 minutes per session, 3 to 4 times a week. The intensity of exercise is usually higher than the target heart rate at the conclusion of phase II. If the intensity is increased, an additional week or two in phase II is suggested in order to monitor the response to increased exercise.

A typical exercise session includes the following:

1. A 10- to 20-minute period of floor exercises
2. A 20- to 30-minute period of continuous endurance activity with emphasis on activities that can be incorporated into daily living
3. A 15- to 20-minute period of recreational activities
4. A 5- to 10-minute cool-down

Floor Exercise

Floor exercises, gradually increasing in intensity, are performed to increase circulation, elevate body temperature—which facilitates muscle contraction—and reduces the possibility for musculoskeletal injury. This period is the warm-up phase. The floor exercise routine is designed to be incorporated into a regimen of activity that can be performed almost anywhere. The emphasis is on muscle endurance, strength, and flexibility, particularly of the lower back. Some typical floor exercises are described in Chapter 13 (Fig. 13–2).

Continuous Endurance Activity

The activities chosen for improving endurance in phases III and IV should take into account the interests of the participants and what the facility can accommodate. Walking and jogging are most popular because they require no additional equipment and are low-level skill activities. Bicycling and swimming are excellent modes of exercise and are very popular, but require special equipment and facilities.

Ideally, a program would include a variety of activities. Because there is no "best" type of exercise, it is important to consider the interest of the majority and how many of these activities can be well supervised concurrently to maintain safety and benefit.

Recreational Activities

An important goal of cardiac rehabilitation is to return the patient to a normal life-style. Therefore, the element of fun should be introduced in selecting activities, as long as safety is not compromised. In some instances activities might have to be modified to achieve that goal. Recreational activities provide an opportunity for fun and camaraderie for the participants, which benefits long-term adherence. These activities are included secondarily for the purpose of training. The objectives of training are derived from floor exercising and continuous endurance activity.

Cool-Down

Following exercise, a 5- to 10-minute walking cool-down is recommended before showering. The purpose of the cool-down is discussed in Chapter 13.

MOTIVATION AND COMPLIANCE

Long-term adherence is the most important factor in the success of any intervention program. Unfortunately, the historical reality of long-term compliance to health intervention programs is not encouraging. Recidivism rates for exercise and other life-style programs range as high as 87%[11,12] with the average about 50%.[13,14] Why is the number of dropouts so high, even among cardiac patients who should be maximally motivated to alter their living habits? To answer this question we need to learn much more about the reasons for noncompliant behavior.

Numerous studies have been conducted in an attempt to identify factors related to noncompliance.[15-17] There have also been attempts to develop test instruments for predicting noncompliant behavior.[18-20] The most encouraging of the test instruments devised for this purpose is a self-motivation assessment test developed by Dishman and Ickes.[18] This particular test has demonstrated both high validity and reliability, and when used in conjunction with percent body fat has identified as many as 80% of nonadherers to an exercise program.[21]

Although a complete list of factors associated with poor compliance has not been identified, a number of life-style and psychosocial variables are important to consider. Life-style factors include smoking, blue collar employment, inactive occupation, and inactive leisure time.[15-17,22] Psychosocial traits account for almost half of the reasons for program dropouts.[13,22] These traits include depression, hypochondriasis, anxiety, introverted behavior, low self-esteem, lack of interest, poor motivation, and family problems. In addition, program variables can affect adherence. Some of these factors are location of the facility, cost, strenuousness of exercise, injuries, and lack of sociability.[12,13,22] Thus, psychosocial factors, personal convenience, and family life-style appear to represent the major impediments to exercise compliance;[12,13,15-17,22] these are summarized in Table 14-4.

Numerous attempts have been made to improve adherence.[12,13,22,23] Oldridge uses the words *motivation* and *variety* to summarize a list of variables that can lead to better attendance and decreased dropout rate[13,24] (Figs. 14-2, and 14-3). In addition motivational strategies, program modifications, and personnel guidelines[5,13] are summarized that will enhance interest and enthusiasm for exercise, as well as long-term program compliance (Tables 14-5 to 14-7).

The information provided by Oldridge[13,24] and Franklin[30] is excellent material for phase II, III, and IV programs. It is also necessary to develop a strategy for good adherence with unsupervised programs. Since the majority of cardiac patients probably do not have access to supervised programs, they must be motivated to continue on their own. Gettman et al.[2] have proposed the following model to improve adherence in the nonsupervised setting:

Table 14-4.   Variables Predicting the Exercise Dropout

Personal Factors	Program Factors	Other Factors
1. Smoker	1. Inconvenient time/location	1. Lack of spouse support
2. Inactive leisure time	2. Excessive cost	2. Inclement weather
3. Inactive occupation	3. High intensity exercise	3. Excessive job travel
4. Blue collar worker	4. Lack of exercise variety, e.g., running only	4. Injury
5. Type A personality		5. Job change/move
6. Increased physical strength	5. Exercises alone	
7. Extroverted	6. Lack of positive feedback or reinforcement	
8. Poor credit rating		
9. Overweight and/or low ponderal index	7. Inflexible exercise goals	
10. Poor "self-motivation"	8. Low enjoyability ratings for running programs	
11. Depressed	9. Poor exercise leadership	
12. Hypochondriacal		
13. Anxious		
14. Introverted		
15. Low ego strength		

From Franklin, B.A.: Exercise program compliance: Improvement strategies. *In* Behavioral Intervention in Obesity. Edited by J. Storlie and H.A. Jordan. Jamaica, N.Y., Spectrum, 1984.

```
MOTIVATION
OPINION AND ATTITUDE
THERAPEUTIC
INSTRUCTORS
VARIATION
AEROBIC
TEAM APPROACH
INVOLVEMENT
OBJECTIVE TESTING
NONCOMPETITIVE
```

Used with permission of Neil Oldridge, Ph.D., Mt.Sinai Hospital, Milwaukee, Wisconsin.

Fig. 14–2. Motivational Possibilities.

```
VARIETY
AEROBIC
RELAXING AND RECREATIVE
INDIVIDUALIZED
ATTITUDE
THERAPEUTIC
ISOTONIC
OBJECTIVE TESTING
NONCOMPETITIVE AND FUN
```

Fig. 14–3. Attributes of A Good Exercise Program. From Oldridge, N.B.: What to look for in an exercise leader. Physician Sportsmed., 5:85, 1977.

Table 14–5. Motivational Strategies

1. Minimize injury with a moderate exercise prescription.
2. Emphasize exercising in a group.
3. Emphasize variety and fun in the exercise program.
4. Include modified recreational games to the conditioning format.
5. Provide music during workouts.
6. Incorporate effective behavioral and programmatic techniques to the conditioning program.
7. Establish a regular workout schedule.
8. Use fitness testing periodically to assess training results.
9. Provide progress charts to record exercise achievements.
10. Recruit spouse support in promoting the exercise program.
11. Recognize individual accomplishments through a system of rewards.
12. Be sure that the exercise leader is capable (Tables 14–6 and 14–7). These are discussed in greater detail elsewhere (Chapter 10).

Table 14–6. Responsibilites of the Exercise Leader

1. Meet the requirements of the exercise test technician.
2. Interpret metabolic data obtained on the participant.
3. Execute the exercise prescription under guidelines established by the physician and the program director.
4. Educate the participant concerning exercise.
5. Evaluate the participant's response to exercise.
6. Interact and communicate with all personnel involved in the exercise program.

Source: American College of Sports Medicine.[5]

Table 14–7. Behavior Strategies of the Good Exercise Leader

1. Show a sincere interest in the participant.
2. Be enthusiastic in your instruction and guidance.
3. Develop a personal association and relationship with each participant.
4. Consider the various motives underlying exercise participation (e.g., health, recreation, social, personal image) and allow for individual differences.
5. Initiate participant follow-up, (e.g., written notes or telephone calls) when several unexplained absences occur in succession.
6. Participate in the exercise session yourself.
7. Honor special days (e.g., birthdays) or accomplishments (attendance, personal achievements) with rewards (e.g., certificates, shirts, trophies).
8. Attend to orthopedic and musculoskeletal problems.

1. Teach the individual how to correctly start an exercise program.
2. Provide some supervision in the early stages.
3. Have the individual report on his or her participation every 2 weeks.
4. Encourage the use of a home program because it may be more convenient.

Gettman et al.[2] found that individuals who exercised in an unsupervised setting improved as much as those in a supervised program if they followed these guidelines. Results from other home programs have also been encouraging[1,3] when the participants have adhered to similar instructions.

In summary the subject of motivation and compliance is very complex. Although our knowledge of the subject has improved as a result of numerous investigations, there is much more that is not understood in motivating people to practice certain behaviors. For more information on motivation and compliance several other sources are suggested.[12,13,15–17,18–20]

HOME-BASED PROGRAMS

Although supervised exercise is advantageous compared to nonsupervised, logistical problems preclude the possibility of everyone having that opportunity. Consequently, the exercise specialist is responsible for providing adequate guidelines when exercise is done at home or in some other unsupervised setting. When this information is made available, home programs have been shown to be both safe and beneficial.[2,3]

The ostensibly healthy individual who is mostly interested in physical fitness should also follow the guidelines presented in this chapter for a correct exercise prescription and training program. For the cardiac patient who must exercise alone, there are additional safety concerns to consider: (1) Undertake a complete evaluation as described in Chapters 3 to 5. This enables the professional staff to establish an individualized program that considers patient needs and interests. (2) Join a supervised program if at all possible for a minimum of 2 weeks. This can help to assess the patient's readiness for regular physical activity. Increased monitoring also provides an opportunity for greater safety.[25–30] This can help to reduce patient anxiety and increase the exercise prescription. Supervised exercise, even for a brief time period, allows the staff an opportunity to observe the patient's mechanics of exercise, which is important in order to lessen the chance of sustaining musculoskeletal injury. (3) It is recommended that some form of home monitoring be undertaken if available. Electrocardiogram signals can be recorded on small, easily portable tape recorders that can be transmitted by telephone to a center where it can be interpreted and feedback

immediately provided to the patient. It is necessary to teach the patient how to palpate the pulse and better ensure adherence to the exercise prescription. (4) The patient who cannot continue in a supervised community program should be in a system where patient contact is maintained. Diaries and record forms should be provided, which are regularly mailed back to the exercise center to be read and discussed with the patient at a later date. A schedule of patient visits with the program staff and personal physician should also be established. Unfortunately, the role of the primary care physician has been ignored in long-term health promotion. This is too bad because it has been shown that physician involvement can be very valuable.[5,31–33] Periodic, supervised exercise classes should be arranged if possible. These visits should include an assessment of progress in order to update the exercise program and evaluate the patient's clinical status.

FACTORS THAT INFLUENCE EXERCISE

There are a number of factors that can cause the exercise precription to be modified. These include weather, altitude, air pollution, medications, meals, time of day, and stimulants.

Temperature and Humidity

Because environmental conditions can affect adaptation to exercise, it is desirable to regulate temperature and humidity when using indoor facilities. Ideal temperature and humidity for exercise is between 40° and 70° F (4° to 24° C) and below 65% relative humidity, respectively.[34,35] At the same time optimal environmental conditions should not be overly emphasized if they are going to result in a patient who refuses to exercise under less than ideal conditions. Consequently, if environmental factors are not optimal, exercise should not be ruled out automatically, but rather should be approached intelligently. Outdoor facilities can provide pleasant surroundings for exercise, especially when weather conditions are acceptable. However, when ambient temperatures are high, in particular when they approach shell and core temperatures (above 90° F), extra precautions need to be observed. As relative humidity increases with rising temperature, precautionary measures become increasingly important. The combination of high temperature and humidity increases the demand on the thermal regulatory and cardiovascular systems and decreases efficiency of performance.[36–40] Heart rates rise precipitously and stroke volume falls as a result of the failure of peripheral cutaneous veins to constrict. Central blood volume is reduced, and peak cardiac output, maximal oxygen uptake, and physical work capacity are all reduced.[41,42] Patients with mild congestive heart failure (CHF) need to be especially careful in hot and humid weather not to develop overt left ventricular failure.[43]

The most significant physiologic problem associated with exercise at high temperature and humidity is interference in the body's cooling process. As ambient temperatures rise and the level of physical activity increases, there is greater heat production and, therefore, a greater need to dissipate body heat. The primary means of heat dissipation is through evaporating perspiration. As relative humidity increases the air becomes more saturated, which reduces evaporation and subsequent cooling. Body temperature and heart rate continue to rise, and physical work capacity is diminished.

Exercise in hot and humid conditions can result in several types of heat injuries. These heat-associated illnesses should be understood and treated properly.

Heat Cramps

Heat cramps are the most common of the thermal regulatory injuries. They are characterized by painful contractions of large muscles, profuse sweating, low salt intake, and possibly potassium deficit. Heat cramps can be avoided by being in good physical condition, having proper water intake, and maintaining electrolyte balance.[44]

Heat Exhaustion

Two types of heat exhaustion can occur, sudden heat exhaustion and dehydration exhaustion. The first occurs in response to sudden exposure to high temperature. If accompanied by exercise the result can be inability of the heart to maintain adequate blood pressure. Both circulation and heat dissipation are diminished, which can lead to cardiovascular system exhaustion. Initially, heart rate and cardiac output may increase as the individual begins to feel warm and fatigued. Sweating becomes profuse, the skin is moist, and the pulse is rapid. The individual becomes uncomfortable, experiences shortness of breath, and may collapse and lose consciousness. The patient usually responds promptly to rest in a shaded area and consumption of fluids. Dehydration exhaustion is different, in that it occurs following a longer exposure with greater loss of fluids, which are not replenished. Sweating is again profuse, and blood volume is reduced, accompanied by circulatory insufficiency. Heart rate rises, and exertion becomes increasingly difficult as dehydration continues. Exhaustion and collapse occur when the body has lost about 5% of its weight in fluid. Treatment should include rest and cooling of the body. Fluids should be administered. Care must be taken to treat dehydration exhaustion because it can result in extensive edema in the legs and may possibly be followed by sudden death if not altered.[44]

Heat Stroke

Heat stroke is the most serious of the heat disorders and can be fatal if not treated immediately. Signs of heat stroke are prostration and sometimes delirium;

hot, dry, and flushed skin; and absence of sweating. Body temperatures may rise to as high as 110° F in extreme cases. The cause of heat stroke is derangement of the temperature-cooling mechanisms in the hypothalamus, similar to that seen in fevers accompanying infectious diseases. Heat stroke is distinguished from heat exhaustion by the hot, dry skin and more profound prostration. Immediate steps should be taken to lower the body temperature; that is, the victim should be immersed in cold water and ice packs or alcohol spray should be applied, while awaiting arrival of medical treatment. Transport to an emergency medical facility is a must.[44]

Maintaining proper electrolyte balance, wearing light apparel, and interspersing exercise with breaks for rest and water are all important steps in preventing the onset of heat illness. Fluids should be taken regularly to replenish loss and stave off increases in body temperature.[44] Avoid fluids with high sodium concentration. Water is best for replenishing fluid loss. Improved physical condition also helps one to acclimatize more quickly.[45–47]

Exercise clothes that are designed specifically to increase sweat by raising body temperature are not recommended. Usually these are made of rubber, plastic, or some synthetic substance that does not allow for evaporation to take place. Their purpose is to augment weight reduction through increased water loss. The physiologic effect of these garments is to restrict cooling and therefore promote greater activity in the sweat glands. The danger of this is that body temperatures can rise to levels that are unhealthy and even dangerous. Furthermore, losing weight in this manner is due principally to a temporary loss of fluids. The lost weight is generally replaced as water intake is resumed.

Saunas, steam baths, Jacuzzis, and hot whirlpools also impose increased physiologic demand, are particularly hazardous for the cardiac patient and should never be used soon after exercise. Even without

exercise these facilities should be used with caution by low-risk patients and avoided by patients with greater risk, epecially those with compromised left ventricular function. The combination of peripheral vasodilation from increased body temperature and the decreased milking action on the veins of the contracting and relaxing muscles from inactivity causes venous return and central blood flow to be impaired. Blood flow to the heart and the brain may be decreased, and episodes of dizziness, fainting, chest pain, or even MI are more likely.

Cold Stress

Cold climates can also create problems for exercise. Adequate clothing is essential for retaining body heat. In extreme cold, body exposure (i.e., hands and face) should be minimized to avoid potential frostbite. Frostbite is especially influenced by the wind chill index and can occur within a few minutes (Fig. 14–4). Outdoor activity in cold weather may seem invigorating but can be particularly risky for cardiacs. Low temperatures increase peripheral resistance at rest and during exercise,[48,49] causing increased arterial blood pressure, myocardial oxygen requirement, and anginal discomfort.[49] Patients with cold-induced angina should be reminded to take nitroglycerin before going outdoors in low temperatures. Physicians should consider a seasonal increase in beta-adrenergic blocking agents in these patients. Cold air can also irritate the respiratory tract and cause aggravated coughing, although there is no evidence that permanent damage occurs. Respiratory discomfort might be alleviated by wearing a face mask over the mouth to warm inspired air. Shoveling snow is particularly risky and should be avoided, because it combines the effect of cold weather with the physiologic responses associated with isometric exercise, pooling of blood in lower extremities from standing, and peripheral vasodilation from too much cloth-

Actual thermometer reading °Fahrenheit								
	30	20	10	0	−10	−20	−30	−40

Est.		Equivalent temperature							
wind	Calm	30	20	10	0	−10	−20	−30	−40
speed	5	27	16	6	−5	−15	−26	−36	−47
in mph	10	16	3	−9	−22	−34	−46	−58	−71
	15	9	−5	−18	−31	−45	−58	−72	−85
	20	4	−10	−24	−39	−53	−67	−81	−95
	25	1	−15	−29	−44	−59	−74	−88	−103
	30	−2	−18	−33	−49	−64	−79	−93	−109
	35	−4	−20	−35	−52	−67	−82	−97	−113
	40	−5	−21	−37	−53	−69	−84	−100	−115

Wind speeds greater than 40 mph have little additional effect	LITTLE DANGER (For properly clothed person)	INCREASING DANGER	GREAT DANGER	DANGER FROM FREEZING OF EXPOSED FLESH

Fig. 14–4. Wind chill chart.

ing, which results in increased body temperature.

High Altitude

The depth and rate of pulmonary ventilation are increased at high altitudes[45,50] from a chemoreceptor response to a drop in arterial oxygen saturation.[51] At sea level blood is approximately 97% saturated with oxygen, although this level decreases at high altitudes and can drop to about 56% at an elevation of 15,000 feet. With chronic adaptation there is a compensatory increase in the number of red blood cells and in the amount of hemoglobin. This may cause an increase in blood viscosity and thereby reduce the oxygen-carrying capacity of the blood.[51]

New capillaries can increase in number by as much as one third with increased viscosity.[52] Maximal oxygen uptake is reduced at high altitudes,[53,54] although maximal heart rate, stroke volume, and cardiac output are not lowered up to 14,000 feet.[53,55] Although increased capillarization reduces the work of the heart,[51] myocardial contractility is not impaired, at least in normals, as evidenced by the absence of ECG changes of any clinical significance during rest and/or maximal exertion.[53,56–58]

Pulmonary edema is another problem associated with high altitude, which may occur in unacclimatized persons and be exacerbated by cold and physical exertion. Although fewer than 5% of those exposed to high altitude are probably susceptible to pulmonary edema, careful prevalence studies are not available. Reduced aerobic capacity, depressed left ventricular function, shortness of breath, dyspnea on exertion, and cough are characteristics of high-altitude pulmonary edema.[59]

Because of the physiologic effects and potential danger of physical activity at high altitude, it is advisable to exercise cautiously at first. Acclimatization occurs with prolonged exposure to altitude, and decreased performance levels return to normal. Physical activity at altitudes above 5,000 feet should be limited in patients with heart disease who normally live at sea level. Myocardial hypoxia can be induced at high altitudes in patients with CHD. When combined with physical exertion, ischemia and a coronary event could be precipitated that would not have occurred at low elevations.[59] The consequences of altitude acclimatization are increased hemoglobin, growth of new capillaries in organs, and increase in the myoglobin concentration of the heart and skeletal muscles. These alterations improve the capacity for transport and utilization of oxygen and increase aerobic capacity toward the normal sea-level value.[51]

Air Pollution

Air pollution is another environmental factor that can affect the physiologic response to exercise. Because certain pollutants are detrimental to cardiovascular mechanisms[60–62] and performance,[62–64] it is advisable to assess air quality prior to exercising outdoors. Air pollution is also a significant consideration for patients with respiratory problems.

Carbon monoxide is the principal air pollutant associated with impaired hemodynamic response to exercise. Carbon monoxide combines with hemoglobin, for which it has greater affinity than oxygen, to form carboxyhemoglobin. Elevated levels of carboxyhemoglobin can precipitate angina at a reduced rate–pressure product,[65,66] increased myocardial ischemia as evidenced by greater ST segment displacement,[60,61] and increased mortality from cardiovascular diseases.[67] Considering the health ramifications of exercising in air pollution, program directors should be familiar with acceptable air quality standards.

Another important pollutant is ozone, which is one of a group of compounds classified as photochemical oxidants. The terms *ozone* and *photochemical oxidants* are often used interchangeably.

High concentrations of ozone are clearly associated with asthma, chronic heart and lung disease, and certain anemias. It has also been well documented that persons who suffer from cardiopulmonary diseases require many hours to recover from ozone attacks. Although it is often thought that photochemical oxidants affect only the sick and elderly, normal healthy persons have also been observed to suffer adverse effects from exposure.[68] Pollutants and unacceptable air quality standards are presented in Tables 14–8 and 14–9.

POTENTIAL RISKS OF EXERCISE

Although regular exercise has been shown to have beneficial effects, increased physical activity is not without certain risks.

Untoward Events

The chance of an untoward cardiac event is reduced if exercise is prescribed as a percentage of maximal attained heart rate. The target heart rate, therefore, is lower than the peak rate, which was attained on the exercise stress test, and the heart rate, at which contraindicating signs and symptoms might have occurred. Untoward events may be reduced further by learning to recognize subjective feelings associated with exercise. Because increases in physical exertion can be perceived accurately,[69–71] exercise intensity can be estimated subjectively by the person who is exercising. With cardiac patients perceived exertion should only be used along with objective estimates of intensity because of the possible appearance of abnormalities when effort is perceived as light.[72] Untoward signs and symptoms are listed in Chapter 13 (Table 13–5).[73]

Table 14–8.   Typical Pollutants and National Air Quality Standards[a]

Pollutant	Effects	Standards
Sulfur oxides	Sulfur oxides come primarily from the combustion of sulfur-containing fossil fuels. Their presence has been associated with increased death rates and property damage.	367 μg/m³ (0.14 ppm) as a maximum 24-hour concentration not to be exceeded more than once a year.
Particulate matter	Particulate matter, either solid or liquid, may originate in nature or result from industrial processes and other human activities. By itself or in association with other pollutants, particulate matter may injure the lungs or cause adverse effects elsewhere in the body. Particulates also reduce visibility and contribute to property damage and soiling.	260 μg/m³ as a maximum 24-hour concentration not to be exceeded more than once a year.
Carbon monoxide	Carbon monoxide is a by-product of the incomplete burning of carbon-containing fuels and of some industrial processes. It decreases the oxygen-carrying ability of the blood and, at levels often found in city air, may impair mental processes. Carboxy-hemoglobin levels above 5% have been associated with physiologic stress in patients with heart disease. Blood carboxy-hemoglobin levels approaching 2% have been associated by some researchers with impaired psychomotor responses.	40 mg/m³ (35 ppm) as a maximum 1-hour concentration not to be exceeded more than once a year.
Hydrocarbons	Hydrocarbons in the air come mainly from the processing, marketing, and use of petroleum products. Some of the hydrocarbons combine with nitrogen oxides in the air to form photochemical oxidants. The hydrocarbon standards, therefore, are for use as a guide in devising implementation plans to achieve the oxidant standards.	160 μg/m³ (0.24 ppm) as a maximum 3-hour concentration not to be exceeded more than once a year.
Nitrogen oxides	Nitrogen oxides usually originate in high-temperature combustion processes. The presence of nitrogen dioxide in the air has been associated with a variety of respiratory diseases. Nitrogen dioxide is essential in the natural production of photochemical oxidant.	100 μg/m³ (0.05 ppm) annual arithmetic mean. The U.S. Environmental Protection Agency is examining other pollutants to determine whether any may be covered by future air quality standards.

[a]Adapted from Clean Air. It's Up to You, Too. U.S. Environmental Protection Agency. Washington, D.C., 1973.

Treating and Preventing Injuries

The following section emphasizes the treatment and prevention of injuries that occur occasionally during those activities that are recommended to enhance cardiovascular fitness.

WALKING AND JOGGING. Walking and jogging (running) are the simplest and probably the most popular of aerobic activities, although they can also be the cause of orthopedic injuries if not done properly.

The best way to prevent musculoskeletal injury from walking and jogging is to warm up adequately, build up distances gradually, wear good shoes, adhere to the exercise prescription, and exercise on firm and even surfaces.

Good flexibility also helps to prevent injury. Tight muscles, particularly of the hip, pelvic girdle, and spinal column increase the possibility of muscular strain and low-back injury. Weak abdominal muscles can

Table 14–9.   Ozone Alert Stages[a]

Stage	Standard and Effect
Advisory	.07 ppm for 2-hour average
	Ultrasensitive people, such as asthmatics, may develop labored breathing and feel dizzy.
	State issues warning that ozone is unusually high.
Yellow Alert	.17 ppm
	Average person feels eye, nose, throat, and lung irritations. Cardiac and lung patients might have trouble breathing. Old and young might feel fatigue.
	State asks public to avoid unnecessary driving and use of electricity. Manufacturing and power plants asked to curb air pollution voluntarily. No open burning or incineration.
Red Alert	.30 ppm
	Coughing. Labored breathing. Chest pains. Severe headache. Fatigue. Cardiac and lung patients in danger. Asthma attacks.
	State orders fleet vehicle traffic curbed or stopped. Parking lots curtailed or closed. Air emissions from certain industries and power plants curbed. Most government agencies and schools closed.
Emergency	.50 ppm
	Possible deaths of infants and persons suffering from heart and lung ailments. Chest pain. Severe cough. Dizziness. Some unable to work. Respiratory infections.
	State orders traffic except emergency vehicles halted. Aircraft flights from the emergency area halted. Manufacturing and power plants curtailed further. Many kinds of businesses ordered closed, including stores and service stations. State says these actions are taken at this level to avoid reaching the .60 ppm ozone "significant harm level" when average persons are affected and death or permanent disablement occur in some.

[a]For the State of Illinois. Courtesy of Illinois Environmental Protection Agency.

also contribute to low-back problems. If minor aggravations occur, heat combined with stretching may be sufficient to continue to work out comfortably. More substantial injuries require immediate ice application to reduce swelling and pain and perhaps aspirin to reduce inflammation. Because of potential side effects, persons taking aspirin should be closely monitored. For example, cardiacs should be aware of the possibility of gastric bleeding. Medical advice should be sought before treating injuries with large doses of aspirin. Sudden increases in exercise intensity and/or duration, as well as wearing shoes with considerable wear can contribute to the occurrence of stress fractures. Insufficient calcium can also be a problem, especially in older athletes and older exercisers. If symptoms are long lasting and if these simple self-treatments are insufficient, then a physician should be consulted.

SWIMMING. In many respects swimming comes as close as any activity to the best type of exercise. Cardiovascular function and muscle endurance in the major muscle groups is enhanced. Swimming is advantageous compared to other activities because of better venous return as a result of hydrostatic pressure and being performed in a horizontal, weight-supported position. However, swimming requires a high level of skill, which makes energy expenditure difficult to quantify. A poor swimmer may be unable to exercise long enough for an effective training stimulus and uses more energy for the same amount of work as an efficient swimmer. An efficient swimmer can exercise at a low level of energy expenditure and a low heart rate.

The most common orthopedic problem associated with swimming is pain in the shoulder caused by pinching of the muscle and bursa between the bones of the shoulder. The best prevention is to increase distance gradually and warm up adequately with exercises for shoulder muscles. If the pain continues reduce the intensity of exercise and change stroke, or both. Ice can help to minimize swelling and aspirin can alleviate inflammation. Nose and ear plugs, as well as goggles are suggested to lessen the risk of eye–ear–nose–throat problems.

BICYCLING. Bicycling is another excellent form of exercise, although certain precautions are necessary to ensure safety and enjoyment. Knee injuries may be as common in cyclists as in runners. The cyclist's problem is often associated with lack of upper leg strength, less joint stability, and improper positioning of the seat.[74] The bicycle seat should be positioned so that the knee joint is almost completely extended on the down pedal. Another common injury in cyclists is that of lower back pain, usually a result of postural problems and weak abdominal muscles. Hip flexibility and abdominal strengthening exercises are useful. Proper seat and handlebar positioning are important. An individual who has not bicycled in a long time should be careful to select a properly fitted bike and should bike with caution until the skill has been remastered. Cyclists should be familiar with and adhere to safety and traffic regulations, be able to deal with minor mechanical problems, and wear appropriate apparel and protective equipment including a helmet.

Other Risks

In addition to musculoskeletal injury, there is also a cardiac risk associated with increased physical activity. Recurrent cardiac injury, with or without exercise, is related to patient prognosis, which can be assessed at entrance into a rehabilitation program[75–78] A review of the literature indicates a fatality risk between 1:116,000 and 1:784,000 patients hours in supervised cardiac rehabilitation compared with a fatality incidence of 0:889,000 patient hours of continually monitored programs.[79,80] Cardiac events that occur in community recreational programs have a risk of fatal events of approximately 1:1,000,000 hours of participation.[81]

In either case, regular exercise for cardiacs in rehabilitation programs, or for normals in community programs is associated with relatively small risk. With cardiac patients, proper treatment with medications, prompt attention to potassium levels, strict adherence to target heart rate, and warm-up before exercise are all important to prevent untoward events.[82]

A record of current medications must be maintained. This needs to include dosages, times taken, and the prescribing physician. The patient should be asked at the beginning of each exercise session whether medications have been taken.

Effects of Common Medications

Although the physician is responsible for prescribing medications, the exercise specialist and cardiac rehabilitation nurse need to understand their effects and how they impact the exercise prescription. Some common medications to be familiar with include:

1. Beta-blocking agents
2. Nitrates (long and short acting)
3. Antiarrhythmics
4. Digitalis drugs (long and short acting).

A comprehensive presentation of medications is found in Chapter 3.

BETA-BLOCKING AGENTS. The primary purpose of beta-blocking agents is to reduce heart rate, blood pressure, and myocardial contractility, thereby reducing myocardial oxygen demand. Since heart rate is decreased, the exercise prescription can be significantly affected. Often, maximal heart rate does not exceed 100 to 125 beats per minute (bpm) in patients on beta-blockers, although effects vary with dosage. Those who supervise exercise classes need to be aware of alterations in the prescription of beta-blockers. Changes in frequency or dosage may necessitate a follow-up exercise test and a new exercise prescription. Abrupt cessation of beta-blockers should be avoided, because it may result in an acceleration of anginal symptoms and possibly precipitate an MI.[83]

NITRATES. Nitrates are prescribed principally for their vasodilation effect and should be kept available for use in the event of exertional angina. The use of nitroglycerin increases physical work capacity by raising the anginal threshold, meaning that a higher rate × pressure product is required before the onset of chest pain. One study demonstrated that nitroglycerin can also reduce exercise-induced arrhythmias associated with ischemia.[84]

Possible side effects from nitroglycerin include dizziness, headaches, and fainting. Since vasodilation can create a hypotensive response, blood pressure should be checked when nitroglycerin is administered. The patient should be observed carefully because of the possibility of fainting. A sitting or reclining position is recommended when taking nitroglycerin for the first time. Nitrate ointments have had renewed popularity and are effective as long-acting agents, which are used as afterload-reducing agents with heart failure.

ANTIARRHYTHMIC MEDICATIONS. Antiarrhythmic medications are administered to reduce myocardial irritability and to lessen the potential for ectopic activity. Antiarrhythmics should be timed for maximal effect when used by patients in exercise programs.

DIGITALIS. Digitalis drugs are used principally to enhance myocardial contractility in patients with ventricular dysfunction. They are also used to control supraventricular tachycardias. Digitalis has the effect of lowering the ST segment of the ECG, the explanation of which is not well understood. Persons who monitor exercise sessions need to be cognizant of this effect and if possible have an ECG record on hand with and without digitalis in order to differentiate between ischemia and medication effect. If possible, digitalis should be stopped 2 weeks prior to diagnostic exercise testing.

Table 14–10 summarizes some common medications and their physiologic effects. A more comprehensive presentation on medications is presented in Chapter 3. Other sources are also recommended.[85,86]

Eating Habits

Proper nutrition is an important adjunct to an exercise program. The basic guidelines for good nutrition are presented in Chapter 15.[87]

The quantity and quality of meals as well as when consumed are all important. Although the amount of food that can be digested comfortably can vary, it is best to refrain from eating a substantial meal for at least 2 hours before vigorous activity. Since digestion requires increased blood supply, diverting blood flow to exercising muscles following a meal can reduce functional capacity, increase heart rate for any work load, cause digestive problems, ECG changes,[88] and possibly provoke anginal discomfort.[49] There are an abundance of good nutritional resources available,[89–93] although much of the information is difficult to understand, contradictory, and without physiologic or clinical basis. The best advice for those with specific nutrition needs is to seek professional nutrition counseling. For additional information on nutrition computer analyses, see Chapter 9.

Stimulants

Substances that act as a stimulant to the cardiovascular system should be avoided, especially before exercise. These include all products that contain nicotine, alcohol, and caffeine. These substances increase the heart rate, decrease the efficiency of the

Table 14–10.   Effect of Drug Interventions on Exercise Regimens[a]

Effect	*Medication*
May increase heart rate	Isoproterenol Quinidine sulfate and procainamide Ephedrine and other bronchodilators and drugs for asthma Thyroid-Synthroid, Thyroid USP Apresoline
May decrease heart rate	Propranolol (Inderal) and all other beta-blocking agents Reserpine Some antihypertensive drugs—guanethidine Aldomet
May decrease blood pressure	Aldomet Ismelin Apresoline Inderal Diuretics: thiazides—Esidrix, Hydrodiuril, furosemide (Lasix) & Ethacrynic Acid (Edecrin) Nitrates—nitroglycerin, long-acting nitrates Elavil, Tofranil, Stelazine
May increase blood pressure	Bronchodilators: ephedrine, epinephrine, aminophylline Nasal sprays, decongestants, Neo-synephrine Thyroid drugs, dexedrine and amphetamines
May increase exercise capacity	Nitrates: nitroglycerin, long-acting nitrates, Nitrol ointment Beta blockers Digitalis: Lanoxin, digitoxin
May affect the exercise electrocardiogram:	
May cause false-positive result	Digitalis: Lanoxin, digitoxin Diuretics causing hypokalemia Tricyclic antidepressants
May cause false-negative test	Beta blockers Antidysrhythmics: Quinidine sulfate and procainamide (by depressing dysrhythmias)
May affect contractility:	
Those that increase cardiac contractility	Digitalis: Lanoxin, digitoxin Isoproterenol (Isuprel) Aminophylline-type drugs
Those that decrease cardiac contractility	Propranolol (Inderal) and other beta-blocking antidysrhythmic drugs: Quinidine sulfate or gluconate (Quinidex, Quinaglute) Procainamide (Pronestyl), Dysinpryole (Norpace)

[a]From H. Miller, Wake Forest University Medical School—unpublished material.

cardiovascular system, constrict peripheral vessels, and adversely affect the cardiac response to exercise and the exercise prescription.[73]

When To Exercise

There is no best time of day to exercise. Some individuals prefer and perform better in the morning hours, while others are better in the afternoon or evening. Such variability is common among humans,[52] even though human circadian rhythms are apparent for sleep, heart rate, body temperature, and excretion of water potassium and ketosteroids.[51] In general, most persons prefer to exercise earlier rather than later, a decision affected by daily routine, job, safeness for exercise, availability of programs, and other responsibilities. Many individuals are physically and mentally tired at the end of the day, which is not conducive for exercise. Evidence suggests that cardiopulmonary capacity is decreased at night, although this is of practical importance only if the work is near the limit

Date_____

Dear Doctor_____:

Your patient has been in the cardiopulmonary rehabilitation program since___/___/___. The patient's clinical history, physical condition and cardiopulmonary status have been reviewed for your input. The following is a summary of these results.

Patients Name_____ Telephone #_____
                 Last   First

Date of admission to the program_____
Diagnosis_____

Current Medications	Dosage	Frequency

Average heart rate at rest_____; during exercise_____
Blood pressure at rest___/___ ; during exercise___/___
Heart rate following 10 minutes recovery_____
Blood pressure following 10 minutes recovery___/___
Electrocardiogram changes during or following exercise_____

Adverse signs or symptoms_____
_____
_____

Adaptation to exercise_____
_____

Musculoskeletal problems associated with exercise_____
_____

Adherence to program_____
_____

Patient Progress Report

	Latest Results	Previous Results
Weight	_____	_____
% Fat	_____	_____
Total cholesterol	_____	_____
Low-density lipoproteins	_____	_____
High-density lipoproteins	_____	_____
Total cholesterol/HDL	_____	_____
Blood sugar	_____	_____

Summary of Patient Progress

_____
_____
_____
_____

Program Director_____

Fig. 14–5. Patient Progress Report.

Name_____

Address_____ Tel. Number_____

_____

Patient Diagnosis_____

Entered Program_____ Current Phase_____

Patient Adherence_____

Attitude Toward Program_____

Heart Rate at Rest_____ During Exercise _____ Recovery_____

Blood Pressure at Rest_____ During Exercise_____ Recovery_____

Electrocardiogram at Rest_____

Electrocardiogram During Exercise_____

_____

Untoward Events_____

_____

Summary of Changes:	Initial Results	Most Recent
Total Cholesterol	_____	_____
HDL	_____	_____
LDL	_____	_____
Triglycerides	_____	_____
Body Weight	_____	_____
Body Fat	_____	_____

Changes in Fitness_____

_____

_____

Date_____ Program Director_____

Fig. 14–6.   Progress report to physician.

Date	Time	Resting	Heart Rate Immediate Recovery During Exercise	Distance Covered	Duration of Exercise	Comments

Fig. 14–7.   Home Recording.

of endurance capacity.[94] It has been observed that heart rate and blood pressure are higher and arrhythmias are more frequent toward the end of the day.[95]

INDIVIDUAL PROGRESS

Progress should be closely monitored in both cardiac rehabilitation and adult fitness. Figures 14–5 and 14–6 are examples of forms that can be used to keep a record of activity and other important information during each exercise session. In addition more comprehensive evaluations, such as those discussed previously in Chapters 4, 5, should be conducted annually or semiannually to assess program effectiveness and to update the exercise prescription. The results of these evaluations along with regular progress reports should be sent to the referring physician and discussed in detail with the patient and family. A progress review with the participant should serve as a motivator and an opportunity to establish realistic goals for the future.

If the person is not in a supervised program, then the information can be obtained through the use of daily diaries (Fig. 14–7), which can be provided at the time of the exercise test and prescription along with self-addressed and stamped envelopes. Instructions are provided to complete these forms and when they are to be mailed, for example, the first of each month. The process should be as simple as possible. Samples of computerized progress reports are provided in Chapter 9.

CONCLUSIONS

Phases III and IV of cardiac rehabilitation and adult fitness programs need to be a long-term commitment. The programs are designed and organized for maximal benefit and safety and to encourage good compliance. The most significant factor of a successful program is good exercise leadership, although equipment and facility considerations are also important.

Supervised and monitored programs are advantageous for cardiac patients. However, programs that are unsupervised and nonmonitored also can be effective.

Adherence to good principles of exercise is a must. The patient must understand environmental factors and the effect of certain medications. Training factors such as eating habits, stimulants, and time of day to exercise are also important in planning the exercise program. Properly blending all these factors is more likely to ensure success.

REFERENCES

1. Williams, R.S., et al.: Guidelines for unsupervised exercise in patients with ischemic heart disease. J. Cardiac Rehabil., 3:213, 1981.
2. Gettman, L.R., Pollock, M.L., and Ward, A.: Adherence to unsupervised exercise. Physician Sportsmed., 11:56, 1983.
3. DeBusk, R.F., Haskell, W.L., and Miller, N.H.: Medically directed at-home rehabilitation soon after clinically uncomplicated acute myocardial infarction: A new model for patient care. Am. J. Cardiol., 55:251, 1985.
4. Kasch, F.W., and Boyer, J.L.: Adult Fitness: Principles and Practices. Palo Alto, Calif., National Press Book, 1968.
5. American College of Sports Medicine: Guidelines for Exercise Testing and Prescription. 3rd Ed. Philadelphia, Lea & Febiger, 1986.
6. Fardy, P.S., Bennett, J.L., Reitz, N.L., and Williams, M.A.: Cardiac Rehabilitation: Implications for the Nurse and Other Health Professionals. St. Louis, C.V. Mosby, 1980.
7. Brock, L.L.: Administrative considerations. In Coronary Heart Disease: Prevention, Detection, Rehabilitation With Emphasis on Exercise Testing. Edited by S.M. Fox, III. Denver, Department of Professional Education, International Medical Corp., 1974.
8. Haskell, W.L.: The allied health professional. In Exercise Testing and Exercise Training in Coronary Heart Disease. Edited by J.P. Naughton, H.K. Hellerstein, and I.C. Mohler. Orlando, Fla., Academic Press, 1973.
9. Fardy, P.S.: Cardiac Rehabilitation for the Outpatient: A Hospital Based Program. In Heart Disease and Rehabilitation. Edited by M.L. Pollock and D.H. Schmidt. 2nd Ed. New York, John Wiley & Sons, 1986.
10. Miller, H.S., et al.: Community programs of cardiac rehabilitation. In Heart Disease and Rehabilitation. 2nd Ed. Edited by M.L. Pollock and

D.H. Schmidt. New York, John Wiley & Sons, 1986.

11. Dishman, R.K.: Compliance/adherence in health-related exercise. Health Psychol., 1:237, 1982.

12. Oldridge, N.B.: Compliance with exercise programs. In Heart Disease and Rehabilitation. 2nd Ed. Edited by M.L. Pollock and D.H. Schmidt. New York, John Wiley & Sons, 1986.

13. Franklin, B.A.: Exercise program compliance: Improvement strategies. In Behavioral Intervention in Obesity. Edited by J. Storlie and H.A. Jordan. Jamaica, N.Y., Spectrum, 1984.

14. Martin, J.E.: Exercise management: Shaping and maintaining physical fitness. Behav. Med. Adv. 4:3, 1981.

15. Oldridge, N.B.: Compliance and dropout in cardiac exercise rehabilitation. J. Cardiac Rehabil., 4:166, 1984.

16. Gale, J.B., et al.: Factors related to adherence to an exercise program for healthy adults. Med. Sci. Sports Exerc., 16:544, 1984.

17. Daltroy, L.H.: Improving cardiac patient adherence to exercise regimens: A clinical trial of health education. J. Cardiac Rehabil., 5:40, 1985.

18. Dishman, R.K., and Ickes, W.: Self-motivation and adherence to therapeutic exercise. J. Behav. Med., 4:421, 1981.

19. Blumenthal, J.A., et al.: Physiological and psychological variables predict compliance to prescribed exercise therapy in patients recovering from myocardial infarction. Psychosom. Med., 44:519, 1982.

20. Dishman, R.K.: Prediction of Adherence to Habitual Physical Activity. In Exercise in Health and Disease. Edited by F.J. Nagle and H.J. Montoye. Springfield, Ill., Charles C Thomas, 1981.

21. Dishman, R.K., Ickes, W., and Morgan, W.P.: Self-motivation and adherence to habitual physical activity. J. Appl. Soc. Psychol. 10:115, 1980.

22. Oldridge, N.B.: Compliance and exercise in primary and secondary prevention of coronary heart disease: A review. Prev. Med., 11:56, 1982.

23. Oldridge, N.B., and Jones, N.L.: Improving patient compliance in cardiac exercise rehabilitation: Effects of written agreement and self-monitoring. J. Cardiac Rehabil., 3:257, 1983.

24. Oldridge, N.B.: What to look for in an exercise leader. Physician Sportsmed., 5:85, 1977.

25. Kosowsky, B.D., et al.: Occurrence of ventricular arrhythmias with exercise as compared to monitoring. Circulation, 44:826, 1971.

26. Vitasalo, M.T., et al.: Ventricular arrhythmias during exercise testing, jogging and sedentary life. Chest, 75:21, 1979.

27. Simoons, M., Lap, C., and Pool, J.: Heart rate levels and ventricular ectopic activity during cardiac rehabilitation. Am. Heart J., 100:9, 1980.

28. Fardy, P.S., et al.: Monitoring cardiac patients: How much is enough? Physician Sportsmed., 10:146, 1982.

29. Meyer, G.C.: Telemetry electrocardiographic monitoring in cardiac rehabilitation: How Long? How often? In Cardiac Rehabilitation: Exercise Testing and Prescription. Edited by L.K. Hall. Spectrum, 1984.

30. Franklin, B.A.: The role of electrocardiographic monitoring in cardiac exercise programs. J. Cardiac Rehabil., 3:806, 1983.

31. Wenger, N.K.: The role of the physician in exercise testing and exercise training. In Exercise Testing and Exercise Training in Coronary Heart Disease. Edited by J.P. Naughton, H.K. Hellerstein, and I.C. Mohler, Orlando, Fla., Academic Press, 1973.

32. Dismuke, S.E., and Miller, S.T.: Why not share the secrets of good health? The physician's role in health promotion. JAMA, 249:3181, 1983.

33. Russell, M.A., et al.: Effect of general practitioners' advice against smoking. Br. Med. J., 2:231, 1979.

34. Yagbu, C.P.: Temperature, humidity, and air movement in industries: The effective temperature index. Am. J. Physiol., 58:439, 1927.

35. Karpovich, P., and Sinning, W.E.: Physiology of Muscular Activity. Philadelphia, W.B. Saunders, 1971.

36. Iampietro, P.F.: Exercise in hot environments. In Frontiers of Fitness. Springfield, Ill., Charles C Thomas, 1971.

37. Damato, A.N.: Cardiovascular response to acute thermal stress (hot dry environment) in unacclimatized normal subjects. Am. Heart J., 76:769, 1968.

38. Dill, D.B., et al.: Physical performance in relation to external temperature. Arbeitsphysiologie, 4:508, 1968.

39. Gilbert, C.A.: Temperature and humidity, radiation, underwater environment, hyperbaric oxygen, and the cardiovascular system. In The Heart. Edited by J.W. Hurst, R.B. Legue, and N.K. Wenger. New York, McGraw-Hill, 1978.

40. Rowell, L.B.: Human cardiovascular adjustments to exercise and thermal stress. Physiol. Rev., 54:75, 1974.

41. Sancetta, S.M., et al.: The effects of "dry" heat on the circulation of man. II. Coronary hemodynamics. Am. Heart J., 56:438, 1958.

42. Sancetta, S.M., Kramer, J., and Husni, E.: The effects of "dry" heat on the circulation of man. I. General hemodynamics. Am. Heart J., 56: 212, 1958.

43. Ansari, A., and Burch, G.E.: Influence of hot environment on the cardiovascular system. Arch. Intern. Med., 123:371, 1969.

44. Man, Sweat and Performance. Rutherford, N.J., Becton, Dickinson, 1969.

45. Buskirk, E.P., and Bass, D.E.: Climate and exercise. In Science and Medicine of Exercise and Sports. Edited by W.R. Johnson. New York, Harper Brothers, 1960.

46. Strydom, N.B., and Williams, C.G.: Effect of physical conditioning on state of heat acclimatization of Bantu laborer. J. Appl. Physiol., 27:262, 1969.

47. Gisolfi, C., and Robinson, S.: Relation between physical training, acclimatization, and heat tolerance. J. Appl. Physiol., 26:520, 1969.

48. Epstein, S.E., et al.: Effects of a reduction in environmental temperature on the circulatory re-

sponse to exercise in man. N. Engl. J. Med., 280:7, 1969.

49. Epstein, S.E., et al.: Angina pectoris: Pathophysiology, evaluation, and treatment. Ann. Intern. Med., 75:263, 1971.

50. Balke, B.: Work capacity at altitude. In Science and Medicine in Exercise and Sports. Edited by W.R. Johnson. New York, Harper Brothers, 1960.

51. Folk, G.E.: Introduction to Environmental Physiology. Philadelphia, Lea & Febiger, 1966.

52. Hurtado, A.: Animals in high altitudes: Resident Man. In Handbook of Physiology, Adaptation to the Environment. Edited by D.B. Dill. Bethesda, Md., American Physiology Society, 1964.

53. Morehouse, L.E., and Miller, A.T.: Physiology of Exercise. St. Louis, C.V. Mosby, 1971.

54. Faulkner, J.A.: Maximum exercise at medium altitude. In Frontiers of Fitness. Edited by R.J. Shephard. Springfield, Ill., Charles C Thomas, 1971.

55. Blomqvist, C.G., and Stemberg, J.: The electrocardiographic response to submaximal and maximal work during acute hypoxia. Acta Med. Scand., [Suppl. 440] 178:82, 1965.

56. Blomqvist, C.G.: Variations of the electrocardiographic response to exercise under different experimental conditions: Deconditioning, reconditioning and high altitude. In Measurement in Exercise electrocardiography. Edited by H. Blackburn. Springfield, Ill., Charles C Thomas, 1969.

57. Harris, C.W., and Hansen, J.E.: Electrocardiographic changes during exposure to high altitude. Am. J. Cardiol., 18:183, 1966.

58. Harris, C.W., Shields, J.L., and Hannon, J.P.: Electrocardiographic and radiographic heart changes in women at high altitude. Am. J. Cardiol., 18:847, 1966.

59. Froelicher, V.F., Jr.: The effect of air travel and altitude on the heart and circulation. In The Heart. Edited by J.W. Hurst, R.B. Logue, and N.K. Wenger. New York, McGraw-Hill, 1978.

60. Aronow, W.S.: Effect of cigarette smoking and of carbon monoxide on coronary heart disease. Chest, 70:514, 1976.

61. Aronow, W.S., et al.: Effect of freeway travel on angina pectoris. Ann. Intern. Med., 77:669, 1972.

62. Pirnay, F., et al.: Muscular exercise during intoxication by carbon monoxide. J. Appl. Physiol., 31:573, 1971.

63. Wright, G., Randell, P., and Shephard, R.J.: Carbon monoxide and driving skills. Arch. Environ. Health, 27:349, 1973.

64. Ramsey, J.M.: Carbon monoxide, tissue hypoxia and sensory psychomotor response in hypoxemia. Clin. Sci., 42:619, 1972.

65. Aronow, W.S., and Isbell, M.W.: Carbon monoxide effect on exercise-induced angina pectoris. Ann. Intern. Med., 79:392, 1973.

66. Anderson, E.W., et al.: Effect of low level carbon monoxide exposure on onset and duration of angina pectoris: A study of 10 patients with ischemic heart disease. Ann. Intern. Med., 79:46, 1973.

67. Cohen, S.I., Deane, M., and Goldsmith, J.T.: Carbon monoxide and survival from myocardial infarction. Arch. Environ. Health, 19:510, 1969.

68. The Health Implications of Photochemical Oxidant Air Pollution to Your Community. E.P.A. Publication No. 450/2-76-016, Research Triangle Park, N.C., Environmental Protection Agency, 1976.

69. Borg, G.A.: The perceived exertion: A note on "history" and methods. Med. Sci. Sports, 5:90, 1973.

70. Borg, G.A.: The perception of physical performance. In Frontiers of Fitness. Edited by R.J. Shephard. Springfield, Ill., Charles C Thomas, 1971.

71. Noble, B.J., et al.: Perceived exertion during walking and running. II. Med. Sci. Sports, 5:116, 1973.

72. Williams, M.A., and Fardy, P.S.: Limitations in prescribing exercise. J. Cardiovasc. Pulmon. Technique, 8:33, 1980.

73. Hellerstein, H.K., et al.: Principles of exercise prescription: For normals and cardiac subjects. In Exercise Testing and Exercise Training in Coronary Heart Disease. Edited by J.P. Naughton, H.K. Hellerstein, and I.C. Mohler. Orlando, Fla., Academic Press, 1973.

74. Nordeen-Snyder, K.S.: The effect of bicycle seat height variation upon oxygen consumption and lower limb kinematics. Med. Sci. Sports, 9:113, 1977.

75. Williams, M.A., et al.: Limitations of exercise testing to screen cardiac patients for early nonmonitored rehabilitation exercise programs. J. Cardiac Rehabil., 4:396, 1984.

76. Starling, M., et al.: Exercise testing early after myocardial infarction: Predictive value for subsequent unstable angina and death. Am. J. Cardiol., 46:909, 1980.

77. Theroux, P., et al.: Prognostic value of exercise testing soon after myocardial infarction. N. Engl. J. Med., 301:341, 1979.

78. Sami, M., Kraemer, H., and DeBusk, R.: The prognostic significance of serial exercise testing after myocardial infarction. Circulation, 60:1238, 1979.

79. Haskell, W.L.: Cardiovascular complications during exercise training of cardiac patients. Circulation, 57:920, 1978.

80. Van Camp, S.P., and Peterson, R.A.: Cardiovascular complications of outpatient cardiac rehabilitation programs. JAMA, 256:1160, 1986.

81. Vander, L. Franklin, B.A., and Rubenfire, M.: Cardiovascular complications of recreational physical activity. Physician Sportsmed., 10:89, 1982.

82. Pyfer, H.R.: Safety, precautions, and procedures in cardiac exercise rehabilitation programs. In Heart Disease and Rehabilitation. 2nd Ed. Edited by M.L. Pollock and D.H. Schmidt. New York, John Wiley & Sons, 1986.

83. Physicians' Desk Reference. Oradell, N.J., Medical Economics, 1986.

84. Gey, G.E., et al.: Exertional arrhythmia and nitroglycerine. JAMA, 226:287, 1983.

85. Froelicher, V.F., et al.: Cardiovascular medications: Their role in cardiac rehabilitation. In Cardiac Rehabilitation: Implications for the Nurse and Other Health Professionals. Edited by P.S.

Fardy, J.L., Bennett, N.L. Reitz, and M.A. Williams. St. Louis, C.V. Mosby, 1980.

86. Lowenthal, D.T., and Stein, D.T.: Drug effects: Exercise testing and training. *In* Heart Disease and Rehabilitation. Edited by M.L. Pollock and D.H. Schmidt. New York, John Wiley & Sons, 1986.

87. United States Department of Agriculture, Select Senate Subcommittee on Nutrition Report, 1980.

88. Simonson, E., and Keys, A.: The effect of an ordinary meal on the electrocardiogram. Circulation, *1*:1000, 1950.

89. Brody, J.: Good Food Cookbook: Living the High Carbohydrate Way. New York, W.W. Norton, 1985.

90. Nidetch, J.: Weight Watchers: Quick Start Program Cookbook. New York, New American Library, 1984.

91. Clark, N.: The Athlete's Kitchen: A Nutrition Guide and Cookbook. Boston, CBI Publishing Company, 1981.

92. Haas, R.: Eat to Win. New York, Signet Books, 1983.

93. Storlie, J., and Jordan, H.A. (eds): Nutrition and Exercise in Obesity Management. Jamaica, N.Y., Spectrum, 1984.

94. Ilmarinen, J., et al.: Study of the circadian variation of different circulatory and respiratory functions at submaximal and maximal ergometer work. Eur. J. Applied Physiol., *34*:255, 1975.

95. Fardy, P.S.: St. Catherine Hospital Cardiac Rehabilitation Program (unpublished observations).

15

CONTINUING EDUCATION AND
BEHAVIOR MODIFICATION

Patient education is initiated in phase I (Chapter 12). The purposes of education in this phase are (1) to clarify the problem to the patient and family so that they clearly understand what has happened, why, and what has to be done and (2) to build on the educational information by introducing the concept of life-style modification and management. Education and behavior modification then become an ongoing process in which appropriate changes in life-style are introduced and carried out. The educational information of phase I must be translated into more positive health behavior or it will have been a wasteful program. The end point of a patient education program is a healthier life-style, not whether the patient tests well on retention of information that is provided during hospitalization.

Life-style modification can be assessed regularly by questionnaire methods (Chapter 4). Occasional home visits by nurses or cardiac rehabilitation staff can also be helpful in patient assessment. To assist with life-style modification, the following should be made available: (1) the classes and materials that have been developed for all phases of the program, (2) individual and group counseling by specialists, (3) coronary support groups, and (4) self-teaching media centers that are available to the patient and family. It must be emphasized that education, behavior modification, and positive reinforcement of the patient are part of a lifelong plan. Many programs are limited in scope and neglect these objectives because of a lack of reimbursement for education.

In addition to exercise the most common and most popular life-style management programs are smoking cessation, nutrition and weight control, and stress management. Each of these subjects is concerned with known risk factors for coronary heart disease (CHD).[1–4]

SMOKING CESSATION

Cigarette smoking is one of the most, if not the most, significant risk factor for CHD.[1–5] Risk from smoking increases both with intensity and duration of the smoking habit.[6–8] Cigarette smoking is also related to other chronic diseases such as cancer, chronic obstructive lung disease, and hypertension.[9–13] Increased risk in smokers is illustrated in Figure 15–1.

Health care costs in smokers are equally staggering. It is estimated that $21 billion are expended on health care annually for smokers,[14] 25% more than for nonsmokers.[14] This amount can be significantly reduced through smoking cessation programs.[14,15] Smokers also have hospital stays that are 114% longer than those of nonsmokers.[14] As a consequence, the American public, especially the payers of health-

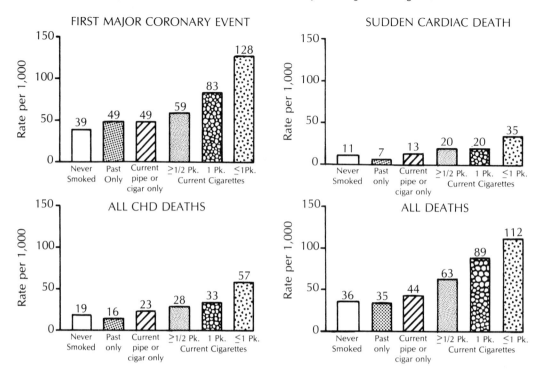

Fig. 15–1. "Smoking status and 10-year, age-adjusted rates per 1000 men for any major coronary event (nonfatal MI, fatal MI, SCD), SCD [sudden coronary death], any coronary death, death from all causes. Data from Pooling Project) Stamier J. Epstein FH: Preventive Med, 1(1-2):31, 1972. Adapted from Inter-Society Commission for Heart Disease Resources: *Circulation*, 42:A67, 1970)" (From Underhill SL, Woods SL, Sivarajan ES, Halpenny CJ: Cardiac Nursing, Phila., J.B. Lippincott Co., 1982.)

care benefits, has demonstrated considerable interest in reducing the incidence of smoking. Smoking cessation programs have varied from group or individual therapy sessions with specific goals and methods to large financial and marketing campaigns undertaken by public and private organizations that are interested in curbing the use of advertising in the tobacco industry. To date the success of these efforts has been mixed. Although the percentage of smokers has steadily declined over the past 20 years[16–19] since the initial report of the Surgeon General,[10] the intensity of smoking has increased among those who have retained the habit or started to smoke,[20] the number of female smokers has changed little,[20] and failure rates of group programs have been unacceptably high.[21,22] Consequently, although some progress has been made (Table 15–1), ample opportunity remains for further improvement.

Numerous stop-smoking programs are available today,[22–25] including, for example, hypnosis, Smoke Enders, sedatives, aversive therapy, nicotine gum, smokeless cigarettes, American Lung Association, Seventh-Day Adventists, books, cassettes, acupuncture. In general, these programs incorporate transfer of knowledge, with techniques of behavior modification, in order to identify the reasons why individuals smoke, as well as how, when, and where individuals are most likely to indulge. Strategies for these programs include financial rewards, group support systems, hypnosis with both negative and positive cues, and a variety of products to facilitate the cessation process. Some programs include more than one of these strategies. For example, a relatively new program in the

Table 15–1.   Changes in Cigarette Smoking Habits in the United States from 1970 to 1980 in Persons Above 17 Years of Age[20]

Year	Total Population	% Smokers	% Male Smokers	% Female Smokers	% Nonsmokers
1970	133,000,000	36.7	43.2	30.9	44.8
1980	161,000,000	32.6	36.5	29.1	46.1

% smoking more than 35 cigarettes per day
  1970
  4.3
  1980
  4.9

United States combines the behavior modification technique with a nicotine gum that is designed to decrease the smoker's dependence on nicotine.[25] This program has had successful trials in Europe[26,27] and is one of the most popular and promising programs on the market.

Regardless of which behavioral techniques might be adopted, professional staff and a support system have to be available to assist the person through this very difficult period. Reasons for smoking are numerous and unless dealt with in a well-directed program of behavior modification, chances for success are slim. Side effects of smoking cessation include nervousness, increased anxiety, depression, increased appetite, weight gain, and irritability.[21] It is essential to understand the implications of these factors, because they can present significant obstacles to success.

NUTRITION MANAGEMENT

The Select Committee on Nutrition and Human Needs of the United States Senate formulated a set of dietary goals for the United States.[28] In summary, the recommendations are as follows:

1. Reduce fat consumption to 30% of total calories.
2. Reduce saturated fat consumption to 10% of total calories.
3. Balance mono- and polyunsaturated fat intake to 10% of total calories each.

4. Reduce cholesterol intake to about 300 mg daily.
5. Increase complex carbohydrate consumption to 48% of total calories.
6. Reduce sugar consumption to 10% of total calories.
7. Reduce salt consumption to about 5 g daily.

These guidelines are suggested for most Americans. They do not apply to those who are in need of special diets and may require special nutrition guidelines.

Modifying eating habits (Table 15–2) can impact on CHD in several ways. Obesity, cholesterol, triglycerides, and hypertension have all been identified as risk factors that can be significantly reduced by adopting appropriate nutrition habits. Although each of these may represent independent risk factors, programs for their reduction overlap in many ways.

Obesity

A universally accepted definition of obesity is needed. Obesity has been defined as being excessively overweight[29]—more than 15%,[30] 20%[31] or 25%[32] above ideal body weight. Part of the problem in selecting a criterion for obesity is an inability to determine ideal weight.[33]

Although ideal body weight may not be precisely defined, the Metropolitan Life Insurance Data are widely used and are acceptable for the majority of the population (Tables 15–3 and 15–4). Although newer Metropolitan Life tables are avail-

Table 15–2.   Summary of Low-Fat
Diet Objectives

1. Reduce the consumption of beef, pork, and lamb.
2. Use poultry, fish, and meat substitutes instead of beef, lamb, and pork.
3. Prepare poultry and seafood without added fat.
4. Increase consumption of meatless meals.
5. Prepare rice, macaroni, and other grains without added fat.
6. Prepare vegetables without added fat.
7. Reduce the consumption of margarine and peanut butter as spreads for breads, rolls, etc. Eliminate butter totally.
8. Use only fat-free salad dressings.
9. Use only skim and low-fat dairy products.
10. Use only low-fat breads and cereals.
11. Avoid commercial baked goods (cakes, pies, cookies, etc.).
12. Avoid egg yolks.
13. Avoid foods high in sodium, and do not add salt at the table.
14. Limit the use of sugar in coffee, tea, and cereal.
15. Substitute fruit toppings for jams, preserves, jellies, honey, syrup, and molasses.
16. Use only recommended dessert recipes.
17. Drink decaffeinated coffee and caffeine-free herb teas.
18. Limit alcoholic beverages.

Adapted from Frye, N., et al.: A Comprehensive Guide to Cardiac Rehabilitation. Sid W. Richardson Institute for Preventive Medicine, The Methodist Hospital, Houston, TX, 1982.

able, the revised numbers have stirred considerable controversy and are not used by many nutritionists and dieticians. Ideal body weight is discussed further in Chapter 4.

The methodology of measuring body fat is described in Chapter 4. Acceptable ranges of body fat are between 10% and 22% for males and 20% and 32% for females.[34] Changes in body fat are more meaningful than body weight, because increased physical activity can result in increased muscle tissue. Because muscle is heavier than fat, exercise training may lead to loss of fat with no change in weight.

Obesity is related to increased risk of coronary disease, decreased cardiovascular function, increased metabolic demands of physical effort, and increased potential for hypertension and diabetes.[35–38] Risk of CHD is also related to changes in body weight, with increased risk associated with higher weight gains.[38,39]

Weight Control

Concomitant with weight loss the following can usually be expected:
- decreased triglycerides
- decreased cholesterol
- decreased blood sugar
- increased cardiac efficiency
- decreased cardiac work
- decreased blood volume
- decreased blood pressure
- improved self-image

Weight reduction for the patient with CHD might need to be modified according to the patient's clinical status. It is important to counsel obese patients that their program should be medically supervised. Particularly distressing to the medical community are programs that consist of fad diets, substantial caloric reduction, fasting, and liquid protein diets. Such programs can result in too rapid a weight loss, potassium depletion, and other electrolyte imbalances.[40,41] These can have serious harmful effects and are occasionally fatal.

A successful weight control program for the cardiac patient consists of a combination of group and individual approaches based on a comprehensive patient evaluation. The program should be individualized to meet specific needs. The basis of the program is behavior modification and management, which includes:

1. Recognition of eating habits.
2. Determination of external cues to eating.
3. Substituting appropriate for inappropriate eating habits.
4. Increasing physical activity.
5. Dealing with psychological aspects of weight gain or weight loss.

Because the physician can have a significant impact on patient health and monitoring life-style,[42,43] a role should be designated for the clinician in weight control intervention. Additional professional staff including dieticians, exercise physiologists, psychologists, and others are also important.

Table 15–3.   Weight Table for Men (pounds)*†

Height‡ (inches)	Suggested ideal weight§	1.1 times ideal weight	1.15 times ideal weight	1.2 times ideal weight
≤60	118	130	136	142
61	121	133	139	145
62	125	137	144	150
63	128	141	147	154
64	132	145	152	158
65	135	149	155	162
66	139	153	160	167
67	143	157	164	172
68	147	162	169	176
69	150	165	173	180
70	154	169	177	185
71	157	173	181	188
72	161	177	185	193
73	164	180	189	197
74	168	185	193	202
75	171	188	197	205
76	175	192	201	210
77	178	196	205	214
78	182	200	209	218
79	185	203	213	222
≥80	189	208	217	227

*From Stat. Bull. Metro. Life Ins. Co., *40*:1–4, Nov.–Dec., 1959.
†Weight—for partially clothed men (allow 2 pounds for clothes if stripped weight is desired).
‡Height—without shoes.
§"Ideal weight"—0.9 times the average weight of men aged 18 to 34 years as obtained from the National Health Survey: Weight by height and age of adults, United States 1960–1962, Series 11, No. 14. For persons with a height less than or equal to 66 inches the relationship between height and ideal weight is given by the formula Ideal weight = 3.5 Height − 92, for persons taller than 66 inches the relationship is Ideal weight = 3.5 Height − 91.

Table 15–4.   Weight Table for Women (pounds)*†

Height† (inches)	Average weight§	Suggested ideal weight‖	1.15 times ideal weight
57	114	103	118
58	117	105	121
59	120	108	124
60	123	111	128
61	127	114	131
62	130	117	135
63	133	120	138
64	136	122	140
65	139	125	144
66	142	128	147
67	145	130	149
68	148	133	153
69	151	136	156
70	154	139	160

*From Stat. Bull. Metro. Life Ins. Co., *40*:1–4, Nov.–Dec., 1959.
†Weight—for partially clothed women (allow 2 pounds for clothes if stripped weight is desired).
‡Height—without shoes.
§"Average weight"—for age group 18 to 34 years.
‖"Suggested ideal weight"—0.9 times average weight of women aged 18 to 34 years as obtained from the National Health Survey: Weight by height and age of adults, United States 1960–1962, Series 11, No. 14.

Regardless of the criterion used to define obesity, the basis for weight control remains the same, that is, establishing eating habits and activity patterns that will result in a metabolic balance. In general, this means increasing caloric expenditure and reducing caloric intake. A carefully designed and regulated plan is devised that takes into account desired amount of weight loss, recommended rate of loss, clinical status of the individual, and other specific needs of the individual.

The rate of weight loss is very important to long-term success. Weight loss should be gradual and include a series of realistic short-term goals, rather than a single long-term objective. Gradual weight loss, 1 to 2 pounds a week, is a safe and effective rate of change and has the advantage of being more permanent than rapid weight reduction.[44] Too rapid weight loss results in loss of lean body mass as well.[40,41] Subsequent weight gain is mostly fat, resulting in more fat per pound of weight.

Unfortunately, the $10 billion-dollar a-year weight loss industry, has bombarded the public with countless programs, which confuse the average person regarding methodology and too frequently compromise the individual's health. Similar to smoking cessation programs and other life-style interventions, it is essential to modify behavior to have lasting benefits. Otherwise, the rapid weight loss of today becomes the rapid weight gain of tomorrow.

Less traditional, but acceptable and effective under carefully monitored conditions, is a program of weight loss through diet supplementation. The advantages of this approach are (1) the instructions are easy to understand, (2) the caloric intake of the program can be carefully regulated, (3) marked improvements are seen quickly, which is often what is necessary to motivate the individual to continue. However, while some of these programs have demonstrated success in achieving short-term weight changes, data on long-term success rates are less convincing. Serious side effects and occasional fatalities have been reported.[40,41] Consequently, the medical community has been wary of the diet supplementation approach and has attempted to inform the public regarding the potential hazards of these programs.

If diet supplementation is to have widespread acceptance in weight control programs, medical supervision is absolutely necessary. In particular, if the caloric intake is restricted to less than 800 calories per day, then a physician must be made directly responsible for the program's conduct because fewer than 800 calories can result in loss of lean body mass, anemia, uremia, ketosis, electrolyte imbalance and possible hypoglycemia and postural hypotension.[40,41] Several products are more acceptable to the medical community because they are generally incorporated into physician-supervised programs (Table 15–5).[41,45,45a]

In any weight loss program, long-term success depends on establishing the behavioral basis for eating habits as well as educating the dieter and those who are likely to influence the success of the dieter about appropriate food selection and preparation. Normally, this instruction takes into account other eating patterns, such as number and size of meals, time of day for eating, chewing habits, and snacking habits.

Under most circumstances, a weight control program should include regular physical activity with diet management.[46,47] A program of vigorous exercise increases caloric expenditure and decreases the size of fat cells.[46,47] If introduced early, before adulthood, there is evidence that regular exercise can also reduce the number of fat cells.[48] This is particularly exciting from a preventive perspective. If regular exercise incorporated in childhood or adolescence lessens the potential for obesity, then a strong case can be made for vigorous physical education in the school curriculum. Types of exercise, as well as benefits from regular activity, are discussed in more detail in Chapters 13 and 14.

Table 15–5. Nutritional Comparison of Leading Dietary Supplements

	Optifast 800	Optifast 70	Medifast 45	NutriMed	COMP. 100	PRO-CAL 100	CareFast	U.S. RDA
Potassium, mg	2350	1955	1000	860	2206	860	2727	..
Sodium, mg	1150	920	920	920	780	920	1200	..
Manganese, mg	4	4	4	4	4	4	4	..
Calcium, mg	1000	1000	600	600	1650	1000	1000	1000
Phosphorus, mg	550	550	350	350	1256	1100	1000	1000
Magnesium, mg	400	400	150	150	400	400	400	400
Zinc, mg	15	15	15	15	22.5	15	15	15
Copper, mg	2	2	2	2	3	2	3	..
Vitamin A, IU	5000	5000	—	5000	7500	5000	10000	5000
Vitamin D, IU	400	400	—	400	600	400	400	400
Vitamin E, IU	30	30	—	30	45	30	60	30
Vitamin C, mg	90	90	—	60	90	90	120	60
Folic acid, µg	400	400	—	400	450	400	600	400
Thiamine (B_1), mg	2.25	2.25	—	1.50	2.25	2.25	2.63	1.50
Riboflavin (B_2), mg	2.60	2.60	—	1.70	2.52	2.60	2.98	1.70
Niacin, mg	20	20	—	20	30	20	40	20
Vitamin B_6, mg	3	3	—	2	3	3	4	2
Vitamin B_{12}, µg	6	6	—	6	9	6	12	6
Pantothenic Acid, mg	10	10	—	10	15	10	10	10
Biotin, µg	300	360	—	300	450	360	300	300
Iodine, µg	150	150	—	150	150	150	150	150
Iron, mg	18	18	18	18	27	18	36	18
Selenium, µg	150	150	—	—	150	—	200	..
Chromium, µg	150	150	—	—	150	—	200	..
Molybdenum, µg	300	300	—	—	300	—	500	..
Calories	800	420	300	300	520	500	600	
Protein, g	70	70	45	45	50	70	50	
Carbohydrate, g	100	30	30	30	79	32.5	95	
Fat, g	13	2	—	0	1	10	5	
Fiber, g	—	—	—	—	—	—	5	

..No RDA requirements yet established for these nutrients.

Figures based on 5 packets per day.

Values for Optifast, Medifast, NutriMed, Complement 100 and Pro-Cal 100 were obtained from manufacturer's labels.

Although weight loss is enhanced by regular physical activity, low-level exercise by itself has little impact on losing weight. Calorie cost of most outpatient monitored exercise programs is estimated at 300 calories per session. Since it takes 3,500 calories to lose one pound of fat, exercising three times a week would require 1 month for a single pound of fat weight loss. Supplementing monitored exercise sessions with home activity such as walking 3 miles daily is suggested. A 1-mile walk is approximately equivalent to 100 calories of energy expended, and 3 miles per hour is a good, brisk rate. Couple this level of activity with 200 calories dietary reduction each day, and the result is 1 pound of fat loss per week, which is a good rate of reduction.

CHOLESTEROL AND TRIGLYCERIDES

Increased levels of cholesterol and triglycerides in the blood are significant risk factors for the development of coronary artery disease (CAD).[1–3,49,50] Recommended levels of cholesterol and triglycerides are less than 200 mg/dl and 80 to 100 mg/dl, respectively.[1,50] Measurement of lipids and the effects of exercise on lipid values are discussed in detail in Chapters 1 and 4.

Obesity is frequently associated with increased levels of cholesterol and triglycerides,[38,51,52] although a stronger relationship exists with triglycerides.[52] It is also possible to have elevated lipids with normal weight. The best way to decrease lipids is a combination of diet management, specifically fat reduction, and physical activity. Lowering lipid values is easier than losing weight for some individuals because it requires no caloric restrictions.

A typical American Diet consists of about 37% calories derived from fat.[53] According to the Senate Select Committee on Nutrition and Human Needs, the fat intake should be lowered to less than 30% of total calorie.[28,53] (Figs. 15–2 and 15–3). Nutrition programs that emphasize low fat consumption (e.g., the Pritikin diet) reduce caloric intake from fat consumption to less than 10% and almost 0% of cholesterol.[54,55] When fat intake is reduced this drastically, it has been shown to have a significant lowering effect.[54,55] Perhaps such a radical approach is necessary for some individuals. More long-term data are required to understand the feasibility and benefits of this kind of program. Furthermore, more effort needs to be directed toward making a stringent diet of this type palatable and appealing for most people.

Reducing the amount of meat consumed and food of animal origin will lower cholesterol in most persons. Because the body manufactures cholesterol at varying levels, the impact of a low-fat diet and physical activity will vary. Nevertheless, sufficient cholesterol is manufactured by the body for cellular function so that its elimination from the diet is not detrimental to health.

Triglycerides differ from cholesterol in that they exist in all sources of fat, animal and vegetable. Substituting polyunsaturated fat for saturated is an improvement, and reducing all dietary fat is even better. Triglycerides are also produced by the conversion of excess calories that are stored as fat. Consequently, they are more sensitive to weight loss than is cholesterol. Triglycerides are also more likely to fluctuate over short periods of time than cholesterol, which is why a 12- to 14-hour fast and refrain from physical activity must precede their measurement.

Lowering the intake of fat in the diet also results in a weight loss in most persons. Since the calorie content of fat is approximately twice that of an equal amount of carbohydrate or protein, weight loss is much more likely to occur when fat intake is reduced. Specific suggestions for lowering fat and calorie intake are listed in Table 15–2.

STRESS MANAGEMENT AND PSYCHOTHERAPEUTIC INTERVENTION

Psychosocial factors are also important in treating and preventing CHD.[56–61]

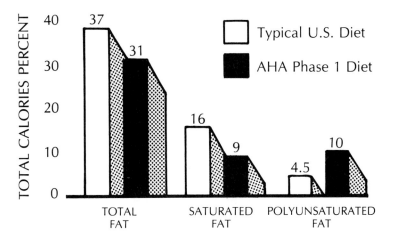

Fig. 15–2.   The typical U.S. diet (data from Abrams, S., and Carrol, M.: Fats, cholesterol and sodium intake in the diet of persons 1–74 years, United States. Advanced Data, Feb. 7, 1981) compared with the American Heart Association's phase 1 diet recommendations. Reproduced with permission. Eating for a Healthy Heart. © American Heart Association.

Stress-related health problems, which are at least partly attributed to modern-day, fast-paced and pressured life-styles, are estimated to cost the American public as much as $60 billion annually.[62] Changes in all aspects of society have resulted in increased stress among both sexes and across all ages.[57,58,63,64] As a consequence, health professionals are confronted with new problems, the cause of which has only recently been recognized.

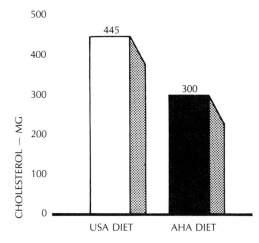

Fig. 15–3.   Dietary cholesterol intake of the typical U.S. diet compared with the American Heart Association's phase 1 diet recommendations. Reproduced with permission. Eating for a Healthy Heart. © American Heart Association.

Stress reactivity is defined as a physical response to external stimuli. When the response is inappropriate, it is associated with dramatic neurohormonal activity, which can result in increased blood pressure, increased myocardial demand for oxygen, increased cardiac arrhythmias, and increased CHD.[57,58,64] Although recognized as a necessary and facilitative aspect of life when experienced in appropriate situations and degrees, excessive stress reactivity has been viewed as resulting in exhaustion and death. Stress may originate from external, social or environmental factors, or may be internal and self-generated. For example type A behavior, which is associated with coronary disease, is an example of self-generated stress. Even though stress has received considerable attention in the past 10 or 15 years, our knowledge of stress and related health disorders and their treatment is still in its infancy.

Measuring stress is complex and imprecise. Although several instruments are available to evaluate stress,[65] interpretation of their findings is fraught with confusion. Instruments such as the Holmes-Rahe Scale of Recent Life-style Changes[66,67] and Rosenman and Friedman type A/type B personality scales [68,69] are controversial,[56,70] even though they are popular, frequently used, and much has been written about them in recent years. Even if stress can be quantified accurately, and sources of stress identified, the question remains if and how response to stressors can be altered.

Consequently, comprehensive programs of cardiac rehabilitation and preventive medicine are concerned with identifying mechanisms to cope with stress and to reduce their potential negative impact. These mechanisms include personal characteristics such as mental attitude, availability of support, self-esteem and being in control of one's life. Other traits are those typically emphasized in stress management, that is, learning to relax, recognizing causes of stress, compartmentalizing stressors into those that can be controlled and those that cannot, developing a sense of self-control, biofeedback, self-hypnosis, rhythmic breathing, and modifying life-style to include better nutrition habits, increased physical activity, and increased sleep and rest.[71–73]

Numerous programs have been developed that utilize techniques to cope with stress and to deal with the effect of stress on physical and mental health. Still, much remains to be learned about successful strategies and methodologies. The health professional must assess the worth of a plethora of available programs and attempt to identify those that will best meet the individual's needs. Cardiac rehabilitation, preventive medicine, and adult fitness programs should incorporate this information, as well as other types of behavior modification, so that the individual has the best opportunity to adopt appropriate life-style management skills.

In addition to the role of stress in CHD, other psychosocial factors associated with postmyocardial infarction (post-MI) and post–bypass surgery should be understood. It is probably advisable that all candidates for cardiac rehabilitation be interviewed by the staff psychologist or social worker and followed when additional consultation is

warranted. The objectives of psychological interview follow:[65]

1. Assist the patient and family in dealing with their emotional adjustment following an MI or surgery.
2. Reassure the patient and family that most of these emotional responses are normal reactions to the present stressful situation and should pass.
3. Identify specific emotional responses that are likely to develop for limited periods of time.
4. Discuss various ways of dealing or coping with these responses.

Specifically, the psychologist or social worker should look for those psychological problems that are characteristic of post-MI patients, such as anxiety, denial, depression, and anger. Figure 15–4 provides an outline that has been developed for dealing with these issues.[74]

These emotional responses can significantly alter family and personal life and the patient's mental health. Parental and job roles, return to normal social and leisure time activity, sexual roles and function, as well as many other aspects of one's life can be significantly changed if these problems are not recognized and professionally treated.

All members of the rehabilitation staff should be familiar with these problems, although they are primarily the responsibility of the psychologist or social worker. This is particularly true if there is expectation of reimbursement for such services.

CONCLUSIONS

Patient education and behavioral self-management should represent an ongoing process through which the professional team along with the patient and family can establish a lifetime plan. While education and behavior programs are not limited to those discussed in this chapter, these are generally considered the most important and common to the majority of rehabili-

A. Objectives
  1. Providing group support and understanding to assist patient and family in dealing with their emotional adjustment following a myocardial infarction.
  2. Reassure patient and family that most of these emotional responses are normal reactions to the present stressful situation and should pass.
  3. Identify specific emotional responses that are likely to develop usually for limited periods of time.
  4. Discuss various ways of dealing or coping with these responses.
B. Specific emotional responses
  1. Anxiety
    a. Manifestations
      1. Inability to concentrate and understand or retain information.
      2. Restlessness or insomnia.
      3. Increased verbalization.
      4. Tremulousness.
      5. Palmar sweating.
    b. Causes
      1. Fear of death or chronic disability.
      2. Uncertainty about illness and prognosis.
      3. Being subjected to "strange" environment and procedures of coronary care unit and rest of hospital.
      4. Changes in usual patterns of daily living.
      5. Restrictions and limitations in activity, diet, etc.
  2. Denial (positive and negative aspects)
    a. Manifestations
      1. Avoids discussing heart attack and/or its significance.
      2. Minimizes severity of condition and its consequences.
      3. May disregard activity and diet restrictions.
      4. Tries to keep interactions on a social, humorous level; may seem overly cheerful.
    b. Causes
      1. Normal defense mechanism to help alleviate anxiety.
      2. Inability to control medical events—focuses on parts of existence he or she can control by ignoring, rejecting, or refusing to believe they exist.
  3. Depression
    a. Manifestations
      1. Sad look, listlessness, and disinterest.
      2. Expressions of pessimism.
      3. Talks with short verbal responses.
      4. Slowness in movement and speech.
      5. Withdrawn.
      6. Loss of appetite.
      7. Crying, irritability.
      8. Expressions of direct or projected anger.
    b. Causes
      1. Patient has become less able to maintain denial, becomes more aware of what has happened, and begins to think about how it will affect his or her future.
      2. May feel powerless, hopeless, helpless, or useless.
      3. Worry about self-image and self-esteem.
      4. Worry about social implications, ie: loss of job, independence, fears of sexual impotence, invalidism, and premature old age.

Fig. 15–4.   Treating Emotional Aspects of Cardiovascular Rehabilitation.

4. Anger
   a. Manifestations
      1. Direct or indirect expressions of hostility toward hospital staff and/or family.
      2. Refuses to follow doctors' orders.
   b. Causes
      1. Frustration.
      2. Resentment of other healthy individuals ("Why me?").
      3. Infantilizing and overprotection of patient by spouse, family, etc.
C. Class discussion and evaluation
   1. Should encourage patient and family to develop good working relationship with personal physician, ask specific questions of him or her, etc.
   2. Encourage patient and family members to discuss fears and anxieties together so that each understands the other and is better able to offer support when needed.
   3. Deal with any questions regarding financial coverage of hospital bills, rehabilitation programs, etc., either in group or individual discussions.
   4. Social worker should be aware of any specific problem areas with each patient and make referral to appropriate resource person, if applicable.

Fig. 15–4 Continued.

tation programs and often provide additional sources of revenues to the program.

REFERENCES

1. Kannel, W.B.: Epidemiologic insights into atherosclerotic cardiovascular disease from the Framingham Study. In Heart Disease and Rehabilitation. 2nd Ed. Edited by M.L. Pollock and D.H. Schmidt. New York, John Wiley & Sons, 1986.
2. Blackburn, H., and Leon, A.S.: Preventive cardiology in practice: Minnesota studies on risk factor reduction. In Heart Disease and Rehabilitation. 2nd Ed. Edited by M.L. Pollock and D.H. Schmidt. New York, John Wiley & Sons, 1986.
3. Blackburn, H.: Progress in the epidemiology and prevention of coronary heart disease. In Progress in Cardiology. Edited by P. Yu and J. Goodwin. Philadelphia, Lea & Febiger, 1974.
4. MRFIT Research Group: Multiple risk factor changes and mortality results. JAMA, 248:1465, 1982.
5. Kannel, W.B.: Update on the role of cigarette smoking in coronary artery disease. Am. Heart J., 101:319, 1981.
6. Aronow, W.S.: Effect of cigarette smoking and of carbon monoxide on coronary heart disease. Chest,70:514, 1976.
7. Tibblin, G., Wilhelmsen, L., and Werko, L.: Risk factors for myocardial infarction and death due to ischemic heart disease and other causes. Am. J. Cardiol, 35:514, 1975.
8. Stamler, J., and Epstein, F.H.: Smoking status and 10-year, age-adjusted rates per 1000 men for any major coronary event (nonfatal MI, fatal MI, SCD), SCD, any coronary death from all causes. Data from the pooling project. Prev. Med., 1:31, 1972.
9. Doyle, J.T., et al.: Relationship of cigarette smoking to coronary heart disease; The second report of the combined experience of the Albany, N.Y., and Framingham, Mass., studies. JAMA, 190:889, 1964.
10. U.S. Department of Health, Education and Welfare: Smoking and Health. Report of the Advisory Committee to the Surgeon General of the Public Health Service. U.S. Government Printing Office, Washington, D.C., 1964.
11. Moser, K.M., et al.: Shortness of Breath: A Guide to Better Living and Breathing. 3rd Ed. St. Louis, C.V. Mosby, 1983.
12. U.S. Public Health Service: Health Consequences of Smoking. 1968 Suppl. Washington, D.C., Government Printing Office, 1968.
13. Finklea, J.F., et al.: Cigarette smoking and hemagglutination inhibition response to influenza after natural disease and immunization. Am. Rev. Respir. Dis., 104:368, 1971.
14. Control Data Corporation: Control Data 1982 Health Claims Data and 1982 Corporate Wide Employee Health Survey. Minneapolis, Control Data Corporation, 1983.
15. Berry, C.A.: Good Health for Employees and Reduced Health Care Costs for Industry 1982.
16. Gillum, R.F., Blackburn, H., and Feinleib, M.: Current strategies for explaining the decline in ischemic heart disease. J. Chronic Dis., 35:467, 1982.
17. Kannel, W.B.: Meaning of downward trend in cadiovascular mortality. JAMA, 247:877, 1982.
18. Warner, K.E.: Cigarette smoking in the 1970's: The impact of the anti-smoking campaign on consumption. Science, 211:729, 1981.
19. Rowland, M., Fulwood, R., and Kleinman, B.C.: Changes in heart disease risk factors, health and prevention profile. United States, U.S. Dept. of Health and Human Services, PHS, National Center for Health Statistics, 1983.

20. National Data Book and Guide to Sources, Statistical Abstract of the U.S. 1985. 105th Ed. Washington, D.C., U.S. Dept. of Commerce, Bureau of Census, 1985.

21. Cutter G., et al.: The natural history of smoking cessation among patients undergoing coronary arteriography. J. Cardiopul. Rehabil., 5:332, 1985.

22. Kannel, W.B., McGee, D.L., and Castelli, W.P.: Latest perspectives on cigarette smoking and cardiovascular disease: The Framingham Study, J. Cardiac Rehabil., 4:267, 1984.

23. Calling it Quits. Dallas, American Heart Association, 1984.

24. Stop Smoking System. American Health Foundation, Mahoney Institute for Health Maintenance, New York Health Promotion Service, 1980.

25. Smokewise. Health Improvement Systems, Inc., Cincinnati, Ohio, Merrell Dow Pharmaceuticals, 1984.

26. Jarvis, M.J., et al.: Randomized controlled trial of nicotine chewing gum. Br. Med. J., 285:537, 1982.

27. Russell, M.A.H., et al.: The effect of nicotine chewing gum as an adjunct to the general practitioner's advice against smoking. Br. Med. J., 287:1782, 1983.

28. U.S. Senate Select Committee on Nutrition and Human Needs: Dietary Goals for the United States. 2nd Ed. Washington, D.C., U.S. Government Printing Office, 1977.

29. Wohl, M.G., and Goodhart, R.S. (eds.): Modern Nutrition in Health and Disease. 4th Ed. Philadelphia, Lea & Febiger, 1968.

30. Van Horn, L., and Cooper, R.: Nutrition and the coronary patient. In Cardiac Rehabilitation: Implications for the Nurse and Other Health Professionals. Edited by P.S. Fardy, J.L. Bennett, N.L. Reitz, and M.A. Williams. St. Louis, C.V. Mosby, 1980.

31. Thomas, A.E., MacKay, E.A., and Cutlip, M.B.: A nomograph method for assessing body weight. Am. J. Clin. Nutr.,29:302, 1976.

32. Tuck, M.L., et al.: The effect of weight reduction on blood pressure, plasma renin activity, and plasma aldosterone levels in obese patients. N. Engl. J. Med., 304:930, 1981.

33. The Modifitness Program: Physician Orientation Manual. Minneapolis, The Delmark Company, Inc., 1982.

34. Lohman, T.G.: Body composition methodology in sports medicine. Physician Sportsmed., 10:47, 1982.

35. Ashley, F.W., Jr., and Kannel, W.B.: Relation of weight change to changes in atherogenic traits: The Framingham study. J. Chronic Dis., 27:103, 1974.

36. Kannel, W.B., and Gordon, T.: Physiological and medical concomitants of obesity: The Framingham study. In Obesity in America. Edited by C.A. Gray. National Institutes of Public Health Publication, No. 70-359. U.S. Department of Health, Education and Welfare, 1979.

37. Rabkin, S.W., Mathewson, F.A.L., and Hsu, P.W.: Relation of body weight to development of ischemic heart disease in a cohort of young North American men after a 26 year observation period. The Manitoba study. Am. J. Cardiol., 39:452, 1977.

38. Alexander, J.K.: Obesity and coronary heart disease. In Coronary Heart Disease: Prevention, Complications, and Treatment. Edited by W.E. Connor and J.D. Bristow, New York, Philadelphia, J.B. Lippincott, 1986.

39. Hubert, H.B., et al.: Obesity as an independent risk factor for cardiovascular disease: A 26 year follow-up in the Framingham study. Circulation, 67:968, 1983.

40. Vertes, V., Genuth, S.M., and Hazelton, I.M.: Supplemented fasting as a large-scale outpatient program. JAMA, 238:2151, 1977.

41. Vertes, V.: Supplemented fasting: A perspective. Drug Therapy, Sept. 1978.

42. Dismuke, S.E., and Miller, S.T.: Why not share the secrets of good health? The physician's role in health promotion. JAMA, 249:3181, 1983.

43. Hjermann, I., et al.: Effect of diet and smoking intervention on the incidence of coronary heart disease. Lancet, 2:1303, 1981.

44. Storlie, J., and Jordan, H.A. (eds.): Nutrition and Exercise in Obesity Management. Jamaica, N.Y., Spectrum, 1984.

45. Genuth, S.M., Vertes, V., and Hazelton, I.: Supplemented fasting in the treatment of obesity. In Recent Advances in Obesity Research. Edited by G. Bray. London, John Libbey, 1978.

45a. Care Fast Weight Loss Clinics. Comprehensive Care Corporation, Irvine, CA, 1986.

46. Franklin, B.A., and Rubenfire, M.: Losing weight through exercise. JAMA, 244:377, 1980.

47. Clarke, H.H. (ed.): Exercise and Fat Reduction. Physical Fitness Research Digest. Washington, D.C., President's Council on Physical Fitness and Sports. Series 5. Vol. 2. 1975.

48. Oscai, L.B.: The role of exercise in weight control. In Exercise and Sport Sciences Reviews. Edited by J.H. Wilmore. Orlando, Fla., Academic Press, 1973.

49. Carlson, L.A., and Bottinger, L.E.: Ischemic heart-disease in relation to fasting values of plasma triglycerides and cholesterol. Lancet, 1:865, 1972.

50. Greenhalgh, R.M., et al.: Serum lipids and lipoproteins in peripheral vascular disease. Lancet, 30:947, 1971.

51. Keys, A., et al.: Coronary heart disease: Overweight and obesity as risk factors. Ann. Intern. Med., 77:15, 1972.

52. Bierman, E.L.: Hyperlipoproteinemia. Current Concepts, A Scope Publication, Kalamazoo, Mich., Upjohn, 1976.

53. Becker, G.L.: Heart Smart: A Plan for Low Cholesterol Living. Supported by Merrell Dow. New York, Pocket Books, 1984.

54. Barnard, R.J., et al.: Effects of an intensive, short-term exercise and nutrition program on patients with coronary heart disease. J. Cardiac Rehabil., 1:99, 1981.

55. Hill, P., Reddy, B.S., and Wynder, E.L.: Effect of

unsaturated fats and cholesterol on serum and fecal lipids. J. Am. Diet. Assoc., *75*:414, 1979.

56. Morgan, W.P., and Raglin, J.S.: Psychologic aspects of heart disease. *In* Heart Disease and Rehabilitation. Edited by M.L. Pollock and D.H. Schmidt. 2nd Ed. New York, John Wiley & Sons, 1986.

57. Buell, J.C., and Eliot, R.S.: Stress and cardiovascular disease. Mod. Conc. Cardiovas Dis., *48*:19, 1979.

58. Syme, S.L.: Social and psychological risk factors in coronary heart disease. Mod. Conc. Cardiovasc. Dis., *44*:17, 1975.

59. Haynes, S.G., et al.: The relationship of psychosocial factors to coronary heart disease in the Framingham Study: Prevalence of coronary heart disease. Am. J. Epidemiol., *107*:384, 1978.

60. Jenkins, C.D.: Psychologic and social precursors of coronary disease. N. Engl. J. Med., *284*:244, 1971.

61. Jenkins, C.D.: Psychologic and social precursors of coronary disease. Part 2. N. Engl. J. Med., *284*:307, 1971.

62. Eighth Report of the Director of the National Heart, Lung, and Blood Institute. Washington, D.C., Government Printing Office, U.S. March, 1981.

63. Rosenman, R.H., and Friedman, M.: Association of specific behavior pattern in women with blood and cardiovascular findings. Circulation, *24*:1173, 1961.

64. Eliot, R.S., and Buell, J.C.: The role of the CNS in cardiovascular disorders. Hosp. Pract., May:189, 1983.

65. Blumenthal, J.A.: Psychologic assessment in cardiac rehabilitation. J. Cardiopul. Rehabil., *5*:208, 1985.

66. Holmes, T., and Rahe, R.: The social readjustment rating scale. J. Psychosom. Res., *11*:213, 1967.

67. Holmes, T., and Masuda, M.: Life change and illness susceptibility. *In* Stressful Life Events. Edited by B.S. Dohrenwend and B.P. Donrenwend. New York, Wiley, 1974.

68. Rosenman, R.H., et al.: Multivariate prediction of coronary heart disease during 8.5 year follow-up in the Western Collaborative Group Study. Am. J. Cardiol., *37*:903, 1976.

69. Friedman, M., and Rosenman, R.H.: Type A behavior pattern: Its association with coronary heart disease. Ann. Clin. Res., *3*:300, 1971.

70. Rabkin, J.G., and Struening, E.L.: Life events, stress, and illness. Science, *194*:1013, 1976.

71. Blumenthal, J.A., et al.: Continuing medical education cardiac rehabilitation: A new frontier for behavioral medicine. J. Cardiac Rehabil., *3*:637, 1983.

72. Thoresen, C.E., et al.: Altering the type A behavior pattern in postinfarction patients. J. Cardiopul. Rehabil., *5*:258, 1985.

73. Chesney, M.A., and Ward, M.M.: Biobehavioral treatment approaches for cardiovascular disorders. J. Cardiopul. Rehabil., *5*:226, 1985.

74. Emotional Aspects of Cardiac Rehabilitation. Unpublished paper, Cardiac Rehabilitation Program, L.D.S. Hospital, Salt Lake City, Utah.

CURRENT AND FUTURE PERSPECTIVES

16

CURRENT AND FUTURE PERSPECTIVES

In spite of recent downward trends, the major health problem of our society continues to be the unnecessary and premature morbidity and mortality from atherosclerotic cardiovascular diseases. Although the causes of atherosclerosis are multiple and to some extent still unknown, physical inactivity appears to be a contributing risk factor. The evidence linking physical inactivity to coronary heart disease (CHD) is substantial, although far from conclusive.[1,2] The downward trend in cardiovascular mortality has occurred during a period of major changes in the public's attitude toward healthier and more active life-styles and a corresponding increase in interest by physicians and other health professionals in matters relating to exercise. This book provides a comprehensive review of exercise testing, adult fitness, and cardiac rehabilitation. In the concluding chapter current and future perspectives regarding the emerging role of exercise in the prevention of cardiovascular diseases and the promotion of better health and well-being are examined from a variety of viewpoints.

THE PUBLIC VIEWPOINT

The public is clearly aware of the emerging role of exercise in our society. Since the late 1960s there has been a virtual explosion of public interest in physical fitness and leisure-time physical activity. Numerous population surveys and public opinion polls have been conducted in recent years to evaluate the public's attitude toward exercise and fitness. Although there may be considerable difficulties in drawing generalizations from these data, a review of the more reliable and relevant national surveys in the United States and Canada has revealed some interesting observations.[3] These findings can be grouped into the following categories: (1) prevalence of leisure-time physical activity, (2) physical activity and age, (3) activity and socioeconomic status, (4) regional differences in activity patterns, and (5) choices of physical activities. Because of their importance to future planning by the health professions, a brief summary of these data is presented.

Prevalence of Leisure-Time Physical Activity

One of the more difficult questions to answer from epidemiologic surveys is the degree of physical activity engaged in by our population. Although there seems to be a general perception that increasing numbers of people are exercising, the studies estimate that less than 20% of the population exercises at a level comparable to that recommended to develop and maintain cardiorespiratory fitness.[3] An additional 35% to 40% of the population engages in some limited forms of physical activities, and 40% to 50% is sedentary. These findings suggest that there is a need for more public and professional education regarding cardiovascular and other health benefits of exercise training as well as the behavioral techniques for developing and maintaining fitness.

Physical Activity and Age

The general conclusion from cross-sectional population studies is that there is a decline in physical activity with age, which is steepest during adolescence and early adulthood.[3] This is especially true for participation in organized sports, and not too surprising, because sports activities are primarily engaged in during high school and college years. The decline seems to level off after age 55 to 60, most likely due to the increased interest in leisure-time activities associated with retirement. It is likely that as the percentage of healthy older adults in our society increases with the decline in cardiovascular disease mortality an even greater proportion of middle-aged and older adults will be exercising in the years to come. The implications to health professionals are obvious. More emphasis should be given to the specific training needs of older individuals, especially those who have physical disabilities and other health problems.

Activity and Socioeconomic Status

Participation in leisure-time physical activity is more prevalent among middle- and upper-class segments of society.[3] The surveys indicate that managers and professionals engage in more fitness activities than other white-collar workers, and white-collar workers are generally more active than blue-collar workers. It is also important to realize that blue-collar workers are less physically active at work than in years past because of technologic advances in industry and agriculture. Data, however, are still insufficient to prove that the increased physical activity associated with increasing income, education, or occupational status has any well-defined health benefits.

Recent emphasis in promoting employee fitness programs by the American Heart Association, the American College of Sports Medicine (ACSM), the Association for Fitness in Business and other organizations will likely have a positive impact on the numbers of working individuals participating in exercise activities. The rationale for health promotion and fitness at the work site is that these programs are likely to be associated with reduced health-care costs, decreased absenteeism, and increased productivity, although well-designed studies documenting these benefits are lacking. Furthermore, the work site has a captive audience, making it a very appealing environment for health-enhancement programs.

Regional Differences in Activity Patterns

The proportion of the population engaged in regular exercise seems to vary from urban to rural communities and among regions in the United States and Canada. Studies indicate a higher proportion of active individuals living in large cities, especially in the suburbs, than in small, rural communities.[3] Also, in the United States, there are more exercisers living in the West fewest living in the South, and an intermediate proportion living in other regions of the country.[3] There is also a similar East–West distribution in Canada.[3] The reasons for these regional differences are not entirely clear, although climatic and socioeconomic factors undoubtedly play a role. Commercial interests in exercise facilities and equipment, coupled with the increasing mobility of the population are likely to even out these regional differences in the future.

Choices of Physical Activity

As the percentage of active adults in our society increases, there is a corresponding shift in participation away from organized sports to conditioning activities that can be carried out on an individual basis. The population surveys indicate that the most popular aerobic activities are walking, swimming, calisthenics, cycling, and jogging.[3] The obvious advantages of these activities are that they are inexpensive, can be carried out at home or close to home, and allow for flexible scheduling. The surveys also indicate that men are more involved in organized athletic events and more vigorous activities than women.[3] Women, however, are becoming physically active in greater proportions than other demographic groups in the general population and are increasingly becoming involved in organized sports. Aerobic dance is much more popular among women than among men.

THE DETERMINANTS OF EXERCISE PARTICIPATION

Although the evidence for the fitness boom is substantial and highly visible in our society, the percentage of individuals actually engaging in vigorous physical activities remains small. National goals established by the Department of Health and Human Services[4] call for an increase in the number of exercisers to 90% of youth and 60% of adults by 1990. Most likely these goals will not be met without active intervention by the health professions. The challenge of the 1980s is to develop effective interventions that encourage sedentary individuals to adopt and maintain regular aerobic exercise habits. Intervention strategies aimed at preventing dropouts from clinical exercise programs including cardiac rehabilitation are also badly needed.

Dishman et al.[5] have carefully reviewed the scientific literature to study the known determinants of and barriers to regular exercise and physical activity. The reasons why people choose to exercise or choose not to exercise are complex and include personal characteristics, environmental factors, and factors relating to the specific exercise activities.

Personal characteristics that may influence exercise behaviors include past and present experiences with exercise programs and other forms of physical activity, health beliefs, and attitudes toward exercise, personality characteristics, biomedical traits, and demographic factors.[5] Previous participation in sports during youth, for example, may have a positive influence on the subsequent exercise behaviors of adults, although other personal or environmental factors sometimes override. In addition, current involvement in adult fitness or cardiac rehabilitation programs is a strong predictor of future participation. Most dropouts from supervised programs occur in the first 3 to 6 months.

Apparent barriers to participation in clinical exercise programs include blue-collar occupations, cigarette smoking, obesity, and type A behavior.[5] In addition, individuals who perceive their health to be poor are unlikely to initiate or maintain a regular exercise program. From these observations it appears that those who are most likely to achieve health benefits from adult fitness and cardiac rehabilitation programs are also the most resistant to participating in them.

Knowledge of and beliefs in the health benefits of exercise seem to be less important motivators to continued participation in exercise programs than feelings of enjoyment and sense of well-being associated with exercise.[5] Individuals who feel good about themselves, feel they are in control of their own destinies, and are self-motivators are most likely to adhere to a program. The perception of self-efficacy or self-confidence is also an important predictor of adherence to physical activities after myocardial infarction (MI). Ewart et al.[6] have shown that treadmill testing 3 weeks after an uncomplicated MI followed by a careful explanation of the results to patient and spouse was associated with improved self-efficacy scores and subsequent maintenance of exercise activities. These data indicate that effective behavioral interventions aimed at improving confidence and sense of well-being are important motivational tools for maintaining an exercise program.

Both social and physical environmental factors are determinants of participation in adult fitness and cardiac rehabilitation programs.[5] Social reinforcement from family members, friends, and other health professionals are all influential in maintaining good exercise habits. Important physical factors include both the perceived convenience of the exercise facility and the actual proximity of facility to home or work site. Frequently, however, the significance of these factors is biased by a lack of interest in or commitment to exercise, with environmental factors being the excuse for dropping out. Interventions that focus on specific behavioral and cognitive strategies have been successful in increasing the frequency of adherence to exercise programs. Examples of successful strategies include written agreements and behavioral contracts, contingency incentives, self-monitoring and self-reward skills, goal setting, and decision making.[5]

There is a great need for additional research on the determinants of exercise habits and the design of optimal intervention programs for ensuring compliance to exercise regimens. It is clear, however, that to be successful, adult fitness and cardiac rehabilitation programs must take into consideration psychosocial, behavioral, and environmental factors that exert influence outside the immediate environment of the exercise facility.

THE PHYSICIANS' VIEWPOINT

The medical profession is undergoing major changes in its approach to medical care not only in terms of organizational, business, and reimbursement aspects of medicine but also its philosophical basis or belief system. Many of these changes are having, and will continue to have, considerable influence on the physicians' role in health promotion, adult fitness, and cardiac rehabilitation. It is interesting to note that attitudes of physicians toward issues relating to exercise and other preventive strategies are, in part, shaped by the public's demand for more information on prevention and health promotion.

The newer health-care systems such as health maintenance organizations (HMOs), independent practice associations (IPAs), and preferred provider organizations (PPOs) are slowly beginning to provide risk-assessment and health-enhancement services along with their more traditional examinations. Overall, however, there is still a lack of consensus among medical professionals on the importance of aerobic exercise in the promotion of health.[7] It is unfortunate that some physicians still believe that health promotion is not their business but rather the business of public health officials and other health professionals.[8] Nevertheless, in spite of these obstacles, there is a growing movement among physicians and hospitals to provide services related to risk assessment, disease prevention, sports medicine, and cardiac rehabilitation.[8]

Although, to some extent, the motivation for these preventive services is in response to public demand, there is also beginning to be a paradigmatic shift in the medical profession away from the traditional, "biomedical" model of medicine toward a more inclusive scientific model. Unlike the biomedical model, which is based on the classic factor–analytic approach that has characterized the Western scientific method for hundreds of years, the new model, called the "biopsychosocial" model by Engel,[9,10] is based on a systems view of life. The implications of the biopsychosocial model for the medical profession's understanding of health and disease are profound. These can best be appreciated by contrasting conceptual differences between the two models.

The Biomedical Model

The traditional view of medicine toward health and disease is a mechanistic one that considers the human body as a complex machine that can only be understood through analysis of its individual components (such as cells, tissues, organ systems).[11] Disease is conceptualized as a breakdown or malfunction in one or more of the body's parts and is best studied using anatomic, physiologic, or biochemical techniques. The physician's role in this model is to identify areas of malfunction and to intervene either physically or biochemically to correct the defects.

From the perspective of the history of medical progress, the biomedical model has enabled remarkable advances to be made in our understanding of the *process* by which various diseases affect the body. The technologies of biomedical science, ranging from molecular biology to sophisticated diagnostic and treatment procedures, have increased our knowledge of disease-induced cellular and organ system malfunction to a level of detail never before imagined. And yet, the *origins* of many of today's chronic diseases such as atherosclerosis and cancer remain largely unknown. By reducing the body into smaller and smaller parts, the biomedical model has forced medical scientists to focus more on mechanisms of disease rather than causes, without appreciating that knowledge of the mechanisms does not necessarily lead to elimination of the causes. The major limitation of the biomedical model, therefore, is its emphasis on expensive technologies for diagnosis and treatment of already existing diseases with little or no emphasis on disease prevention or health maintenance.

Nowhere is this approach more evident today than in cardiovascular medicine, where technology has become the dominant force governing the practice of cardiovascular physicians and creating a "booming medical industry" in the process.[12] In coronary artery disease, for example, the quantitative aspects of the disease process are examined using noninvasive and invasive techniques that permit exact localization of lesions and their functional consequences. Treatment interventions are then designed to physically correct the lesions (coronary bypass surgery, coronary angioplasty) and pharmacologically manipulate other manifestations of the disease process. The exciting technologic aspects of these procedures coupled with the enormous financial rewards to physicians and industry have overshadowed the effects of some physicians, public health officials, and others to promote disease prevention.

There is, however, a growing awareness among some physicians and others that the technologic solutions to many of today's major health probems, including atherosclerosis, are accelerating health-care costs far beyond manageable levels. In addition many of the present solutions to already existing diseases are palliative at best and not curative, with frequent recurrences of disease manifestations and further complications. As a result, attention is now being shifted toward the study of disease origins and ultimate prevention of disease. With this new focus of attention, however, comes the realization that the biomedical model of disease may no longer be adequate to solve the major health problems of the 20th century.

The Biopsychosocial Model

The new scientific model that is being proposed is not just a replacement for the more traditional biomedical model but rather an extension of it that incorporates the psychological, social, cultural, and ecologic determinants of an individual's health status.[9,10] All of the advances of modern medicine, which are based on analytic studies of the human body and its component parts, are retained in the new model. The new model, however, by taking a systems approach, focuses attention on the individual person as a dynamic living system and not just the sum of its parts.

Figure 16–1, reprinted from Engel,[10] illustrates the biopsychosocial model as a hierarchy of systems. Each level in the hierarchy is an organized, dynamic system incorporating all lower level systems while, at the same time, serving as a component of the higher level systems. The individual person in this model is represented by a

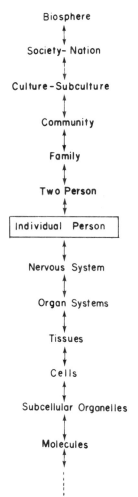

THE BIOPSYCHOSOCIAL MODEL
(Systems   View   Of   Life)

Biosphere

Society- Nation

Culture-Subculture

Community

Family

Two Person

Individual   Person

Nervous System

Organ Systems

Tissues

Cells

Subcellular Organelles

Molecules

Fig. 16–1.   Engel's biopsychosocial model.[10] Reprinted, by permission of The New England Journal of Medicine 306; 802, 1982.

midlevel system with the more traditional organismic systems below and the more complex social systems above. Unlike the biomedical model, each subordinate system in the hierarchy can be influenced by higher level systems, a feature that essentially does away with the outdated concept of mind–body dualism introduced by Descartes in the 17th century and a fundamental concept of the biomedical model.[11] The biopsychosocial model permits a more realistic appreciation of the role of mental processes in the preservation of health or the development of disease. Finally, each system in the hierarchy has distinctive features and interrelationships requiring scientific methodologies unique to that level. The implications for medicine are that a multidisciplinary approach may be the only way to solve many of today's complex medical problems.

The applications of the biopsychosocial model to the conceptual aspects of CHD are illustrated in Figure 16–2. In the classic, or reductionist, approach to atherosclerosis, diagnostic studies, treatments, and research investigations are usually directed at the organ system level, tissues, cells, or subcellular components in the progressive downward search for the ultimate molecular and genetic defects responsible for the disease manifestations. In the new model the patient as a whole person is the focus of attention, which in addition to numerous host factors and subordinate systems, is influenced by all higher level systems. Because the patient does not exist in isolation but rather as a component part of these higher level systems (environment), it is easy to appreciate the importance of various psychosocial factors in the development and progression of atherosclerotic disease manifestations. The model also facilitates a better understanding of the challenges and eventual solutions to reducing the morbidity and mortality from coronary disease by focusing as much or more attention on the higher social systems that

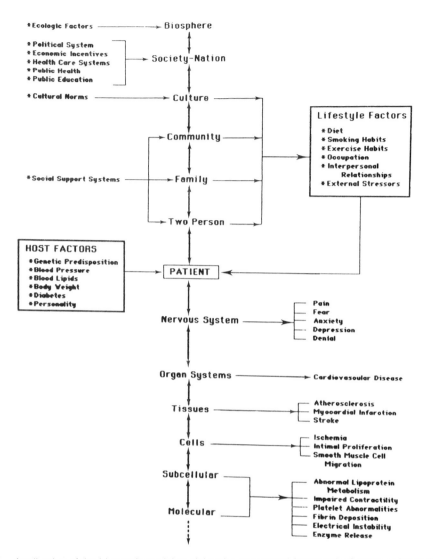

Fig. 16–2.   Application of the biopsychosocial model to the conceptual framework of coronary heart disease.

influence the patient's life-style and health behaviors.

Scientific models are, at best, approximations of reality or truth. The biomedical model has become so ingrained into the belief systems of physicians that its limitations are easily overlooked. The biopsychosocial model appears to be more inclusive and, therefore, a better approximation of natural phenomena. As such, it is more likely to become accepted by physicians and other health professionals in the years to come. Although the dominant force in cardiovascular medicine today is still reductionism, there is emerging evidence for a "new-wave" movement in medicine, which is concerned with more humanistic issues relating to health and disease and, therefore, more supportive of preventive health practices and wellness.[11]

THE SPORTS MEDICINE PERSPECTIVE

The emergence of recreational and therapeutic exercise in our society has led to a proliferation of professional activities associated with exercise—athletic training, adult fitness, cardiopulmonary rehabilitation, exercise testing, and exercise research—to name just a few. In broad general terms these various activities can be designated as "sports medicine." Unlike any other medical specialities, however, sports medicine includes physicians in all specialities as well as nurses, physical therapists, exercise physiologists, athletic trainers, and many other health professionals.

In actuality sports medicine is much more than a medical specialty, because it encompasses all medically related activities associated with sports and exercise. Dr. Allan J. Ryan, one of the founding fathers of sports medicine and long-time editor-in-chief of the journal *Physician and Sportsmedicine*, describes four general categories of sports medicine.[13]

The first involves the medical supervision and care of professional and recreational athletes. Included in this aspect of sports medicine are team physicians, orthopedic surgeons, athletic trainers, and other exercise specialists. Services provided by these individuals are primarily directed toward maintenance of or improvement in athletic performance.

A second category of sports medicine concerns the application of exercise-training techniques and sports to the physically and mentally handicapped population, also called "adaptive physical education."[13] To some extent this aspect of sports medicine overlaps with physical and rehabilitation medicine, whose practitioners include physiatrists, orthopedic surgeons, neurosurgeons, physical therapists, and nurses. In a broader sense, however, there is a growing interest in promoting recreational and competitive athletic activities for the physically and mentally handicapped outside the institutional setting. Two examples of this "wellness" movement for the handicapped are the popular Special Olympics for mentally retarded and the increasing number of athletic events organized for wheelchair athletes.

The third aspect of sports medicine involves the prescription of exercise for the general population. This is an area that is becoming more and more important because of the increasing public demand for accurate information on exercise. Practically all medical specialties including pediatrics, obstetrics, family practice, internal medicine, psychiatry, and many others are beginning to recognize the importance of exercise and are providing patients with information on starting and maintaining exercise programs. In addition many other health professionals (e.g., exercise physiologists, physical educators, fitness specialists, physical therapists, and nurses) are helping the public become more physically active. So-called "sports medicine clinics" are cropping up all over the country in hospitals, health spas, shopping centers, and recreational resorts. Unfortunately, standards of excellence have not been uniformly followed in setting up and operating these facilities, and as a result there is no way of ensuring that these clinics are providing adequate services. The recently published 3rd edition of the Guidelines For Exercise Testing and Prescription by the ACSM[14] should contribute significantly to the development of acceptable standards for exercise prescription, testing, and certification of exercise program personnel.

The final category of sports medicine activities concerns the therapeutic use of exercise in the treatment and rehabilitation of sick or injured patients. Cardiac rehabilitation is the classic example of this aspect of sports medicine, although therapeutic exercise programs also exist for patients with pulmonary disease, arthritis, cerebrovascular disease (stroke), diabetes mellitus, and many other physically disabling conditions. Although physicians are frequently responsible for the overall operation of these various rehabilitation programs, the day-to-day application of exercise therapy to patients recovering from illness or injury is usually the responsibility of a certified exercise specialist or physical therapist. Explicit behavioral objectives for the training and certification of these exercise personnel have been published by the ACSM.[14]

Although not a specialty per se, sports medicine does bring together individuals from many diverse backgrounds who share a common interest in exercise. The ACSM has become the umbrella organization representing the many professional interests of these individuals. Through its committees, regional and national meetings, and its journal, *Medicine and Science in Sports and Exercise* the ACSM plays an important role in providing scholarly programs and educational materials to the many practitioners of sports medicine. Because of its importance to the overall quality of sports medicine activities across the country, the ACSM needs the support of all its members. In addition individuals who are just starting careers with an emphasis in sports medicine are strongly urged to support the ACSM and contribute to its many activities.

THE FUTURE OF CARDIAC REHABILITATION

For more than 30 years, cardiac rehabilitation has been evolving as a multidisciplinary science and service dedicated to restoring the cardiac patient to "optimal physical, social, emotional, psychologic, and vocational status."[15] During the same period the overall management of patients with cardiovascular disease, CHD in particular, has improved dramatically.

Whereas in the 1950s, acute MI patients remained in bed for weeks at a time, patients today are out of bed several days after hospital admission, going home 7 to 10 days post-MI, and are back to work as early as 3 weeks post-MI. Because of the emphasis on early ambulation as well as early revascularization, the deconditioning effects associated with prolonged bed rest are no longer a problem for most patients. Accordingly, the emphasis in phase I cardiac rehabilitation is shifting away from a primary focus on physical reconditioning to a focus much more oriented toward patient education and behavioral management.[16]

To be sure, exercise training is still a fundamental component of all phases of cardiac rehabilitation. Nevertheless, it is not possible to justify exercise training per se as a realistic intervention for reducing the risk of reinfarction and death[17] or significantly improving left ventricular function and perfusion.[18] The evidence for these particular benefits of exercise training after MI is at best only marginal.[19] Furthermore, it is unlikely that additional large-scale studies evaluating cardiac rehabilitation programs will be forthcoming because of the high cost and complexity of these studies.

The lack of proof that cardiac exercise programs reduce morbidity and mortality after MI has caused concern among members of the medical profession, the health insurance industry, and government agencies responsible for funding Medicare payments. Many are questioning the need for organized cardiac rehabilitation services, especially the reimbursement for monitored exercise programs. At a time when accelerating medical costs are spiraling out of control, there appears to be a threat to the continued funding of cardiac rehabilitation.

For health professionals working in cardiac rehabilitation, these concerns may seem somewhat overstated and unjust, since these individuals are frequent witnesses to the remarkable improvements in functional capacity and cardiovascular risk behaviors achieved by their patients. Unfortunately, their observations may be biased by a closeness to the program and its participants, their own personal belief system, and financial considerations. For these reasons many cardiac rehabilitation personnel are not likely to provide an objective assessment of the cost-effectiveness of their programs.

It is clear, however, that cardiac rehabilitation services are striving to meet the needs of the cardiovascular disease population in an efficient, cost-effective manner. With the increasing regulation of health-care services by the federal government, it is not unreasonable to expect that a government sponsored technology assessment of cardiac rehabilitation, as suggested by Davidson,[20] will be initiated in the future. It is also possible that the results of an assessment will not be in the best interests of current programs. One can only hope, however, that, as more information becomes available regarding the effectiveness and limitations of cardiac rehabilitation services, new programs will be structured that maximize the benefits to the patients.

CONCLUSIONS

Cardiac rehabilitation as a discipline appears to be in a state of transition. The future role of this "technology" in the overall management of patients with cardiovascular diseases will depend on a number of different issues. Most important of these is the evolving treatment of acute cardiac events. If, in fact, methods for early reperfusion of ischemic myocardium after acute coronary thrombosis can truly minimize infarct size and relieve ischemia, there may be a decreasing need for phase I and monitored exercise treatment services and more emphasis given to patient education and behavioral management.

Second, issues relating to the most cost-effective methods for delivering cardiac rehabilitation services must be resolved in order to reach the majority of patients in need of these services. In addition, programs will need to be restructured to accommodate the changing life-styles and work patterns of the participants. Finally, effective behavioral interventions need to be developed that encourage patients to maintain their healthy life-styles after leaving the more formal phases of cardiac rehabilitation.

In 1985 the American Association of Cardiovascular and Pulmonary Rehabilitation (AACVPR) was formed in order to bring together professionals from many disciplines having a mutual interest in cardiac and pulmonary rehabilitation. The purpose of the organization, as stated in the bylaws,[21] is as follows: "Recognizing that cardiovascular and pulmonary rehabilitation is a multidisciplinary field, the American Association of Cardiovascular and Pulmonary Rehabilitation is dedicated to the improvement of clinical practice, promotion of scientific inquiry, and advancement of education for the benefit of health-care professionals and the public." In addition to planning regional and national meetings, the AACVPR has designated its official journal to be the "Journal of Cardiopulmonary Rehabilitation."[21]

Looking to the future, it is anticipated that there will be continued debate and controversy regarding the appropriate role for rehabilitation services and personnel in the evolving management of patients with heart disease. It is hoped that cardiac rehabilitation professionals will be sensitive to these concerns and challenged by them to provide the scientific basis for the necessary reorganization of existing services in order to best serve the public need.

REFERENCES

1. Siscovick, D.S., Laporte, R.E., and Newman, J.M.: The disease-specific benefits and risks of physical activity and exercise. Public Health Rep., *100*:180, 1985.
2. Kannel, W.B., Wilson, P., and Blair, S.W.: Epidemiological assessment of the role of physical activity and fitness in development of cardiovascular disease. Am. Heart J., *109*:876, 1985.
3. Stephens, T., Jacobs, D.R., and White, C.C.: A descriptive epidemiology of leisure-time physical activity. Public Health Rep., *100*:147, 1985.
4. Department of Health and Human Services, Office of Disease Prevention and Health Promotion: Prevention '82. D.H.H.S. Publication No. (PHS) 82-50157. Washington, D.C., U.S. Government Printing Office, 1982.
5. Dishman, R.K., Sallin, J.F., and Orenstein, D.R.: The determinants of physical activity and exercise. Public Health Rep., *100*:158, 1985.
6. Ewart, C.K., Taylor, C.B., Reese, L.B., and DeBusk, R.F.: Effects of early postmyocardial infarction exercise testing on self-perception and

subsequent physical activity. Am. J. Cardiol., *51*:1076, 1983.

7. Wechsler, H., et al.: The physician's role in health promotion—A survey of primary care practitioners. N. Engl. J. Med., *308*:97, 1983.

8. Dismuke, S.E., and Miller, S.T.: Why not share the secrets of good health? The physician's role in health promotion. JAMA, *249*:3181, 1983.

9. Engel, G.E.: The need for a new medical model: A challenge for biomedicine. Science, *196*:129, 1977.

10. Engel, G.E.: The clinical application of the biopsychosocial model. Am. J. Psychiatry, *137*:535, 1980.

11. Capra, F.: The Turning Point. Science, Society and the Rising Culture. New York, Simon & Schuster, 1982.

12. America's $39 Billion Heart Business. US News and World Report, p. 53, March 15, 1982.

13. Roos, R.: A conversation with Allan J Ryan, MD. Physician Sportsmed., *14*:193, 1986.

14. American College of Sports Medicine: Guidelines for Exercise Testing and Prescription. 3rd Ed. Philadelphia, Lea & Febiger, 1986.

15. Hellerstein, H.K., and Ford, A.B.: Rehabilitation of the cardiac patients. JAMA, *164*:225, 1957.

16. Blumenthal, J.A., Califf, R., Williams, S., and Hindman, M.: Cardiac rehabilitation: A new frontier for behavioral medicine. J. Cardiac Rehabil., *3*:637, 1983.

17. May, G.S., et al.: Secondary prevention after myocardial infarction: A review of long-term trials. Prog. Cardiovasc. Dis., *24*:331, 1982.

18. Froelicher, V., et al.: A randomized trial of exercise training in patients with coronary heart disease. JAMA, *252*:1291, 1984.

19. Shephard, R.J.: The value of exercise in ischemic heart disease: A cumulative analysis. J. Cardiac. Rehabil., *3*:294, 1983.

20. Davidson, D.M.: Cardiac rehabilitation: A technology in need of assessment? J. Cardiac. Rehabil., *3*:876, 1983.

21. Wilson, P.K.: American Association of Cardiovascular and Pulmonary Rehabilitation. From the president. J. Cardiopul. Rehabil., *5*:304, 1985.

Index

Page numbers in *italics* indicate a figure, "t" following a page number indicates a table.

393